The Behaviour and Welfare of the Horse, 2nd Edition

Andrew F. Fraser MRCVS, MVSc

Formerly Professor of Surgery (Veterinary)
Memorial University of Newfoundland
Canada

and

Formerly Editor-in-Chief, Applied Animal Behaviour Science

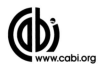
www.cabi.org

CABI is a trading name of CAB International

CABI Head Office
Nosworthy Way
Wallingford
Oxfordshire OX10 8DE
UK

CABI North American Office
875 Massachusetts Avenue
7th Floor
Cambridge, MA 02139
USA

Tel: +44 (0)1491 832111
Fax: +44 (0)1491 833508
E-mail: cabi@cabi.org
Website: www.cabi.org

Tel: +1 617 395 4056
Fax: +1 617 354 6875
E-mail: cabi-nao@cabi.org

A catalogue record for this book is available from the British Library, London, UK.

Library of Congress Cataloging-in-Publication Data

Fraser, Andrew Ferguson.
The behaviour and welfare of the horse / Andrew F. Fraser. -- 2nd ed.
      p.
   Rev. ed. of: The behaviour of the horse / Andrew F. Fraser. c1992.
   Includes bibliographical references and index.
   ISBN 978-1-84593-629-7 (hardback : alk. paper) -- ISBN 978-1-84593-628-0 (pbk. : alk. paper)
   1. Horses--Behavior. 2. Animal welfare. I. Fraser, Andrew Ferguson. Behaviour of the horse. II. Title.
   [DNLM: 1. Behavior, Animal. 2. Horses. 3. Animal Welfare. SF 281 F841b 2010]

SF281.F73 2010
636.1'083--dc22

                                                  2009040515

First edition (1992) ISBN-13: 978 0 85198 7 859

Paperback ISBN-13: 978 1 84593 628 0
Hardback ISBN-13: 978 1 84593 629 7

Commissioning editor: Sarah Hulbert
Production editor: Tracy Head

Typeset by SPi, Pondicherry, India.
Printed and bound in the UK by Cambridge University Press, Cambridge.

Contents

About the Author

In his youth, Andrew F. Fraser worked as a horseman. He then received his veterinary education in Glasgow, Scotland, and Guelph, Canada. He was an agricultural veterinary practitioner in Britain, North America and Jamaica for 14 years. He served as the Veterinary Director at the Newfoundland Pony and Horse Sanctuary, Trinity Bay, Newfoundland – a facility for aged or infirm horses. He has retired as Director of Animal Care and Professor of Surgery (Veterinary) at the Memorial University of Newfoundland, Canada, was previously a Professor in the Department of Clinical Studies, Western College of Veterinary Medicine, Saskatchewan, Canada, and Senior Lecturer in the Department of Surgery, Royal (Dick) School of Veterinary Studies, University of Edinburgh, Scotland.

He has been a pioneer in the scientific study of applied animal behaviour and was the original editor-in-chief of the journal *Applied Animal Behaviour Science* for 16 years. His ethological books include *Reproductive Behaviour in Ungulates* (1968, Academic Press), *Farm Animal Behaviour* (1974 and 1980, Bailliere Tindall), an edited volume entitled *Ethology of Farm Animals* (1985, Elsevier) and, with D. Broom, *Domestic Animal Behaviour and Welfare*, 4th Edition (2007, CAB International). He is the author of *The Native Horses of Scotland* and *Days of the Garron: The Story of the Highland Pony*. His further books on horses, published by Creative Publishers, include *Horse Twilight* (1990), *Founding Horses* (1991) and *The Newfoundland Pony* (1992). The first edition of *The Behaviour of the Horse* was published in 1992 by CAB International.

Andrew Fraser has developed a specific interest in the behaviour and well-being of horses, having owned numerous horses during his life. He currently resides in Newfoundland.

Preface

Since publishing the first edition of this book, applied research on domestic animal behaviour has become married to practical animal welfare science. These two disciplines have gained status and relevance from each other. The impetus for such development appears to be no more than a civilized advance in our appreciation for the animals we use. In the meantime, there has been more enlightenment acquired about the natures of our animals from the greatly expanded body of scholars in these joint disciplines, which have retained their scientific principles.

The horse has, of course, retained an eminent place among livestock with respect to care. There is particular public concern for its well-being in all aspects of its existence. It was therefore an obvious decision to combine the topics of equine behaviour and welfare in an updated version of the original edition. In doing so, some portions of text in that publication which rationalize welfare have been incorporated. Other additions include new information and some items contained in two recent monographs by the author. The latter are *Humane Horse Care* and *Carriage Horse Welfare*, published privately by the Canadian Farm Animal Care Trust in very limited editions. The principal objective in this second edition has been to focus on matters that are determinant in the recognition, establishment and maintenance of the horse's well-being.

Over recent decades, a body of information on horse behaviour has become established by publications from expert sources. These endeavours to accumulate knowledge of the horse's manner of living and its nature, and its means of dealing with its domesticated conditions should not cease; so much has still to be learned, understood and acted upon. The point has now been reached where advised actions in support of the horse's basic well-being become evident in various new ways that fit its behaviour and circumstances. Such a policy of favourable action for the animal is actual welfare. Applied ethology has an inherent purpose in determining factors of animal welfare. This text now connects both issues, recognizing the character and dynamics of the horse and seeking, where possible, to accommodate these with suitable care and husbandry by either implication or prescription.

A.F. Fraser
Newfoundland, Canada
August 2009

Acknowledgements

During the past 15 years the author has been able to make periodic observations on horse welfare at the 10-ha Hopewell Horse and Pony Sanctuary, Newfoundland. This land was initially leased to the author by the Crown Lands Department of the Government of Newfoundland and Labrador, and the author expresses his full gratitude for that generosity. Several people facilitated these observations at the sanctuary, including Mr M. Green, Mr B. Martin and Mr R. Walsh, to whom much appreciation is conveyed.

In the past 12 years, other instances of pony care and breeding in Newfoundland and Iceland provided opportunities for observation; they also supplied helpful data on pony husbandry and reproduction. The Department of Agriculture in Iceland kindly gave detailed records on pony breeding results for several years. All those who helped the author with information on these indigenous, insular ponies are thanked appreciatively.

Professor D. Bieger of the Memorial University of Newfoundland is thanked for his friendship and his informative sessions on neuroethology. The author also wishes to thank Mr T. Hughes, President of the Canadian Farm Animal Care Trust, for his encouragement to produce the two monographs referred to in the preface. Special gratitude is expressed to Christina Rees for her considerable work in transcribing and editing the text of this book. The author also expresses gratitude to Allison Rees, Ian Fraser and Stefanie Smith for their valuable assistance in various aspects of this project. Additionally, the author thanks Melanie MacDonald and others, who provided their credited illustrations. Finally, the author expresses much gratitude to Sarah Hulbert of CABI, whose sundry positive endeavours launched and steered this project into print.

Introduction

The horse continues to keep its special place in the human world. Its status has been changed from 'farm animal' to 'companion animal', but many would argue that it was always exactly that. It has been a companion to humankind from the start. The horse moves with the times: new breeds emerge, for example the Newfoundland pony, and one new horse type of a 'toy breed', namely the American miniature horse. The horse and human have gone together as civilization and its cultures have evolved.

With the modern search for proper relationships between humans and sentient creatures, the associate horse can be the model animal to study for clarification. Its ways reveal its nature and manner of living. As a deserving animal, the horse's welfare is of importance to society, and when its own ways are recognized in full, it becomes clear that its welfare can be assured by tending to these with appropriate animal care.

The horse's essential nature is displayed in its behaviour, and when this is examined objectively and meaningfully it is an exercise in applied ethology (Jensen, 2002). This scientific method is used to learn about domestic animals' functional characteristics and significant dynamics. The objective is to comprehend the activities of the animals and their kind, then eventually put the knowledge to use in rational animal management. In the pursuit of applied ethology, various forces are at work and provide this subject with its form. Now that it has been academically established for approximately 40 years (Fraser, 2008a), it has attained much relevance in the determination of animal welfare in practice, well-being and health.

Well-being

As a fairly fresh concept, animal well-being emerges comprehensively as a state of healthy life. In animal management it is, in essence, the condition of optimal health. It has various physical, behavioural and physiological manifestations in animals. In the individual subject, its establishment and maintenance constitute the humane objective when veterinary attention is directed at animal disease or disorder. Without receiving much specificity before, it is central to the art and science of veterinary medicine and surgery. To put it quite simply, an animal's well-being is its state of being well, plus its expressed sense of this. It reflects comprehensive health in the animal. Health is made evident in an animal's compound fitness. Physiological and behavioural indicators of soundness are as important as physical signs of health and well-being.

Animal welfare has fairly recently been introduced to veterinary education and the animal sciences as a specified subject. This ensures that humane factors in animal use are reinforced by scientific education. Animal care has also emerged, at the same time, as a specific discipline embracing welfare. Welfare is what much of veterinary medicine is about, through its delivery of preventative measures and the relief of suffering animals. When welfare gives support to animal life, it is the well-being within that life that benefits.

The essence of an animal is made up of three factors: namely, its physical characteristics, its behaviour and its natural needs. In other words, its nature is a part of the wholeness of its identity. The animal's nature provides a rational indicator of the employment it deserves, especially in domestication, with all of its restrictions. This is the essential right to live for its allocated period, under conditions that are in keeping with its nature. While this is not an absolute right, due to exceptional circumstances of reality, the support of animal well-being can serve as the basic principle in animal care and use. Clearly, this calls for recognition of the animal's particular nature. It is here that applied ethology steps in, for it is not sufficient merely to have general knowledge of animal behaviour; it is the particular behavioural nature of the specified subject that is needed in order to arrive at a moral contract with it, as we make use of it.

Empathy

In the application of behaviour knowledge for a given animal, there is a need for some rational sympathy for the subject. This is needed to clarify the animal's action in human comprehension. Professor Bernard Rollin, who is a philosopher at the University of Colorado, where he contributes to the College of Veterinary Medicine and is the Director of Bioethical Planning, acknowledges this and states that the necessary change in perceptual ability may often require what he calls a 'gestalt shift' in the observer. By this, he evidently means a quite sudden and fairly radical alteration in a person's point of view, to form a new realization. For those without a pre-existing empathy with the living subject, such a change of view is needed to acquire appropriate sympathy for the subject. Some sympathy for the animal, in its given condition, is a guiding light in the determination of a code for its humane management.

Full recognition of the animal's nature forms the foundation for the morality of its given use and conditions of care. In such a moral determination, philosophy, common sense, general knowledge, scientific facts and the interpretations of applied ethology should all be in harmony. Negotiating such harmony, in the widest of discussions without boundaries, is not an easy task, but the emergence of animal welfare as an academic discipline has done much for the progress that is being achieved.

With regard to the horse, it can be said that this animal has always enjoyed some moral status, although this continues to be refined in principle and practice. Perhaps the horse serves as a model on which to base analogous considerations for other domesticated and utilized animals. Horses are dependent on human care. Our obligation to horses is beyond question. Perhaps this matter can be summed up with a statement stating that public opinion has already given horses a specific right: it is a right to humane treatment in human use. The phenotypic characteristics of the horse as a strong, kinetic animal have established its use. The horse also has a suitable nature to go with its function. By facilitation the expression of the true equine nature in work, sport and recreation, a moral principle in equine use is observed. With the enlightening of society, such standards will change and evolve continuously.

Ethics that relate to the use of animal life may have an influence on some practices with horses, such as defined ethics of use. Animal scientists and veterinary practitioners should be aware of developments in the new field of animal bioethics and be receptive to informed public opinion on ethical issues. One matter receiving increasing appreciation is the property of sentience in the more highly developed species of animals. Most notably, the horse has the property of tangible sentience and affective properties. Acknowledgement of the latter adds to the case of due welfare (Fraser, 2009a,b).

Sentience

Among animals, sentience is the factor that influences behavioural variations and also affects states of awareness and emotion. Sentience is a property of many animals that have advanced sensory development. Sentience was not recognized in the natures of neural-developed species until fairly recent times. The force and implication of this factor compel moral duty towards sentient-developed life. Their sensitivities and feeling existences elevate the higher animals beyond pedantic argument to a rightful place in human consideration. As Rollin states, 'Animals have a right to enter the scope of moral concern and to be morally considered by any person who weighs his actions morally'. If a creature is alive and has demonstrable interests, it falls within the scope of morality and is clearly deserving of some moral consideration. Balcombe (2009) points out the moral significance of using animals that can express evident pleasure: this feature of pleasure expression is a product of developed sentience. Horses can express pleasure in their vocalizations. This takes the form of a low bumbling sound.

Recognition of sentience in an animal that is used in domestication raises some questions about the obligation incurred by society through such use. It is argued that such an animal is deserving of maximal humane consideration, because of its sentience on one hand and because of a human moral duty on the other. This makes the horse a moral object in domesticated use. The horse, it is further argued, has a right to such consideration. This cogent argument moves the debate on animal rights from a hypothetical position to a very practical one. The salient factor of sentience cannot be dismissed from this issue.

The Issue of Rights and Ethics

In this era when the idea of animal rights has intruded into the human conscience, there is an obligation to review the status of the horse in its modern, domesticated position. A consideration of its well-being would appear to demand such a review. For this purpose, it is essential to refer to the expert opinions of academic philosophy. The principal figure in this field is Professor Rollin. From the publication in 1985 of his book *Animal Rights and Human Morality* and his other publications, such as two edited volumes, in 1990 and 1995, of *The Experimental Animal in Biomedical Research*, Professor Rollin has shown why animals must be the object of moral concern. His compelling case is that such moral concern leads us directly to animal rights. He argues quite simply that with greater animal use, the greater is an obligation to care for them and to have respect for them. Such respect affords them a right.

While an animal, of itself, cannot possess some absolute right, human society can give it the grant of certain rights. That there is logic in doing so is a proviso. Such logic would be based on knowledge of the animal's behaviour and the substance of its well-being. Warbel (2009) has pointed out that applied ethology brings out ethical issues relating to animal use. For the horse's well-being, a rational application of ethics, based on modern equine knowledge, is justified. This monograph aims to give all pursuers of humane horse care and horse well-being suitable information on a spectrum of relevant matters on equine living in general.

Animal Care

Occasional reference is made in the text to animal care as a feature of husbandry for the horse in need of special attention or improved health. The term has become used for a standard of animal husbandry that emphasizes welfare. As a specific term, animal care was initially used with reference to the technical custody of laboratory animals and for health purposes; the responsibility for this was increasingly placed in veterinary and technical hands. A scientific discipline evolved which gave the animal freedom from infection. Stability of well-being resulted. In principle, emphasis was placed on preventative measures and humane husbandry to protect animals from their various characteristic diseases.

This disease-free objective was transferred to general livestock in time. Health schemes emerged to reduce the incidence of clinical conditions in contained populations of livestock. Preventative measures in animal husbandry, parasite control, vaccination programmes, and improved feeding and hygiene are the main features. These result in significant health improvement.

Proper care of all the utilized animals calls for similar protocols. Animals used for food production, for companionship and for recreation can all have a better existence with the benefits of good husbandry, ethical treatment and preventative veterinary medicine. Animal care is the route to responsible and humane animal use at all levels. This is applied animal welfare for horses also.

Terminology

The terminology that is necessary in this field comes from various sources. Throughout the text of this book there are references to physical parts and regions of the horse. Figure I.1 is provided here to illustrate the 'points' of a horse, as these are identified in their standard terms. The special terminology used in the text is given and defined in the glossary. Certain terms in the text relating to equine behaviour and welfare that have not been used previously in either of these conjoined disciplines are taken from medical and other sources, in order to describe particular features not recognized in this field before. Where these are first used in the text, their definitions are immediately given and they also appear in the glossary.

Objective

The horse's behaviour is not viewed here in isolation. Since behaviour is effectively comprehensive bodily function, its creative neurology, physiology, endocrinology and anatomy receive some attention in the text to underpin the equine dynamics described. An effort is made to take a dimensional picture of the horse's apparent

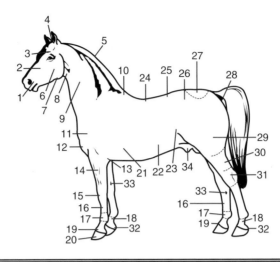

Fig. I.1. Points of the horse. Drawing by Stefanie Smith.

nature and the fitting of this into its domesticated circumstances. Managemental needs, in support of the horse's well-being, can be better recognized from such a standpoint. A clearer perspective of equine welfare can emerge from such considerations, given fairness in the assessment of balance between the horse's natural manner of living on one hand and its forms of use, plus its custody, on the other.

Some specific matters of veterinary relevance are addressed where these are of importance in protecting equine subjects from foreseeable clinical conditions. Many of these conditions attend the common behavioural events in the course of a horse's life. Veterinary medicine should provide major support for horse welfare and can do this best when combined with knowledge of the discipline of horse behaviour. Its behaviour contains its otherwise invisible nature, which is the core of its being.

1 Development of Equine Behaviour

Behaviour and Evolution

When the behaviour of the modern domestic horse is studied, both objectively and realistically, ethology is being applied to a subject that is not entirely a product of natural selection. Variations have been used in the creation of breeds by generations of horse breeders. The general objective was to get various horse types into purpose-built categories, defined as breeds. Nevertheless, this animal's great inheritance is its natural past, which deserves appreciation because that is the source of much of its behaviour today (Clutton-Brock, 1999).

The norms of horse behaviour today are the natural heritage of a very long history of evolution in a world without human control. Horses were subjected to nature's control as they developed as a species for some 8 million years before their domestication. During those times there was natural selection, in which some individuals were ultimately more successful at living and breeding than other individuals, depending on their genes. This is the process of differential reproduction, whereby evolution occurs as a result. Ethology has an interest in natural selection. Both behavioural and physical (i.e. visible) characteristics of a living thing (phenotype) must be distinguished from its genetic make-up (genotype). Evolution can only produce its changes if phenotype and genotype are both involved. Adaptations can occur for the good of the individual; an adaptation is a difference in a trait that increases the fitness of its carrier.

It has long been appreciated that selection of some kind plays a part in determining which individuals are able to survive. It was made clear by Darwin that the evolution of a species occurred by selective processes (Jones, 2001). These processes determine which individuals are most able to survive and reproduce their kind, and so able to participate actively in the continuation of that form of life.

It is evident that what is selected is the whole make-up of the living organism, including its variations and genes, and its behavioural fit into its ecological niche. The state of overall fitness is achieved, largely, through behaviour, structure and niche, and their constant interaction with each other. Applied ethology is interested in the animal's dynamic wholeness. The applied ethological perspective of evolution is therefore both holistic and traditional. It recognizes that behaviour and structure have their particular environmental needs and their own particular motivational components for survival (Lorenz, 1965).

Innate Behavioural Patterns and Environment

Ethological wholeness includes many interrelated systems, which are the products of early development, or epigenesis. Fixed behavioural patterns, as the products of epigenesis, show how highly endowed animals, such as horses, are equipped with behavioural requirements for many circumstances. These behavioural endowments are common to all individuals in a given species. Sometimes, inherent behavioural variations are attributes possessed only by certain individuals or types of horses. Fixed patterns are not variations but are 'fixed' in the given species – possibly as end points of evolution, serving as cornerstones in the long-term support of the species.

Niche factors must be taken into consideration as part of the animal's wholeness and continuity. In horses these factors include systems of husbandry, space, seasonal factors, nutrition and methods of use. The factors of niche aid the continuing success of the species over many generations by allowing the germplasm to accurately duplicate the attributes of the parents. Continuity is aided by the availability throughout the ages of environmental niches to which the species is adapted. Environmental aids ensure that once the attributes of a species have proved themselves effective the species will persist. Complementing niches must remain in domestication for the preservation of the horse (Price, 2002).

Changes in form or type

Novel features in a species can arise as the result of genetic changes, such as mutations, occurring during cell division in the reproductive process. Such a variety might or might not be suited to the parental niche. It could be forced to achieve wholeness in an alien niche (e.g. in adjacent territory). As a new niche brings about isolation, the mutant character would be perpetuated in homozygous form. This type of event would allow the new form to continue to reproduce unchanged. This has happened to horsekind. The domestic horse is one equine species, with close relatives (Table 1.1). The present array of horse types suggests that this has occurred periodically, giving us ponies, heavy horses and 'hot-blooded' horses, for example (see Fig. 1.1 for varietal extremes). Through mutation, the latter type of horse, notably the Arabic, became more reactive and more athletic compared with the 'cold-blooded' type. Archetypal characters (both physical and behavioural) are retained in a mutant. Many of the attributes of the antecedent and well-established stock would persist as attributes of the mutant. This genetic inheritance contributes to the success of the mutant form as a derivative with archetypal attributes. The origin of archetypal behavioural attributes lies in the phenomenon of epigenesis, whereby fixed designs are accurately and actively able to continue their developmental functions through other generations. The newborn foal, transferred suddenly from an intra-uterine environment to a completely new environment to which it must quickly adapt, illustrates the nature of evolved and 'fixed' developmental behaviour, the latter being a constant in foal survival (Robinson, 2007).

Initial learning

The mare and its newborn react to one another reciprocally. The smell and taste of the uterine membranes and fluids attract the parturient mare to lick the foal clear of membranes and clean of fluids. While doing so, the sensorium of the foal is being 'imprinted' with the mare's image. Thereafter, it efficiently recognizes and remembers her form. Similarly the mare quickly identifies her progeny and accepts it as something to be protected. The evolved and innate abilities to learn quickly are thereby well illustrated in both neonate and adult.

In evolution, parents care only for their own offspring, and reproduction occurs only between members of the same species. Such attachments in horses depend on the critical timing of first impressions in the neonatal foal (Bateson and Horn, 1994). The timing of the sensitive period is found to be closely matched to the period during which the possibility of error is very small, such as before the newborn has a chance to meet members of any species other than that of the mother.

The neonate foal relates to its mother not as a complex organism but as a unitary stimulus. Parturient mares isolate themselves from the herd before parturition. Usually, the first large moving object seen as a distinct phenomenon by the newborn foal is its own dam. Although the newborn can be quite easily confused by other large moving objects, it receives, through touch, 'thigmotaxic' stimuli. Through contact of its muzzle with the ventral surfaces of the dam's body, it learns the identity and location of this vitally important region and eventually finds the dam's udder and food (see Fig. 1.2). The mare's behaviour is modified to increase the efficiency of her task of watching over the foal, thus granting her reproductive success (see Fig. 1.3).

Attributes and variations

Discontinuity can be seen in the behavioural differences between species. For example, horses, unlike cattle, show an active contribution by both partners

Table 1.1. Classification of equine species.

Classification	Species	Common names
Order Perissodactyla (odd-toed ungulates)	*Equus caballus*	Horse (domestic)
Suborder Hippomorpha	*Equus asinus*	African wild ass (and domestic donkey)
Superfamily Equoidea Family Equidae	*Equus burchelli*	Common zebra

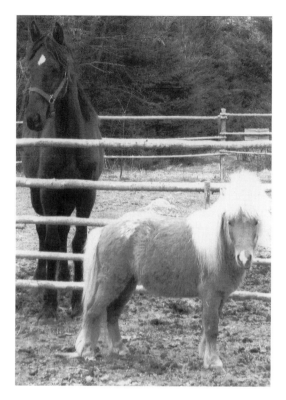

Fig. 1.1. Varietal extremes. Friesian yearling filly behind American miniature horse. Photo: R. Butler.

of a pair during mutual grooming, and the incisor teeth are used for this purpose. In contrast, in mutual grooming in cattle, one partner is active and one is passive, and the tongue is used. Horses rise up forequarters first, while cattle raise their hindquarters first. Such examples lend support to the concept of discontinuity or independence in the evolution of such behavioural attributes. However, discontinuity in the evolution of behaviour *within* a species (rather than between species) can represent mutational change, which can provide the nucleus for a new type.

Much of the behaviour of all animals is concerned with learning and discovering the attributes of themselves and their environment. Play and exploration operate in this function. When all the attributes are established, they have a prominent part in enabling the individual to pursue its life history. These attributes contribute to the organism's constitutional 'wholeness'. Attributes, such as variations in colour, hoof size and gait, are not recognized as having any marked survival value. In nature they could then be lost without any adverse effect on species survival. Mankind, in caring for domestic horses, supplies their niche with certain items such as food, shelter and protection. The outcome has been that many attributes have been conserved that otherwise would have been lost,

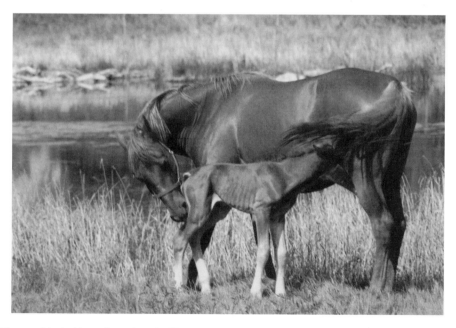

Fig. 1.2. Mare and foal with tactile reciprocity. Photo: A.F. Fraser.

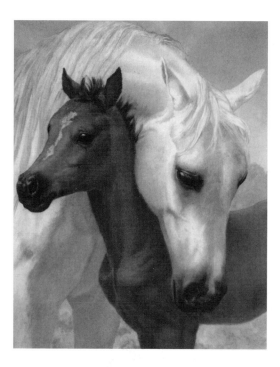

Fig. 1.3. Mare with reproductive success. Anonymous artist.

with a by-product of a study in applied ethology. The wildness factor is actually a faculty that gives the horse the potential to live in a wild state. When it is closely and chronically confined, such a condition has a dysphoric effect on many horses. A state of dysphoria would be an excellent element for an abnormality in behaviour to flourish.

Domestic selection

Variation under domestication leads to the realization that many mutations are non-adaptive in the usual sense of the word applied to natural environments. However, if the possessors of such mutations are complemented by man's agency, they can survive and reproduce, perhaps indefinitely, as non-adaptive mutants. Many variations, such as colour, play no essential part in leading to the survival of the newborn during the critical postpartum period. The true unit is the species as a whole, including variations, as well as the environmental niche and incidental factors within that niche.

Although attributes that have been selected lead on to further evolution, a species is essentially stable. For the complete success of the species, however, it must be aided by features of the environment. In the achievement of this environmental fit, a prominent part is played by behaviour. Behavioural attributes therefore have an active role in bringing about evolution.

Breeds with non-adaptive characters have appeared and have been kept true by continuous human selection. In contrast, it can be suggested that natural selection is non-human selection of attributes that nature periodically throws up through chromosomal mutation, as between the Przewalski and the domestic horse.

Inherent capability in learning

Learning is an example of an evolutionary system of great adaptive significance. Selection will favour the ability to learn and acquire insight through experience. It has been observed that untrained adult horses, on the first attempt to halter them, react negatively and vigorously to this form of control. They will persist in struggling against the handling and leading attempts using a halter up to the end of a 'breaking-in' session of, say, 15 min. If the animals are released at this point and again subjected to a haltering session after an interval of several days, they respond differently. On this occasion they do

such as the hoof size of the Clydesdale and the colour of the Appaloosa. There are specific (i.e. of the species) as well as varietal (i.e. of breed or type) attributes. Distinction must be made between sets of behavioural attributes. Varietal attributes differ between breeds (i.e. cold-blooded, warm-blooded and hot-blooded), but in behavioural anomalies they have no difference (Flannigan and Stookey, 2002). Figure 1.4 illustrates a hot-blooded type.

Without a difference between varieties of heavy and light horses in dealing with their stereotypes, an interesting fact emerges from this study by Flannigan and Stookey. A stressfulness inherent in the severe immurement of the horse seems to target a specific neurological frailty factor in this species. Its establishment seems to precede the time of human selection of variant types, which is a practice typical of domestication. If this equine factor is pre-domestic, it stems from its early wild state; the horse may have a behavioural core that is still suited to wildness. After thousands of years in stables, the horse seemingly retains a wildness factor in its behavioural constitution. While this may be regarded by most horse users to be a common belief, it is useful to have that opinion supported

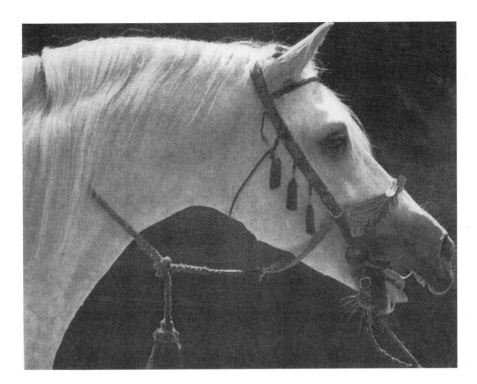

Fig. 1.4. Hot-blooded stallion. Photo: S. Hlalky.

not show the negative reactions of the first session and many are found to accept the control of the halter. Clearly, some learning has taken place in the meantime, which is of adaptive significance.

Two schools of thought can be identified with regard to the issue of genetic effects versus environmental influences on behaviour. This conflict has been variously described as instinct versus learning, nature versus nurture, or endogenous versus exogenous determination of behaviour. A compromise synthesis is now generally recognized, in which all phenotypes are seen to be derived from the interaction of an organism's genetic potential with its environment. Behaviour, of course, is as much a phenotype as any physical characteristic. In relation to this the following equation is recognized as a general law:

Genotype + Environment = Phenotype (behaviour, physiology, morphology, chemistry, etc.)

Although the relative contributions of genotype and environment may vary considerably, neither one is ever without input. Even when behavioural phenotypes, such as temperament, differ with regard to the interaction between experience and genotype, some contribution from each factor always takes place.

A suitable way of recognizing the interaction of genetics and environment in the production of behaviour is to realize that behaviour is not contained in complete form within genes. Genetic codes for behaviour do not have the capability of independent manifestation as behaviour without an environmental backdrop. The genetic nature of behaviour, even that which is 'fixed' in the animal, is like a template. Through this, a clear pattern can be produced only if the proper tool – such as stimulation – can be applied to it and only if there is proper material – such as an appropriate environment – to take up the pattern.

Clearly the genetic basis of behaviour varies in degree of specificity. Some behavioural templates are precise and detailed while others are vague in outline and more general in form. A precise genetic basis of behaviour is seen in newborn foals; for example, the pattern produced by the template of postnatal behaviour is sharply outlined. Several primary and co-essential stages can be recognized in the comprehensive repertoire of foal behaviour during the formation of the neonatal–maternal bond. Secondary neonatal functions are less precise.

Action patterns

Genetic specification relating to behaviour is dependent upon the importance of the item of behaviour in question. Behaviour that is most imperative has a template more precise and detailed than is the case for behaviour relating to matters of lesser priority. For example, fight-or-flight reactions are very precise forms of behaviour. This is in accord with their role in states of emergency. On the other hand, the behaviour of play, while characteristic in form, is very variable and imprecise in its display; this is in accord with its typical occurrence during phases of environmental neutrality. Play, nevertheless, uses environmental substrates for its production, and animals will sometimes use inanimate objects as outlets for play behaviour. Clearly the genetic control over behaviour is variable.

One broad area of behaviour that contains many items of precise and detailed activities is reproduction, which is the basis of evolution. Those behavioural features on which evolutionary forces depend are the most 'fixed' in form. Such fixation is the substance of behavioural phenomena termed 'fixed action patterns'. In the broad fabric of behavioural display, some characteristic units of behaviour present a pattern. The fixed action pattern became adopted as the name of the basic unit of ethology and was given three definitive properties, as follows:

1. Each had its own causal factors.
2. The component parts of the behaviour pattern appeared in a definite sequence.
3. Once triggered by a stimulus, the behavioural display continued without regard to continual stimulation.

It is therefore a form of stereotyped behaviour (Mason and Rushen, 2008). Even the most stereotyped behavioural patterns are graded in degree from time to time, and many can be controlled by environmental changes. Behaviour often shows a gradation in all its characterizations. When behaviour has form and regularity and has consistent features that are recognizable and definitive, it merits special recognition. The terms 'fixed action pattern' and 'modal action pattern' are therefore used in describing behaviour that has characteristic features as follows:

1. Structural (being made up of individual component acts).
2. Taxic (having a relationship to the environment as regards its direction).

3. Temporal (relating to the timing of other events).

Many action patterns are recognizable by their form and their orientation, jointly. Action patterns, as behavioural processes, are the means whereby the environment can influence the animal. Their great role in evolution is now clear.

Homeostasis and survival

In addition to reproductive success, the establishment of homeostasis through feeding and related behaviour is vital to survival (Robinson, 2007). At the level of the individual animal, it is of the highest importance and takes the form of behaviours directed towards maintenance. It is now better appreciated that maintenance behaviour is very extensive and comprehensive. Formerly, this was considered to be limited to the basic needs for life. The needs of the living animal are continuous; however, they include more than those most basic items such as food, water and shelter. The integration of activities is represented in the unitary behaviour that gives the individual and its species much of its ethos. It is suggested that maintenance is the essence of homeostasis (see Table 1.2).

In domestication, homeostasis is dictated by husbandry systems. This is done by manipulating methods of management in such ways that animal self-maintenance is facilitated. This is the objective in traditional animal husbandry and good animal care. Given its freedom in an appropriate environment, the domestic horse is still able to care for itself. The survival successes of feral and liberated horses speak volumes on the innate behavioural resources of these animals, which have been retained through hundreds of generations of domesticated breeding and selection. Perhaps now, more than ever before, the evolutionary heritage of domesticated horses can be appreciated (Bateson, 2003). The recognition of inherent behaviour, either precise as a pattern or variable as a process, should form the basis of a modern ethical approach to horse husbandry (Christiansen and Forkman, 2007).

Appraisal of Behaviour in Horses

Progress has been made in studies of social, sexual, perinatal, parturient, maternal, developmental, maintenance and abnormal behavioural systems in

Table 1.2. Equine forms of maintenance behaviour.

Category	Varied features	Function
Reaction	Reflexes, responses in general, fight or flight	Defence
Ingestion	Grazing, drinking, chewing, browsing	Nutrition
Body care	Rubbing, rolling, scratching, nibbling	Hygiene
Motion	Natural gaits, play, comfort shifts	Exercise
Rest	Drowsing, idling, lying, sleeping	Restoration
Association	Affiliation, bonding, herd unity	Companionship
Exploration	Attention, curiosity, wandering	Learning
Territorialism	Affinity for home base and home range	Security

horses. Special concepts relevant to domesticated animals, such as behavioural well-being, have evolved in applied behavioural studies. The transfer of the findings of all animal behaviour studies into practice is a continuous challenge to practitioners and students. In order to know the nature of their animals, they must be able to appraise behaviour (Budiansky, 1997).

Although veterinary clinicians and animal scientists tend to develop their own procedures for behavioural assessments of animals, a general appraisal of a horse's reactivity and a good history should be included in a behavioural examination of any case study, whether this involves one individual or a group (Gore *et al.*, 2008).

The horse's attitude, disposition and temperament should be assessed before any handling of the animal is performed. The animal's perception and awareness of its general environment should be noted. In particular, the subject's appreciation of sense-directed stimuli must be determined. Sensations such as vision, sound and position must be appraised. Eye movement, involving the lids and orbit, is an important singular feature. In the horse, the upper eyelid showing contraction or elliptical change can indicate temperament. Again, a high degree of exposure and mobility of the orbit is an indication of anxiety, while a very fixed orbital position may indicate some distress.

The horse's willingness to move and the nature of its posture and gait are important considerations. Evaluation must also be made of various reflex responses, both general (such as the response to sound) and specific (such as the response to a local stimulus, e.g. pressure on a given site on the body). Reflex responses to localized stimuli, such as tapping below the jaw, may also be noted if there is a need to determine significant reactivity. Within

an adequately extended examination period, acts of normal behaviour should become noticeable. These might include behavioural items of self-maintenance, such as feeding (or response to an offering of food) and body care. Illness, in general, can inhibit grooming and stretching reflexes. Acts of body care, such as 'comfort shifts', evacuation and self-grooming, in long behavioural examinations are especially significant because such behaviour often ceases as a first sign of illness.

General Features

Behavioural appraisals are of value in judging fitness from illness. General reflexes should not be studied only as isolated phenomena but as actions of the whole animal. Pandiculation (holistic stretching after arousal or rising) is an action pattern of common occurrence seen in healthy foals and, to a lesser extent, in adult horses. Differences in responses occur between breeds (Ligout *et al.*, 2008; Lloyd *et al.*, 2008).

In a study of posture in the course of behavioural appraisal, it must be remembered that many postural abnormalities are not shown unless the horse is at rest or minimally disturbed in its usual stable. For this reason, patient and quiet observation of the animal may be necessary before any abnormality of posture can be detected. As a rule, the behavioural examination is best performed in a quiet space or enclosure, with limited light, where distractions will be minimal. Tranquillization should be avoided; parts of the examination, such as forced running, which could stimulate the animal, should be postponed until the end.

In determining the suitability of a horse for a given role, its characteristic behavioural repertoire is of paramount importance (Seaman *et al.*, 2002).

For this to be determined with reliance, a broad range of behavioural responses and performances should be appraised. Again, in the course of convalescence from an illness, the behaviour of self-maintenance returns to the animal's behavioural repertoire. An extended period of behavioural examination of the animal in its bedded premises is usually necessary for convalescence to be appraised by the behavioural method. Some outdoor methods allow the behaviour of horses to be studied in test situations without demanding 'artificial' conditions imposed upon them. These tests can allow critical appraisal to be made on a horse, or horse group, with minimal manipulation, allowing behaviour to occur in a fairly spontaneous manner. Such methods include the use of recorders on the horse, passing through a chute or a simple maze. Even fearfulness can become evident in this method (Lansade *et al.*, 2008).

Appraisal methodology

In assessing important aspects of behaviour, effort is made to keep the assessment objective precise and, if possible, to arrive at a numerical measurement. Examples include measures of behavioural traits, temporal factors and temperament scores. In addition to these, dominance levels, conspecific interactions and time budgets are areas where scores are used in appraising horse behaviour.

Open- and closed-field tests

The 'open-field test' is a basic ethological method (Lehner, 1996). It has great potential in quality and quantity of observations and results. It is also consistent with both humane principles in ethological experimentation and general appraisal of temperament and health. In the open-field test, which in some instances could be more aptly termed the 'closed-field test', the animal is liberated into an enclosure that permits extensive movement, such as an arena, a paddock or a large pen. The total ground area or floor space can be subdivided by actual regions or imaginary dividing lines, making a number of territorial subsections. The animal's movements in the area, within a given period of time, are determined. Special note is taken of the part or amount of enclosure covered and explored and the animal's general responses, including changes in reactivity. Scores can be determined for 'open-field' (or closed-field) appraisals of social interactions, such as

'dominance hierarchy'. While the open-field test is principally applied in experimental situations to one animal, equivalent methods of behavioural assessment can be applied under natural and practical situations to groups (Martin and Bateson, 2007).

Horses are frequently studied behaviourally by records of their paddock use. These records are often made on 'plans', which can show the paddock use in such maintenance activities as feeding, resting and evacuating. These studies reveal the level of organization of behaviour practised by horses, even in field confinement. Even when they are chronically confined in restricted paddocks, horses attempt to use allotted space in the interests of body care, social determination and self-maintenance generally. Studies on these features provide clues to optimum management and convenient husbandry consistent with welfare.

Deprivation tests

Another test method of great potential value in assessing the importance to the horse of certain features of behaviour is based on deprivation of opportunity for given time periods. By temporarily depriving an animal of any behavioural activity that is normal and common, it is possible to determine the importance of that activity to the animal, by observing its activity when the behavioural opportunity is restored. Behavioural needs can then be determined by this method (Lehner, 1996).

Specific tests

Other tests are now used increasingly in horse ethology to varying extents. The outlines of such tests are as follows.

A STIMULUS–RESPONSE TEST This method has been profitably used in noting the effects of 'teasing' on oestrus display, or determination of libidinal sensitivity in the stallion, for example.

INCIDENT FREQUENCIES These have been put to good use investigating avoidance and aggression within social behaviour and the stability of specific behaviour in such circumstances as leadership. In addition, this method can draw attention to behaviour that is apparently abnormal and warrants improved definition and diagnosis.

Table 1.3. Varieties of oestrus manifestations in mares.

Character of oestrus	Common duration	Nature of behavioural display	Urinary ejaculations
Normal heat	> 3 days	Frequent and complete	Numerous and copious
Weak heat	< 3 days	Occasional and incomplete	Absent
Silent heat	> 3 days	Occasional and partial without stallion; aggressive with stallion	Absent

FREE CHOICE To estimate the preference of an animal for given features of husbandry, it can be allowed to make a choice between differing circumstances.

ETHOGRAM RATINGS Such studies indicate the normal balance among all the individual components of major behavioural catalogues (ethograms). With these proportions established, excesses or reductions have become recognizable. Ethograms give reasonable evidence of normative behaviour.

NATURAL SITUATIONS Sometimes an individual animal can be assessed behaviourally to best advantage in its normal biological situation. For example, the vitality of the newborn foal can be determined by a behavioural study of the animal at its birth site. The action patterns that unfold in the young animal in such characteristic and predictable ways serve to show the vitality of the individual neonate. Both the order and the time of behavioural events give a general picture of the foal's viability and the progress of its postnatal maturation (Morresey, 2005).

Head lifting and shaking occur first, quickly followed by rotation of the body to sternal recumbency. Rising attempts soon follow, and a first, fully upright stance is normally attempted within 30 min and attained within 1 h. The first successful suck of the active neonate foal is achieved when it is between 1 and 2 h old. Delays in the behavioural schedule of development are indicative of imminent clinical problems resulting from dysmaturity in the newborn (Russell and Wilkins, 2006).

Certain reactive behavioural activities are common to adult horses and can be used in the appraisal of temperament. These include threat displays, challenges and dominance activities, which are best seen in natural situations (Keeling and Gonyou, 2001).

Breeding soundness should be based to a considerable extent on evidence of normal reproductive behaviour. Such behaviour often hinges on the occurrence of overt oestrus. The primary character of oestrus is, of course, receptivity to mating. The intensity of oestrus may vary considerably in mares. The appraisal of oestrous behaviour is therefore essential in horse breeding, although the normal female mating state obviously has both behavioural and physiological elements (see Table 1.3).

Critical Appraisal of Behaviour

While the behaviour of a normal and healthy horse is clearly the concern of many people, it is often the veterinary surgeon or the animal scientist who is required to understand abnormal behaviour. Increasingly veterinary clinicians have their attentions directed towards such behaviour-based conditions as distress, discomfort, pain and deprivation of needs. These conditions are stressful, and stress is a heterogeneous group of dysfunctions, the manifestations of which are many. Appreciation of this fact makes the veterinary scientist better able to guide horse users in the optimum and acceptable conditions of maintenance and care. This newer role for the veterinary scientist depends largely on the use of applied ethology and the appraisal of abnormal behaviour as an aid to diagnosis. At the present stage it is impossible to deal with this topic comprehensively, but one can consider a number of clinical circumstances in which diagnosis can be established on the basis of a horse's behaviour. Greater veterinary involvement in applied ethology has been urged to support the disease aspects in the discipline of welfare (Willeberg, 1997; Christiansen and Forkman, 2007; Fraser, 2008b).

The postural characteristics of the horse are among the commonest behavioural features to undergo change in diseased conditions. It is therefore essential to appreciate normal posture as a basis for recognizing postural abnormalities for

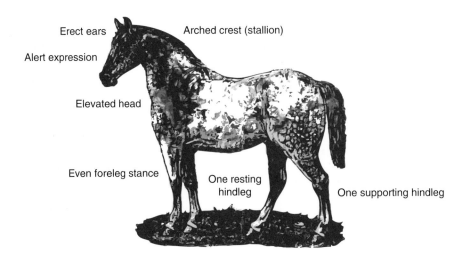

Fig. 1.5. Postural signs of well-being.

clinical purposes (see Fig. 1.5). The following are the main circumstances under which horses adopt abnormal postures:

1. Mechanical conditions involving loss of support of stability by the animal.
2. Nervous conditions in which there is a reduction in adequate neural function to maintain muscular tone.
3. Painful conditions that make it impossible for the animal to maintain its natural posture. In addition, there can be permanent adaptive changes to pain, which the animal may have acquired as a result of prior experience of any disabling circumstances.

These three circumstances are further considered below.

Mechanical conditions

Mechanical conditions influencing postural behaviour are many, and the following few examples are given as illustrations. For example, fracture of the metacarpus in the horse makes it impossible for the animal to take any weight at all on the affected leg. Fracture of the humerus also leads to lack of mechanical support and a grossly altered posture. Severance of the flexor tendons in the horse leads to a sinking of the fetlock and a turning up of the toe. Congenitally contracted tendons in foals also make normal posture impossible. Limb injuries in horses can respond in many cases to therapy and rehabilitation, allowing normal limb function to be restored (Back and Clayton, 2001).

Nervous conditions

Nervous conditions that can create abnormal postures include radial paralysis following, for example, prolonged recumbency during anaesthesia. A lesion in the cervical vertebrae causes the condition of 'wobbler' in the horse, the main characteristic of which is a stiff neck (Gore *et al.*, 2008).

Painful conditions

Painful conditions causing abnormal posture in horses include suppurative arthritis and osteomyelitis of the fetlocks. The latter condition causes a tucking under of the hind legs. Gonitis (inflammation of the stifle joint) occurs principally in horses, causing them to point to the ground with the toe of the affected hindlimb. Arthritis also leads to abnormal posture in other animals; for example, pigs with arthritis will arch their backs, presumably to minimize skeletal and abdominal pain (Broom and Fraser, 2007).

Permanent adaptive changes to pain may arise in a condition such as laminitis. On rare occasions, animals that have experienced laminitis for some period of time can learn to go almost on 'tip-toe' with the forefeet. This position appears to minimize pain. The adoption of this posture also means that the hind legs of the animal are brought further forward.

The behaviour of a horse in pain has certain specific features that are recognizable. The facial expression in pain is often quite characteristic; usually there is a fixed stare within the eyes. The eyes are not as mobile within the orbit as in the healthy horse, and the eyelids tend to be slightly puckered. The ears are usually held slightly back and fixed in this position for long periods. In addition, the affected horse may have dilated nostrils. These facial signs collectively give a horse a facial appearance of concern. In pain, the animal is often seen to turn its head to one side or another, looking at either flank.

In colic or abdominal pain, the horse shows various abnormalities of posture (Herdt, 2007). With persistent pain they may show unusual recumbent behaviour, while at other times they may adopt an unusual stance. Horses may back into a corner of a loose box, and may be observed standing, pushing their heads against a wall when an uncomfortable or painful condition is present. Abdominal pain may cause the animal to lie down frequently, rising repeatedly after short intervals. In between these periods of recumbency, a horse with colic may scrape at its bedding with a forefoot, while slowly pivoting around on its hind legs. It has been reported that Thoroughbred horses suffering azoturia sometimes scrape up mounds of wood shavings provided as bedding and then stand with their back legs on these mounds (Mills, 1991).

Locomotion and Mobility

When the locomotor behaviour of a horse is to be examined, it should be singled out and observed in good light, moving about on a clean, dry and level surface. The horse should be led by hand at different gaits when special examination of locomotor behaviour is being carried out. It can then be allowed to run freely to observe free action (see Fig. 1.6).

Lameness is defined as impaired movement or deviation from normal gait. More frequently, in the veterinary context, lameness refers to abnormal gait caused by painful lesions of the limbs, feet or back, or to mechanical limb defects. Neurological deficits that produce lameness are usually defined separately after their differential diagnosis.

Abnormalities of both posture and gait should immediately arouse suspicion of multifocal, diffuse or systematic distribution of lesions in the nervous system (Oliver and Lorenz, 1993). Some alterations of mental state, such as depression, disorientation or hyperexcitability, may also accompany some locomotor signs.

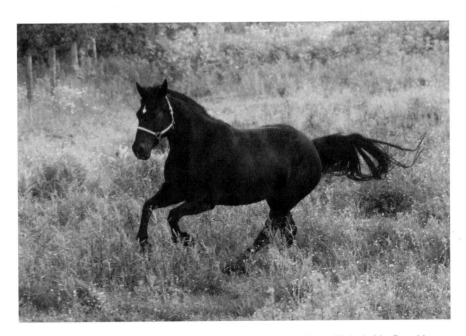

Fig. 1.6. Spontaneous running in a horse freshly turned out into pasture. Photo: Melanie MacDonald.

Development of Equine Behaviour

Several metabolic and other systemic disorders have secondary effects upon the central nervous system (CNS), including serious locomotor deficits, although their primary pathophysiology is not within the locomotor apparatus. Nervous signs are often mediated through the central nervous system and are often intermittent, always generalized and produce a wide spectrum of inconstant neurological signs. These include confusion, seizures, tremors, vision disturbances and episodic weakness (Palmer and Rossdale, 1976; Radostits *et al.*, 2000).

Ataxia means uncoordination of muscular action or gait. Signs of this include wide-based stance, swaying movements, falling, rolling, dysmetria (imprecise gait) and exaggerated abduction of the limbs on turning. Ataxia is one of the most common clinical signs in nervous diseases. Another drastic dysfunction of locomotion is paralysis. Paralysis is defined as loss of motor or sensory nerve function; paresis is partial paralysis. Respiration should be given particular notice for signs of any respiratory disorder.

Assessment of gait should take account of every aspect of gait, such as length of stride, whether too long or too short. A painful skeletal lesion gives a short stride with a reduced support phase and is often unilateral. The commonest form of this is a 'limp'. In the wide range of clinical veterinary textbooks, there is extensive detail on all clinical dysfunctions affecting equine mobility.

Inherent and Acquired Behaviour

The issue of instinctive or innate behaviour versus acquired, learned behaviour in horses is controversial. Reaction and other adaptive responses appear to be basically pre-programmed, or genetically encoded, but are subject to behavioural modification by neural organizations, endocrine systems and physical features. Inhibitions and reinforcements become established with experience and opportunity. Choices emerge with environmental challenge and experience. Maintenance and reproductive motivations, e.g. hunger, thirst, comfort, motion, association and sexual motives, switch and change priorities. Feeding and reactive and reproductive behavioural motives, in particular, are modified by the experience and environmental circumstances of a horse.

Lorenz (1965) and other early ethologists described instincts or innate forms of behaviour in various vertebrates. Innate behaviour is that element of behaviour that has been inherited. This inherited basis of behaviour may be modified during the life of the animal, according to its experiences with its environment. The evolved genetic basis ensures that the animal is equipped with a repertoire of adaptive responses that can be utilized without essential prior experience. The precise nature of innate behaviour allows us to recognize readily that such behaviour can be elicited in the proper circumstances without prior experience. Many of the neonate's functions are predetermined. Some innate behaviour may not be revealed until the animal is adult and mature, as, for example, in most kinds of maternal behaviour. The adult horse's characteristic sexual behaviour is largely determined by genetic factors. However, it is important to recognize that, even with this fixed foundation, innate behaviour can become modified by experience.

Release of Innate Responses

Much of the 'priming' of innate behaviour is done by the endocrine system, and the coordination of action patterns is dependent on activation of nerve centres, e.g. the hypothalamus. The releasing of innate actions requires specific stimuli, which are essentially sign stimuli or 'releasers'.

Certain theories exist in connection with releasers. A releaser is defined as any specific feature in an animal's environment that prompts an innate response. Behavioural characters that are peculiar to the equine species can thus be set in motion by certain stimuli. The theory of the innate releasing mechanism (IRM) has grown from this hypothesis. The IRM is considered to be a physiological mechanism, built into the animal and inactive until such time as it becomes appropriately stimulated. The appropriate stimulus in the environment is considered to be the key which unlocks the appropriate action pattern.

In this theory, releasers act upon the IRM by issuing a simple sign stimulus. One particular type of releaser that plays an important part in determining behaviour is the social or sexual releaser. Such a releaser may be an animal's odour, shape, sequence of movements, variety of sounds or general display; it serves the specific function of eliciting a particular response in another member of the same species. The role of such releasers is considerable in the mating and nursing behaviour of horses (Kiley-Worthington, 1999).

Imprinting

'Imprinting' is a special form of behavioural linkage. A very modified concept of it has been applied to the horse. In its first recognized form it was an avian phenomenon, but it has mammalian analogies. It was first noted by Lorenz, who described it in the hatchlings of ducks and geese. He divided the clutch of eggs laid by a greylag goose into two groups: one hatched by the goose, the other incubated. Those hatched by the mother followed her around in the first day; she was the first moving object they saw. Those hatched in the incubator were exposed only to Lorenz and they learned to follow him. In the translation to English, this specificity of following was termed 'imprinting'. Lorenz placed both broods under a box. In the presence of both the goose and Lorenz the box was removed, and Lorenz and the goose then moved away in different directions. The incubated goslings following Lorenz and those hatched by the goose followed her.

Such imprinting from original experience occurs during especially sensitive time periods in development. They may have long-lasting effects upon subsequent behaviour, whether in chicks or other infant animals (Horn, 1985). In imprinting, the animal's genetic programming causes it to be maximally sensitive at the critical period to a moving object, so that it can speedily learn the strong habit of following that object. This strong following habit does not seem to be built up over a duration of time or with practice. The animal's following behaviour is apparently developed completely in one episode.

The goslings not only followed Lorenz, they also followed each other in linear formation and kept specific distances between themselves. The distance they kept from Lorenz was reduced as he reduced his height by crouching or swimming as he led them. The following response itself may be an innately patterned motor response released by the moving image that has been recognized. This is the result of a sensory stamping on imprinting (as a coin is imprinted with an image) as a memory template in the nervous system. Such a memory image and resulting behaviour might be further modified during or after the critical period by counter-learning experiences and exposure to different environmental influences. The influence of the template fades in time, particularly in mammals. Some obscure influences of imprinting can persist for extended periods of time in such areas of behaviour as mating orientation. Male animals, for example, may attempt to mount individuals of an alien species with which some degree of imprinting may have occurred in a critical period of development.

At the critical time the mother quickly learns the identity of her newborn and relates to it like a particularly vulnerable extension of herself. In contrast, other young, even if evidently similar, are rejected; hostile behaviour is exhibited to the alien, and such behaviour in mares may amount to extreme aggression in many cases. When the maternal critical period has passed, adoption of fostered young by learning is more protracted and less certain. Such phenomena explain the characteristic behaviour of the mare after foaling. Her maternal behaviour is strongly and quickly motivated to establish parental care (Clutton-Brock, 1991).

Other critical periods occur and these are typically at key biological points. An example is at puberty, when sexual orientation is enhanced by learning during strong motivation. Young stallions that do not gain appropriate orientation at this critical time often have some delay in learning the motor skills of mounting and mating.

Adaptive Behaviour

Environmental features provided by the husbandry system exert influences that determine whether the horse can adapt behaviourally to the system. Various environmental circumstances have been studied. Changes in behaviour, and ultimately in physical conditions, result directly or indirectly from environmental adaptation. The adaptive mechanisms of horses living under various environmental conditions have shown differences in response to housing, enclosure and the immediate environment. Some responses are maladaptive and some vary between breeds and individuals. Adaptation is evident in respect of thermoregulation and ingestion (Herdt, 2007).

The level of temperature at which the so-called cold-blooded type of horse is able to maintain a normal body surface temperature (the thermoneutral zone) seems to be roughly from −10°C to +20°C. Warm-blooded horses, on the other hand, can maintain a normal body surface temperature in ambient temperatures of about +5°C to +30°C. These ranges are artificial, however, because they presuppose no wind or rain. Air movement and precipitation compound the effects of low temperatures and minimize the effects of upper temperatures. Under extremes of temperature, both types of horses use behavioural methods in attempting to control their temperatures. The most easily recognizable evidence of adaptive behaviour in horses is the movements directed towards thermoregulation and related aspects of body care. These include sheltering, shade-seeking, inactivity, etc. An early behavioural adaptive change during high temperatures is a reduction in food intake. This may arise not only from the shade-seeking activities of the animal but also from a reduced desire for food. Consequent results are an alteration in grazing behaviour and a general decline in all activity. Such an alteration in behaviour indicates a welfare problem (Dawkins, 2004).

Taste and imitation play important parts in grazing behaviour, and this ensures that the requisite elements are consumed by a horse in appropriate quantities and suitable type to maintain health (McGreevy, 2004). Adaptive seasonal changes in eating indicate that grass palatability has been altered. Seasonal palatability varies markedly on 'unimproved' pasture. Horses generally prefer grass that is high in leafiness, greenness and nitrogen content. Sugar, organic acids and fats are preferred, whereas tannins and alkaloids are avoided. Variation in food choice by ponies is explained by the abundance of plant species at different stages of the growth season. As a rule, a drop in the percentage of time spent feeding on a species of grass can be attributed to a dearth of that grass or to the growth of a preferred one. The exceptions to this rule occur in summer and autumn, when certain leaves, such as beech, are increasingly consumed by horses.

Acid grasslands attract more horses in winter than in summer, probably because of the availability of other grasses in summer. In winter there is more exposure of grassland, as the cover of fibrous plants dies away. In the Camargue, in southern France, a long-term study of horses there shows a marked seasonality in the use made of plants. Deep-water rushes, which are high in protein, form the main summer food, while perennials and legumes are dominant in the diet at other times.

Much contemporary controversy centres on the extent of behavioural adaptation that has taken place in farm animals because of the restrictions of husbandry. Opinions have been commonly expressed in support of a notion that adaptation is inevitable in the face of continuing husbandry pressure. Some believe that many generations of selection for productivity have resulted in animals being docile to a level that would be disastrous in the wild but essential under domestication.

Docility is, however, adaptive behaviour and is chiefly the result of selection and individual management, where there is the capacity for such adaptation. The influence of domestication is not detrimental to animal well-being if the techniques of domestication allow the animal to adapt to a humane system (Riolo *et al.*, 2001).

Innate behaviour and expression are two different factors. While the phenotypic expression can be environmentally modified, the brain circuitry and chemistry of the genetic programme will persist in the animal despite it being domesticated. Clearly there has been the assumption that much adaptation in respect of domestication has taken place over recent centuries. This assumption of general behavioural adaptation in domestication leads on to two contingent assumptions. First, a general potential for further (and possibly faster) adaptation must exist to cope with any change in husbandry. Secondly, adaptation to confinement has been largely achieved already, through exposure to conventional husbandry.

The main assumption and the two contingent assumptions have failed to take certain facts into account, including the following:

1. Species attributes are characteristic and fixed in the species and are liable to quick change only by mutation in an individual.
2. Varietal (or breed) attributes are the features on which domestic selection has been concentrated.
3. Behaviour is phenotypic.
4. Adaptation is not inevitable.

In the adaptation controversy, there has been a failure to make a distinction between varietal (i.e. of the breed) behavioural attributes – some of these have flourished and others have disappeared as a result of selection – and specific (i.e. of the species) behavioural attributes – most of which have persisted. Specific behavioural attributes, and in particular those of maintenance, must persist of necessity since they are bound in with much critical physiology. It is important to recognize the fact that (genetic engineering apart) while domestic selection can eliminate some behavioural varietal traits and propagate others, it cannot create any totally new genetic attributes.

Many domesticated changes in horses have undoubtedly occurred by full use of fortuitous mutation, such as heaviness or smallness. By exclusion of variability much refinement of characteristics has also been achieved in breed features. This has been done using genetic material already present. Deliberate elimination of innate behaviour has not been a major objective and no claim of its significant removal can be made with scientific justification.

No convincing proof has been advanced showing the elimination of any equine behaviour essential to survival. On the contrary, much evidence shows that such behavioural potential still exists in highly bred domestic horses not subject to survival pressure. Today's horse keepers and horse breeders are clearly left with products of evolution and are obliged to act as curators, not as creators. As Kilgour and Dalton (1984) famously concluded: 'Domestication has not greatly altered the species-specific behaviour patterns of farm animals'.

It will be evident that the degree of natural equine adaptability is high but that the capability for unnatural adaptation is limited. While the horse can acquire certain behavioural methods of adapting to its circumstances and environment, it can readily acquire maladjusted forms of behaviour. Husbandry factors can give rise to behavioural anomalies, and many items of anomalous behaviour are of diagnostic value in the identification of defective husbandry.

The relationships between husbandry systems and behavioural factors are complex but are interrelated and interdependent. The animal's experiences establish many habits which facilitate its routines of living. This process of habit formation is notable in horses. Undesirable husbandry can also establish bad habits in the animal's behavioural repertoire. The acquisition of both types of habit is therefore a result of husbandry and reflects on its quality. Horses change their behaviour as a result of learning from their experiences and from their husbandry. Learning is therefore a part of each animal's development. The animal depends on learning and memory to cope with the circumstances of the environment that it experiences, not only at the moment of the experience but also in later circumstances of a similar nature. Such learning develops through various processes. Two principal processes of learning are classical conditioning and operant conditioning.

Conditioning

A response is termed conditioned when a stimulus, other than the natural or originally effective one, can bring about the response. The normal, or originally effective, stimulus is termed the unconditional stimulus. Classical conditioning is a form of learning which typically speeds up responses. The unconditioned stimulus acts as a primary reinforcer to the behavioural response. The conditioned stimulus is therefore a secondary reinforcer. Reinforcement is the result of the reward or the return obtained by the responses. Some stimuli achieve positive responses; some trigger negative activities. For this reason, it is sometimes convenient to recognize positive and negative reinforcers which may, in their own turn, be unconditioned or conditioned, i.e. primary or secondary. In mating, for instance, it could be said that the unconditioned stimulus is the general form of the stationary mare, but it is observed that many other stimuli, in time, elicit full behavioural response in the stallion. In the case of stallions under restrained husbandry, leading the animal out towards the customary service area will act as a sexual stimulus. When conditioned stimuli have been established, they can be very effective in stimulating the animal's responses.

The classical procedures in conditioning are those that involve repetition of the same sequence of stimuli. Routines of husbandry are suited to the establishment of conditioning. Sometimes an animal will be conditioned not to make a response that it already makes. This undoubtedly occurs when unfavourable circumstances are associated with activity. Undoubtedly conditioning of this negative type is fundamental in the establishment of inhibitions, which are known to be a necessary part of training. On the other hand, conditioned responses can be further stimulated or reinforced when the unconditioned stimulus follows after a conditioned one. The animal, when stimulated to certain behaviour by conditioning, can have its behaviour reinforced by subsequent reward from the natural, or unconditioned, stimulus. In this way the term reinforcement often implies a consummatory act. A reduction in motivation is a usual sequel to a consummatory action, and such reduction is therefore a further implication of reinforcement.

In conditioning a state of generalization is common. In generalization, actions occur in response to a variety of stimuli that are unrelated or have only a loose connection with the primary stimulus. The numerous daily routines of animal husbandry create many generalized states of conditioning, such as the sound of food preparation.

Examples of positive conditioning are numerous. Stud horses become sexually activated when led out by their grooms for breeding; horses at grazing run to a trough when someone appears with a bucket. The examples of negative reinforcement would include most avoidance behaviour, such as the avoidance of persons associated with aversive stimulation. In the following examples the reward is avoidance of undesired experiences. Horses may run from the approach of a handler as a result of negative reinforcement. They may avoid a horse trailer as a result of fearful learning. It is good behavioural management, therefore, to reduce painful and frightening incidents, particularly in the young animal's first experiences of significant events such as control, loading and handling. Classical conditioning supplies many learned refinements to the behaviour of reactivity.

Operant Conditioning

A major type of learning is instrumental or operant conditioning. It is, in effect, trial and error learning and is the learning that occurs from the numerous empirical activities that are generated by exploratory and investigative behaviour. Operant conditioning is also called instrumental learning or conditioning, since the behaviour is the instrument by which the reward, or reinforcement, is obtained. Training animals is an operant task: the trainer must wait until the animal produces the desired activity. This is then rewarded promptly as a reinforcement. This process of learning can be speeded up by 'shaping' the behaviour through training. In the course of their training, horses are very dependent on operant conditioning for learning behaviours that are not natural, innate actions. In their training for circus performances, horses are taught before feeding to operate within the circus environment in the desired ways. When appropriate behaviour is shown, a food reward, or verbal reinforcement, is given. Reinforcement leads to improvements in learning and to the establishment of new behaviour. As learning proceeds in operant conditioning, the animal makes fewer empirical actions until, eventually, it performs proficiently.

Horses show many responses that coincide with peaks of daily routine work or the absence of such activity. Stabled horses become very active, vocal and even agitated when feeding is due or overdue, or the preparations for feeding are underway and can be heard. They quickly learn to associate specific sounds with certain husbandry routines; a great repertoire of conditioned reflexes quickly becomes established in most horses in this way and by the use of the human voice. Skilful exploration of conditioning can allow the experienced horse handler to exercise a good deal of control over the behaviour of the horse by use of oral sounds, words, whistling, etc.

Habit

Habit is one way in which behaviour becomes altered as a result of developmental experiences. These experiences integrate components of behaviour into efficient patterns that become constant in form. Habituation is the elimination of responses that are not imperative or biologically meaningful. Thus habituation of horses to the many circumstances of their use is clearly a very important factor in their training and in their overall welfare (Appleby and Hughes, 1997).

Horses acquire many habits through routine learning. Learning adds to the repertoire of an animal's inherent behaviour. If its learning is deficient, an animal will remain deprived of some of the functions possessed by others and, as a result, it is likely to be a less adaptable individual. One influential aspect of the behaviour of horses reared with others is in their strong imitative (allelomimetic) tendencies. The individual is influenced by the reactions, grazing and drinking activities, eliminative behaviour or movement of others. The force of this is evident when a horse is placed in isolation; out of sight of any of its kind, its characteristic habits soon become disrupted. Its intake of food and water declines and it makes constant efforts to join other horses if it can possibly do so. Some isolated horses are found to decline all food and drink when first isolated, even though both food and water may be immediately available.

Experience

The effects of early experience on adult behaviour are strong. When horses are raised as orphaned animals, their later behaviour differs from the reactive characteristics of most normally reared horses; they are often difficult to restrain and to train, for example. At the same time, foals reared exclusively in their mother's company usually adopt the reactive tendencies of the mother and acquire the mother's temperamental characteristics. Foals reared without human contact before weaning may have difficulty in accepting handling by humans in their later life. They appear to be insecure under human control. Acquisition of undesirable behavioural states can be avoided by early handling. Ideally, this should begin with bodily restraint of the day-old foal. Through this it learns that there is no danger in being contained by human force and that short separation from its dam is not traumatic. A foal should be touched all over to learn acceptance of human contact. Sessions of touching, bodily restraint and brief separation from the mother allow the foal to learn to accept and adapt to human control over its behaviour. After it is weaned, such early experience aids in its handling (Zentall, 1996).

During the paediatric period the total effects of experience are compounded. The development of emotions, the opportunity to pursue exploratory behaviour, the social experiences of the young animal and the development of its physical and physiological apparatus all combine to influence the animal's reservoir of acquired behaviour. Post-weaning environmental experiences also play their part in developing the behaviour of the subject in subsequent adult life. Experimental processes continue into this period and senses also continue to develop (Houpt, 1991). Any impaired development is serious. A deterioration in foal behaviour is often the result of bacterial infection. With accurate diagnosis, most can respond to antimicrobial therapy (Owen *et al.*, 1983; Quinn *et al.*, 2000).

A study of the many factors capable of affecting the behaviour of a horse must include the various early experiences that can permanently affect the behaviour of that individual, even into its adult life. Environmental factors and social forces have a much more powerful and durable influence when applied in early life than similar ones experienced in adult life (Forkman, 2002). The immature animal is more prone to acquire habits than the adult animal. Social and traumatic experiences tend to have more effect the earlier in life they are experienced. Horses are seen to benefit from as great a variety of environmental stimulations as possible in early developmental life. An infantile store of experiences is accumulated from environmental effects.

Investigatory activities, from which much learning is derived, continue throughout life, though they tend to be more obvious in the young animal. Good habits are dependent on familiarity with a wide range of husbandry features that provide optimal conditions for the animal. Exposing foals to essential husbandry procedures, such as haltering, can prove to be helpful in their adaptations. Many routines become established as the basic pattern of management, and it is very desirable to allow the animal to acquire experience of these routines before these become enforced procedures. Much learning in young foals is by observation, and they learn more readily by watching their mothers than by watching others. Their mothers, of course, permit close investigation by their own young. Grazing horses, again particularly young ones, learn from others such things as food selection and location, paths and routes, watering places and shelters. Needless to say such learning is of critical importance in the ability of the young horse to integrate successfully with its environment and home range. Visser *et al.* (2003) found that learning ability in young horses was variable between horses but very consistent in individuals.

Intelligence

Studied attempts have been made to make appraisals of animal intelligence on the implicit assumption that animals and their behaviour could be better understood through proper comprehension of their intelligence. The assumption was faulty. Although intelligence in mankind is well understood and in many cases affects human behaviour, it cannot be assumed that intelligence in animals is of an identical nature. It can now be recognized that intelligence in horses is more general than specific and that its role in behaviour is apparently a supportive one based on essential sensory perception. Nevertheless, animal intelligence does exist, although it is difficult to define. It is not a critically important factor in behaviour, although properties of intellect can be found in equine behaviour, in which judgements are very appropriate.

While various methods are often used to attempt to measure intelligence in animals, it would appear that the length of time that an animal can remember a specific training signal or command can be taken as some measure of intelligence. Horses learn many techniques in maintaining themselves. They use operant conditioning very readily to make optimum use of their environments. Some horses learn with greater facility than others, and variation in intelligence is shown in this way.

Intelligence is demonstrated when the horse learns to ignore irrelevant stimuli, just as it also becomes sensitized to significant stimuli. This permits the behavioural developments that make discrimination possible. The animal's integration with its domestic environment is facilitated by this ability to compare and contrast, based upon intelligence. Most horses can accurately discriminate between stimuli and evaluate them, e.g. they can differentiate sounds, visual features of special significance, the identities of people and so on. This ability appears to improve with experience (Domjam, 1998).

Discrimination is established when the animal responds only to imperative stimuli. Discrimination between similar stimuli, such as fast-moving objects, is not improved by prior experience but by the capacity to perform complex discriminations. Discrimination of identity, for example, depends on prior experience of the stimuli or of similar situations; experienced mares show better maternal discrimination and neonatal care than inexperienced ones. Foal care improves with experience rather than with age. Young foals quickly learn to discriminate the characteristics of their mothers, and mares quickly learn to discriminate their own young from those of others.

Constant confinement and restriction of activity can defy intelligence and affect horses. While a horse's physical condition may be preserved in the stable, its emotional (nervous) condition is likely to be adversely affected by chronic restriction. In many cases, if the restrictive husbandry is constant, the animal's natural activities become redirected, so to speak, into anomalous action patterns. To

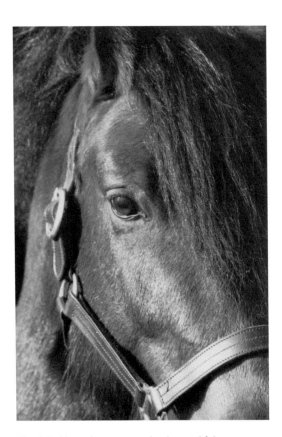

Fig. 1.7. Normal eye expression in watchfulness. Photo: Melanie MacDonald.

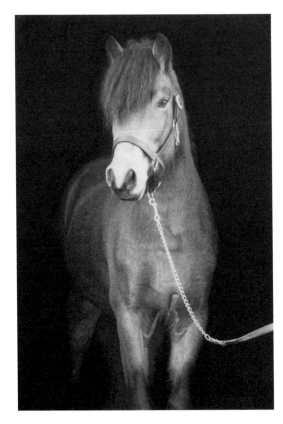

Fig. 1.8. Colt showing full attention. Note orientation of body, dilated nostrils, pricked-forward ears and watchful eyes. Photo: Melanie MacDonald.

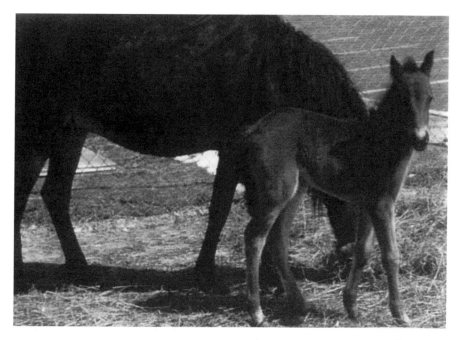

Fig. 1.9. Foal watching and learning. Photo: A.F. Fraser.

put this more simply, restriction affects their behaviour and creates bad habits, which become ingrained. In constant close confinement, horses can suffer affective dysfunctions. The typical dysfunctions usually occur in mouthing (Sambraus, 1985), marking time and reacting, but affective states can also appear in adverse features of temperament or disposition.

A traditional form of restriction used on horses is in the form of 'breaking-in' for human use. The term says much about the animal's affected spirit. Such evoked submissive responsiveness in the horse is achieved forcibly. Today there is increasing awareness of the alternative method of inducing compliance in the horse by humane manipulation of the animal's nature. Induced compliance is preferable to imposed submission. Compliant horses are able to develop in their conventional tasks by using intelligent responses.

Intelligent horses show much attention to events in their vicinity – that is their means of learning (see Figs 1.7–1.9).

Welfare Addendum

The equine nature is expansive from its massive inheritance and its cumulative experiences. Its immediate circumstances create an additional factor in the determination of its behaviour. As a result, no two horses are exactly alike in general conduct. Every horse is unique in its nature: in its character, temperament, personality and individual behaviour. It follows that horse welfare is axiomatic, that the management of each horse should be in accord with its particular individualism and, therefore, that knowledge of equine behaviour in general is fundamentally required in modern horse care.

2 Sensory Faculties and Behavioural Roots

The end points of sensitive evolution in horses can be seen in their sensory faculties of reflex actions, sensitivity to underfoot conditions, effective flight, shyness, specific gregariousness, emotionality, food preference, kinetic learning ability and self-important memory. These faculties rest, of course, on the sense of vision, hearing, smell, taste and touch. The equine senses are reviewed here in summary form to show certain links with behaviour and matters of welfare. In addition, the underlying systems in the horse's sensorium require to be appreciated for their fundamental role in the outputs of overt behaviour (Pilliner and Davies, 2004).

Sensibilities

Vision

The horse has its eyes located on the lateral aspects of its forehead. Some breeds have a slightly more lateral orbital location than others. The horse has a high degree of panoramic sight due to this anatomical feature. In the horse, panoramic vision provided scanning capacity, which was undoubtedly a key feature in its early survival. Vision is one of the most important considerations in defence. The eyes of the horse are so arranged that it is simultaneously able to see almost entirely to its rear and completely on both sides (Timney and Keil, 1992). Types of early forms of predators, with which it obviously coped, were considerable. This evolutionary type of adaptation in sight has some disadvantages under modern circumstances. It is unable, for example, to focus its eyes close enough to see objects very keenly if less than 0.6 m (2 ft) from its face. The horse has particular difficulty with visual 'accommodation', i.e. focusing on objects directly in front of it. When it concentrates to focus its eyes forward to its maximum ability, it appears momentarily to lose the ability to observe consciously to the rear and to the sides. The newborn foal has poor accommodation (see Fig. 2.1).

In circumstances in which the horse was subject to predation, the advantages of rear vision are obvious. Most breeds of horses have their eyes so laterally placed that their rear vision is only blocked by the width of the horse's own body. This vision, together with its keen awareness of sudden movement and its preparedness for quick flight, must have made the horse difficult to apprehend by predators when it was a hunted animal. These peculiar advantages and disadvantages of the horse's vision explain a good deal of its behaviour (see Fig. 2.2).

As a result of having its eyes set on the sides of its head, the horse has monocular vision, i.e. it has the ability to see separate things with each eye at the same time. It may be able to see an object with one eye only for a while, until adjustment of view brings the object into the view of the other eye as well. One significant effect of this is that minor objects, as they come quickly into view, appear to jump suddenly into the horse's conscious vision before the second eye catches up with the first eye to observe a given object properly. It is this visual characteristic that explains why they are sometimes less likely to shy from moving objects than they are from minor stationary objects. Moving objects sail into view, while stationary ones jump into it with the animal's own motion. Alteration of head position may be required to bring a stationary item into view clearly. The smaller the item the more likely the horse is to have this object come unexpectedly into its vision, causing it to shy away from it.

Some defects in forward vision are compensated by flexibility of the neck. The horse actually uses movements of its head and neck to help focus the eyes. This is done by raising its head up and down, or tilting the head to one side or the other. The retina of the eye, the part of the interior lining that receives the image, is slightly curved and not entirely a flattened 'ramp', as was formerly believed.

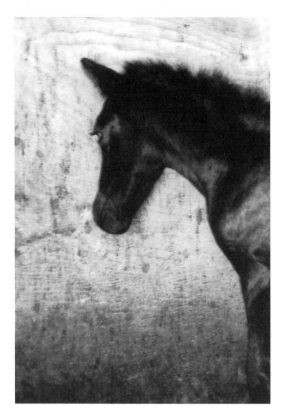

Fig. 2.1. Newborn foal with poor eyesight exploring its environment. Photo: A.F. Fraser.

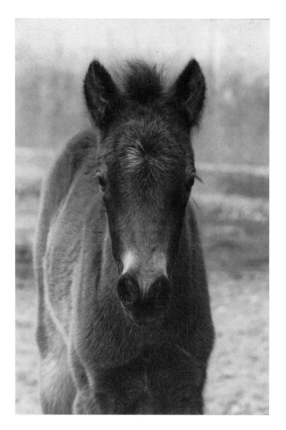

Fig. 2.2. Foal with lateral position of eyes, giving good panoramic vision but limited forward bifocal sight. Photo: Melanie MacDonald.

Although it has remarkable all-around sight, the horse is unable to see objects above the level of its eyebrows or at its mouth. Such limitation is by no means exclusively equine. Horses usually lip offered food before catching it with their teeth.

The poorly developed muscular body around the pupil of the equine eyes is an anatomical factor that contributes to focusing difficulty. In many other higher forms of life, this body is quite strong and is able to pull or release the lens so that it may quickly change in thickness and so act in focusing. However, head movement overcomes some of these focusing problems. If the horse raises its head it can see things at a middle distance much better, although its long-range vision is relatively poor. If it lowers its head, close objects come into sharper view. By moving its head in a lateral direction to one side or the other, the horse is capable of focusing on specific items. In addition, the horse has the capacity for interocular transfer of sights as a means of learning (Hanggi, 1999a,b).

Some breeds, notably the Arabian, have prominent eyes, which allow them to have slightly better visual scope than the majority of other horses. Among mountain and moorland breeds of ponies, there is a degree of frontal vision. This is a feature of their adaptation to the native environments. With good frontal vision the horse has its eyes set over a slightly narrow nose bridge, allowing the eyes effective anterior viewing scope. In such individuals the narrower nose below the eyes helps to facilitate forward binocular vision. Such horses have slightly better frontal vision than others. As a result they are better able to focus, have improved images on their eyes and react better within their environments. They can also perform certain tasks that require good eyesight better than other horses might manage.

Horses with an adequate degree of frontal vision are able to utilize binocular vision, a valuable asset in adaptation. This is the kind of visual property that gives the animal the advantageous ability to focus easily on objects directly in front of it. The horse with this capability is obviously at an immediate advantage in dealing with mountainous and complicated terrain. It helps mountain and moorland ponies to cope with the numerous small obstacles in their environment, such as rocks and marshes. Binocular vision permits highly efficient selection of nutritious herbage. It can also assist in jumping. As a horse approaches a difficult jump, it will strut for a stride or two if given the opportunity, in order to better see the jump and 'gather' itself for effort.

When the horse puts its face perpendicular to the ground, its best forward or frontal vision is obtained. This involves flexion of the neck at the poll. Poll flexion is a common form of head carriage seen in many horses with high-stepping action. This style gives the best possible vision of the ground immediately ahead. At slower rates of travel, such as the slow trot, this is a suitable style of going. When the horse is running and is required to see objects at a greater distance, it is obliged to raise its head. When it does raise its head for this purpose, it loses both side and ground vision to some degree. This can generate alarm when the ground area is rough or alien. It is pointless and inhumane to scold or punish a horse for a sight mistake or problem of vision. Horses can have various causes for poor sight due to ocular disorders, such as opacities and growths. These can be in addition to their natural peculiarities. Horses have plenty of such peculiarities and consideration should be given to them when vision is difficult or in question.

Hearing

Horses have a good sense of hearing. This is essential for appropriate behaviour when bond formation is being encouraged by vocalization between breeding mares and stallions and between brood mares and foals. The range of equine hearing exceeds the human range, and verbal commands are readily perceived. The extensive mobility of the horse's ears enhances this sense; they are essentially sound receptors with independent direction. They can direct sounds around a lateral arc of 180°, and move singly or in unison. The ears can swivel or become pricked-up forward to direct the ear tunnels towards the sound sources. Ear mobility is used to improve acuity in the sense of hearing, although some ear movements are protective, as when the horse lays its ears back as it prepares or threatens to fight. To concentrate on a distant source of sound, horses may turn their bodies in the given direction, allowing the sound waves to bounce off the slopes of the shoulders and upwards towards their ears.

Harsh noise can cause very anxious behaviour in any horse that is unaccustomed to it. A lack of harsh noise is especially important in breeding premises, to eliminate stress. An apparent feature of stress in some animals is termination of the brain's hormonal link with the gonads, causing the sex organs to suffer poor function with the loss of brain (hypothalamic) support, leading to diminished motivation (Hogan, 2005).

Olfaction and taste

The sense of smell is important to the horse. The olfactory receptors that generate the sense of smell are located in the mucous membrane in the upper part of the nasal cavity. The receptors in the olfactory mucosa bind with any odorous molecules entering the aerosol form. Through sniffing actions, the horse can promptly intensify the current of air in the nasal passage, creating more intimate contact between an odorous substance and the receptors in the mucosa. The receptor cells are modified neurons having two processes. The main process forms the olfactory nerve, which goes to the brain, while the other process extends over the surface of the olfactory mucosa. In smell, the airborne odorous substance enters the nose, comes in contact with lipid and protein material in the membrane and interacts with the microscopic hair-like structures on the receptor cells.

When good fit takes place between the odour molecule and the receptor site, there is efficient depolarization in the nerve cell, which forms an electrical potential. The action potential travels through the olfactory nerve to the olfactory bulb and then to the cortex for processing into the sense of smell. From the olfactory bulb, outgoing axon processes make up the olfactory tract of the brain. This tract passes to other brain regions and, in particular, is involved with a great many connections making up the rhinencephalon (part of the limbic system) to become a more compound sense with strong associations, some of which are social or sexual (Hubbal et al., 2009).

Horses have very good senses of both smell and taste. They may respond adversely to strange, unnatural odours or taste. The senses of smell and taste help them in food selection. Even when there is an abundance of other, established grazing available, horses show a strong preference for the first growth of grass from any newly seeded areas of pasture. Smell is also vital in a wide range of reproductive and social situations. While being a typical herd species, horses show a marked preference for certain individuals of their own species. Two horses encountering each other for the first time display keen olfactory attention in nose to nose contact. Further exploratory behaviour at introduction involves an olfactory investigation of the other's head, body and hindquarters, using their acute sense of smell to detect individual odours (McDonnell, 2002).

Taste is important to horses for appropriate food selection. Like smell, the sense of taste is the result of interactions of chemical stimuli with receptors located on the surface of a mucous membrane. In this case the receptors are taste buds on the tongue. Olfactory cells in the nasal membranes can combine the senses of smell and taste. Both senses need to be considered together. They share a common feature: as chemical senses, they are dependent upon contact with chemical substances for stimulation. This is in contrast with the other senses, which are dependent upon energies of light, vibration or pressure.

The taste buds are end organs in the mucous membranes of the mouth. The majority of them are located on the anterior two-thirds of the tongue. In taste, monosodium glutamate seems to facilitate the binding of chemical stimuli with molecules on the membrane of the tongue over the taste receptor. Molecules are transduced into a gustatory impulse conveyed to the brain and to a level of consciousness. Some differences occur in taste detection and preference for items of food. Taste preferences involve conscious selection of items for ingestion. Houpt and Wolski (1982) reported that, of 29 pasture species, horses and ponies preferred timothy, white clover (but not red clover) and perennial ryegrass. Dandelion was the most preferred herb.

Accessory olfactory system

The horse has a supplemental olfactory system in the form of the vomeronasal organ (VNO). This is a tubular structure on the floor of the nasal cavity; it communicates with the mouth via the nasopalatine canal. It does not exist in the human but it is present in a broad range of animals, being well developed and very functional in the horse. The lumen of the tube alternately constricts and expands under stimulation, causing it to act as a pump. This organ, as a purely anatomical structure, was first described by L. Jacobson in the early 19th century. The function of the VNO is as an accessory olfactory system that detects pheromones. The system makes use of the behavioural phenomenon of flehmen, notably in the horse, among many other ungulates (Meredith, 1999).

A pheromonal protein first stimulates the olfactory epithelium and this activates the pumping mechanism of Jacobson's organ. When the male comes in contact with the non-volatile 'protein' of the vaginal secretion, this is transferred to the nasal cavity and drawn into the lumen of the vomeronasal organ. This organ relays its impulses to a centre in the hippocampus that controls sexual behaviour. In particular, Whitten's hypothesis is that:

> Whole urine and 'peptide' is drawn into the lumen, where it generates potentials that are transmitted to the accessory olfactory bulb and thence to the hippocampus and the lateral hypothalamus...flehmen...could be a means of holding a lake of urine over the orifice of the vomeronasal organ while the pump takes samples. It could also even act as a venture to clear the site for the next sample.

This seems to be an eminently tenable theory regarding the function of the VNO and the accessory olfactory system of the horse (Whitten, 1985; Booth and Signoret, 1992).

Touch, somatic sensation and pain

The horse is very sensitive to touch and pain. The receptors in this sensory system are the nerve fibre ending plus the specialized non-neural cells associated with it. Each sensation is associated with a specific type of receptor. Distinct receptors respond to heat, cold, touch, pressure, joint position and pain. Somatic sensation occurs mainly through touch and pressure from mechanical forces on hairs, the skin and deeper subcutaneous tissues, and through rotation of joints. Temperature changes also stimulate this system. In pain, a stimulus affects receptors at the ends of certain small neurons (Cunningham and Klein, 2007).

The touch-pressure receptor organ is the pacinian corpuscle, located in the skin. The nerve terminal of the corpuscle is surrounded by layers of cells and extracellular fluid. When a mechanical force disturbs these layers and fluid, a potential is generated and the receptor fires an electrical stimulus.

Receptors in joints and ligaments are activated by mechanical forces such as stretching, twisting or impact. The combined stimulation signals the nature of joint movement. Action potential frequency along nerves from the receptors to the central nervous system indicates various features, e.g. extension, flexion or twisting. With temperature stimuli, the agitation in the skin causes changes in protein molecules which alter membrane permeability. This causes a generator potential in the nerve ending, leading to an action potential in the nerve and ultimately the temperature sensation (Heidemann, 2007).

Pain generally results in the release of 'pain mediators' (bradykinin, prostaglandins and others), acting on specific 'pain receptors'. Pain receptors generate electrical potential in response to traumatic stimulation such as tissue-damaging pressure, intense heat, irritating chemical substances and skin abrasion. Electrical firing from the receptors increases as the severity of the stimulus intensifies. Specific pain pathways go to pain centres. The cortex creates the perception of pain and makes the horse aware of the strength and position of the pain stimulus. Non-specific pathways for pain travel to the brainstem (and a part of the thalamus) to arouse reactivity. These non-specific pathways are also connected with the limbic system, which plays a major role in integrating autonomic and endocrine responses, plus the behavioural processes of aggression and defence, which feature in responses to pain (Bracher et al., 1998).

In response to the pain reflex, escape or withdrawal efforts are made. In addition, a range of physiological changes occurs from the effects of the activation of the sympathetic nervous system by the limbic system (Brooks, 1981). These sympathetic effects are exhibited in fear or rage, fight or flight. A pain stimulus gives rise to a painful sensory experience in conjunction with a behavioural response and an emotional component. These elements are very durable in a horse's memory. In particular, the experience of pain includes some emotional components of fear, anxiety and unpleasantness. The complex nature of pain is due to the combination of sensory experience followed by a reaction. The pain reaction includes such emotional responses as fear and a behavioural reactive component in such situations as extreme trauma, in addition to the classic physiological changes historically described by Cannon (1953).

Memory

The horse, as it matures, acquires very good memory. This memory seems to be selective for unpleasant events, but a well-trained horse remembers its training all of its life. This lasting memory tends to fix habits, both good and bad. Fixation of the latter can create behavioural problems. Considerate handling when young can be the basis of good temperament in later life, and this facilitates its tuition in training. The horse has a great capacity for retaining knowledge of past experiences through its good 'long-term' memory process in the hippocampus and its links within the limbic system. Memories of pain and fear are the strongest, and persist long after the unpleasant event has passed. Memories of such episodes are virtually impossible to eradicate from a horse, and its behaviour may continue to be affected by painful memories of certain situations. This great capacity for long-term memory is the main feature of its learning. When a horse can perform a new act, the memory of that action will probably remain with the horse for the rest of its life. An increasing usefulness in a horse can be created by building up its achievements to become ingrained habits. If a horse is hurt or is punished while doing something that is inherent to its nature, it will be very difficult, if not impossible, to eradicate this negative experience from its memory at a later date.

Learning

A horse can learn what is wanted of it by rewarding the desired action and subsequently presenting the reward only on the production of that same action. Repetition is important, as is consistency in teaching. Teaching a horse is like 'shaping' its behaviour. A start is made by rewarding, through encouragement, each successive activity that approximates the action desired. People who are good at horse teaching try first to get a horse to do something similar to the desired action. Then they increasingly reward only that behaviour that is close to the desired action. The skill of the horse teacher lies in recognizing small, progressive responses and rewarding each of them. Even the smallest progress may be the key to the desired performance. As lessons become completed, the desired responses alone will be reinforced by reward. Verbal praise and appreciative patting serve as rewards for desired behaviours, but small items of food work best (Jahiel, 2004).

In an attempt to eliminate some undesired behaviour such as biting or kicking, an unpleasant corrective must be paired repeatedly and exactly in time with the misbehaviour. This is very difficult to achieve. Even the slightest delay of the corrective nullifies the intended lesson. Experience shows, however, that punishment is not successful in horse education. Punishment at a later time after some misconduct is not only pointless, it is also inhumane and damaging to its well-being.

Good riders know that in the synchronized relationships between horse and rider, there is no need for crude mechanics, such as a fierce bit, to control a normal horse. Modern experts work with the horse's natural reactions, supplementing and moulding their responses with carefully chosen lessons. In a short time, this can produce a well-trained and a well-integrated animal, capable of producing responses considerably different, eventually, from its natural, untrained activities.

Intelligence

Forms of intelligent behaviour can be observed commonly in working horses. Impressive displays of intellectual properties have often been witnessed: for example, in the way horses could predict what was next wanted of them and in their ability to negotiate the most complex mazes of streets in towns. While various methods are often used to attempt to measure intelligence in animals, it is now reasonably assumed that the length of time that a horse takes to learn specific actions can

be a measure of intelligence. Promptness in learning may be real evidence of intelligence in horses. The compound of its temperament plus intelligence often determines a horse's reactions, which collectively make up its general behaviour. The way horses respond to imperative circumstances around them, when free to do so, is affected by their own temperament and individual intelligence (Table 2.1).

Emotionality

When horses form pairs they seem able to read each other's intentions and to function almost as one bonded unit. Pairs of horses in states of intimate understanding have been termed 'empathic pairs' (i.e. emotional bonding). Very specialized forms of close association occur in some pairs of horses that have become closely bonded to each other. It would be possible to describe this as a special equine feature of emotionality (see Fig. 2.3). Although some horses have more equine intelligence than others, their emotive quality and their sociability allows them to work intimately together in teams.

With such emotionality goes a degree of vulnerability. For example, emotional tensions in horses can affect their digestion. Under difficulty in adapting to their circumstances or the type of work, some horses become so emotionally affected that their digestive processes become noticeably impaired. The texture of their dung changes and it is evacuated much more quickly after consumption, since

Table 2.1. Principal ways of dealing with imperative factors in behavioural well-being in horses.

Behavioural category	Homeostatic features	Maintenance values	Roles in well-being	
			Short range	Long range
Fight	Aggression, agonistic acts and play	Self-assertion	Suppression of competitor	Control over resources of various kinds
Flight	Submissive withdrawal	Avoidance of threatful situations	Self-protection	Security of individual Stabilization of hierarchies
Feed	Search, selection and ingestion of food Consumption of water	Self-maintenance in respect of visceral needs Self-sufficiency in nutritional needs	Ingestion to repletion Suppression of hunger	Building up body reserves and storage

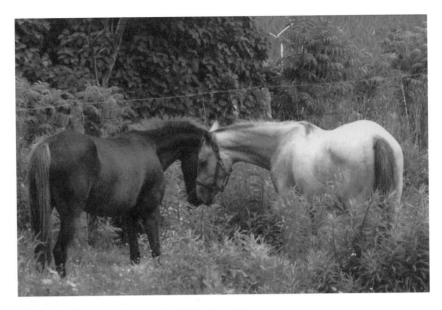

Fig. 2.3. Empathetic pair of friends. Photo: Melanie MacDonald.

the digestive upset causes food to pass out of the body before it is properly digested. When the horse becomes relaxed and accepts its conditions, its digestion can return to normal. This change can occur in a short time.

Horses can exhibit clearly the emotion of affection. This is not limited to the obvious affection between mare and foal. Young foals with regular playmates show it to each other in the 'head-overlay' display of affection (see Fig. 2.4a). This show

(a)

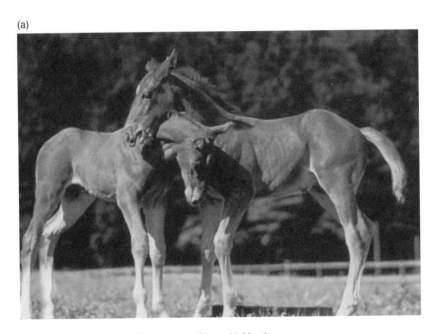

Fig. 2.4. (a) Affectionate head overlay with associate. Photo: H. Hastie.

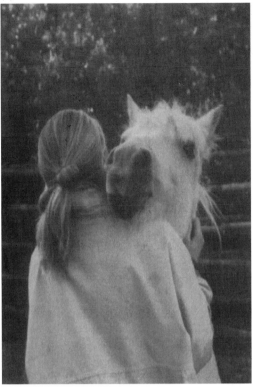

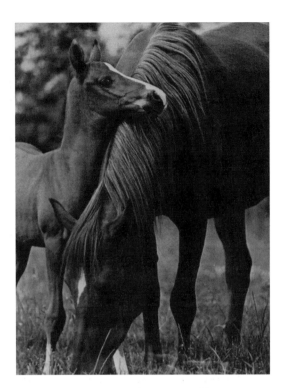

Fig. 2.5. Head overlay by foal on mare. Photo: A.F. Fraser.

Fig. 2.4. *Continued.* (b) Head overlay with handler. Photo: J. Woodman.

of affection takes the form of extending the head and laying it over the neck of the object of affection. It can be seen less commonly between older horses. The display can be shown to human subjects when, in this case, the horse puts its head over the shoulder of the person (see Fig. 2.4b). The action is evidently analogous to a hug and the component of emotion is beyond doubt. It would not be exhibited to a person, of course, if the level and style of care being provided by that person were inferior. If this display can be regarded objectively, it is further evidence of the high level of sentience in the horse. A less demonstrative sign of friendliness in horses is when physical contact occurs readily between them. Some stabled horses tied in adjacent stalls may draw back at night and put their hindquarters in mutual contact for long spells.

Sometimes foals will attempt the head overlay on the necks of their mothers, giving rise to some peculiar actions (see Fig. 2.5). The significance of this display of emotionality is that it is present from

a very early age and is not attained with maturation. Clearly foals are sentient beings like adult horses in general.

Equilibrium

The sense of position in equilibrium is due largely to impulses carried from the vestibular portion of the auditory nerve arising from impulses in the inner ear. The inner ear, as an excavation within the petrous temporal bone, contains the osseous labyrinth, within which there is fluid derived from the cerebral spinal fluid. Fluid movements establish sensations of position and balance, i.e. equilibrium. The inner ear's vestibular part functions mainly in the determination of balance. Its nerve supply is the vestibular branch of the eighth cranial nerve. The vestibular portion is made up of parts of the osseous labyrinth known as the vestibule and the three semicircular canals. Each of these canals connects with both ends to the vestibule and is arranged so that each is on a different positional plane, being at right angles to each other. One canal is approximately horizontal, another is approximately vertical and transverse to the head, while the third is upright.

The receptor system in the semicircular canals operates in relation to head movement. When the head is moved, the fluid filling the semicircular canals bends the hair cells of the canal system. The degree of bending causes stimulation. These hair cells are therefore stimulated during any motion of the head. The sense of position and equilibrium is chiefly derived from such stimulation. This sense determines balance and also directs the continuous and various reflexes concerning the maintenance of body position in motion. In the horse, the sense of balance is obviously developed to a remarkable degree. This is evident in such activities as carrying weight at speed with sharp changes in direction. Most equestrian recreation depends on the horse's keen sense of balance. When the horse is allowed to select its own head position, it knows how to move its head and neck in cantilever fashion to ensure that it preserves balance.

Behavioural Roots

The discipline of domestication, acting over millennia, has given us the types of livestock we now use for products or association. Any return to a pre-domesticated lifestyle would create suffering for most of the animals in human care. They have been developed along physical, physiological and behavioural lines in the domestication process. In contrast with equivalent wildlife forms, our domestic animals can be regarded as developed, for human purposes at least. Their behavioural suitability is a primary development.

With horses, as with the other domestically developed animals, all behaviour is rooted in the neurotransmission of the central nervous system and the endocrine chemistry of its outposts. Some overview of this root system helps to illustrate the firm basis of equine behaviour in general. Some of this firmness is responsible for fixed individuality of spirit on one hand and the various exact locomotor functions on the other. In addition, the instinctive patterns in reproductive behaviour constitute many firmly organized modes of activity (instinct here is regarded as an inherited action of a complex nature). Many abnormalities or anomalies in equine behaviour also show remarkable firmness and similarity of form within each type. Firmness and consistency of behavioural output characterizes horses, both individually and collectively.

Neurological organization

It has been said that the role of the nervous system in health and disease is so important that every logical and conceivable scientific approach should be used to improve its understanding. This is particularly true for any behavioural study. It should not be merely a matter of simplicity versus complexity, but rather what contribution both can make to overall comprehension. Behavioural needs and anomalous behaviour in horses are growing problems, calling for modern understanding. Neuroethology can be a fresh approach to the problems in our understanding of brain mechanisms for facilitating plasticity and adaptation to the environment.

Some awareness of neurological controls is helpful in an appreciation of horse behaviour, as these relate to the diverse psychological functions of perception, learning, memory, thinking, problem-solving and performance. The nervous system's essential function of electrical communication depends on neurons, which conduct information towards the central nervous system. These are classed as follows in three types:

1. Sensory or afferent neurons.
2. Motor or efferent neurons (which conduct information out from the central nervous system).
3. Interneurons or internuncial neurons (those that are contained completely within the central nervous system and whose function it is to distribute and integrate information within the latter). Implicit in this definition of interneurons is that they both receive information from and transmit it to other neurons.

The horse is an animal whose central nervous system consists of distinct regions. In spite of the diversity of regions and centres in the brain, the variety of tracts in the spinal cord and the array of peripheral nerves, the nervous system functions as a whole and all parts are interconnected through neuron linkage. It is estimated that no more than seven nerve cells are required to link any one part with any other part of the entire sensorium.

The nervous system's main parts are the central nervous system and the peripheral nerves. The central system has its own major divisions, namely the brain and spinal cord. The cerebrum, cerebellum and brainstem constitute the main parts of the brain. In addition there are special parts such as the cerebral cortex, the basal ganglia, the reticular formation and a range of regions, such as the hypothalamus. Specialized nuclei, such as the locus ceruleus, are also recognized in abundance. One notable system, which is a collection of specialized brain parts, is the limbic system. The brainstem is an important bottleneck in the processing and integration of behavioural output. Its notable structure is the reticular formation.

Reticular formation and connections

The reticular formation's functions include the production of general arousal in the central nervous system. The reticular formation embodies a mechanism by which states throughout the central nervous system are regulated. Some of these regulations are diurnal, e.g. one state is sleep and another is wakefulness. Between these two are many degrees of alertness and inattentiveness. All are expressions of some pattern of activity in the reticular formation (Cunningham and Klein, 2007).

The reticular formation is a place of convergence for information of widespread origin; this constitutes its role in ascending systems and also in a context of descent. Neurons in the rhombencephalic reticular formation can respond to inputs from secondary sensory cell groups in the spinal cord. They may also respond to a message from the cerebellum or from the neocortex. A large number and variety of messages converge on the reticular formation, which has to process this excess of neural matter and then dispatch impulses via reticulospinal fibres, which terminate either on intermediate neurons or directly on motor neurons.

Cerebral cortex

The cerebral cortex, although acting as a unit, has certain localized regions where sensory impulses are received and subjected to redirection. These specialized areas of the cortex are primary sites for sensory reception, the nervous activity subsequently spreading over a greater area. The cortex has a multitude of cells and neural paths, each one communicating with many others. This extremely complex relay system permits tremendous variability in the way that nerve impulses may be channelled.

The cerebral cortex possesses four main sensory areas into which projectory fibres discharge:

1. The somasthetic or body sense area.
2. The visual area.
3. The auditory area.
4. The olfactory area.

All of these are important in the reception, interpretation and execution of nerve signals. The cortex is of fundamental importance in determining behaviour.

Somasthetic area

This area is sited in the parietal lobe of the cortex and receives nerve impulses from many parts of the body, particularly its massive surface.

Visual area

Nerve fibres are collected from the retina of the eye into the optic nerves and are distributed within the cortex to the extensive visual area at the occipital part of the cerebrum. Cogent recognition of set situations and the selection of releasers that activate action patterns take place in the visual area.

Auditory area

This is located in the temporal lobe of the cerebral cortex. The area receives nerve impulses concerned with auditory sensations from the thalamus. The fibres of the hearing nerve end in the pons, from which region other fibres pass to the thalamus and then to the cortex.

Olfactory area

The sensory area dealing with smell plays a much more important role in breeding behaviour than has generally been recognized. An olfactory region is located in the hippocampus, which receives projection fibres from the centre in the olfactory bulb. This centre deals with olfactory reflexes. The fibres of the olfactory system originate with nerve cells located in the mucous membrane of the nasal passage and terminate within the olfactory bulbs.

It seems that areas of the cortex are designed to correlate dynamically with receptive areas on the body's surface. The neural importance of the superficial area and central nervous areas changes according to the major activities of an animal; for example, it seems that the appropriate area of the cortex is more receptive to stimulation from the genitalia during breeding times.

The limbic system

The limbic system (see Fig. 2.6) is a determinant and integrator of strategic and tactical functions. It is involved in displays of emotional behaviour and acts as the central representative of the autonomic system. It consists of an interconnected group of brain structures within the cerebral borders (limbus: a border) and includes portions of the frontal lobe cortex, temporal lobe, thalamus and hypothalamus, together with certain midbrain parts that act as function generators (Broad *et al.*, 2002).

Neuron pathways connect these brain regions in segmental integration. The component parts of the limbic system, therefore, have many connections with each other and with other parts of the central nervous system. Information from the different afferent and efferent routes influences the limbic system and its peripheral arm, the autonomic system. The activity of the limbic system can result in a wide variety of autonomic responses and of body movements that comprise purposeful behaviour. In the hypothalamus – the main output stage of the limbic system – a rage response can also be caused by destruction of certain parts. Certain other hypothalamic areas elicit behaviour that has a strong 'emotional' component. For example, the medial hypothalamus exerts inhibition on the circuits producing fight-or-flight behaviour. Upon receipt of appropriate environmental stimuli, the temporal lobe inhibits the medial hypothalamus, allowing activity in the integrated limbic system to increase, with resulting emotional behaviour (Heimer, 1978).

The structures involved in the control of emotional behaviour are predominantly located throughout the limbic system, and the main controlling centres for consummatory behaviour are located here, within the hypothalamus in particular. Much consummative behaviour, of course, relates to maintenance, the ongoing operation of which relates to behavioural homeostasis. Limbic matters therefore clearly relate to homeostasis, which is the essential business of self-maintenance.

The limbic system represents a device for providing the animal with a means of coping with the environment. Parts of the limbic system are concerned with primal activities related to food and sex; others are related to emotions and feelings; and still others combine messages from the external world. The limbic system is a fundamental regulator of survival responses. On the basis of behavioural analysis, this regulation seems to be inhibitory in nature. Each of the limbic system structures is highly specialized and is tuned to

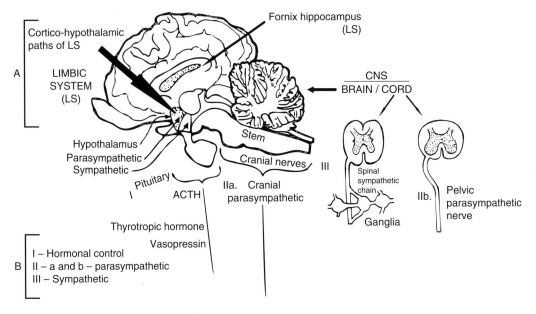

Fig. 2.6. The autonomic nervous system with its outlets. I, the pituitary; IIa and b, parasympathetic nerves; III, sympathetic chain.

specific changes in the internal or external environment. The hypothesis is that, however specialized, the structures of the limbic system regulate basic, primitive activities. Acting through suppressive mechanisms, the limbic system allows new directions in behaviour to occur. For example, the circumstances under which the hippocampus acts to regulate the activities of other brain regions seem to be conditions of uncertainty. Life becomes uncertain when old patterns of responding fail to produce the anticipated rewards or when old habits fail to pay off. This suppression prevents the animal from continuing in its old ways of responding and from over-reacting in general. The limbic system, more than any other brain part, creates the animal's own characteristic output of emotionally tuned behaviour.

The hippocampus and the amygdala are two main components of the limbic system. Other limbic components include the fornix at the free edge of the cerebral mantle. Various parts of the forebrain convey neural activities to the hypothalamus through the limbic system, so that by one route or another, the important hypothalamus is in receipt of impulses from optic, olfactory, acoustic and tactile sense organs. The limbic system also contains neural centres such as the amygdala, which control aggressive behaviour in its various forms. The frontal cortical areas play a role in coordinating the signals from the limbic system that are to be integrated with the activities of the 'cognitive brain', i.e. the majority of the neocortical surface. Horses have plenty of cognitive behaviour. The limbic system makes possible the suppression of established ways of responding in order to allow behavioural modifications based on information from the internal environment via neocortical tissue (Isaacson, 1982).

The hippocampus is a prominent component of the limbic system (Fig. 2.7) and is concerned significantly with emotion in behaviour. It is connected to the hypothalamus via a tract called the fornix to generate a physiological output into behaviour that expresses emotion.

The hypothalamus requires special identification. It can be regarded as an extended part of the limbic system since it is its terminus. It has an executive role as the hormone system's initiator and is also the autonomic system's controller.

The importance of the limbic system in well-being is a major one, although it operates subconsciously. It helps the horse to absorb its circumstances and adjust to these to its limit. It is a very old neural system in terms of evolution and was once regarded as the 'nose brain' because of its strong involvement with the olfactory region, particularly in non-mammalian vertebrates.

Basal ganglia

Three large subcortical nuclear groups are collectively called the basal ganglia and account for 5% of the brain mass. The basal ganglia nuclei participate in the control of movements together with the cerebellum.

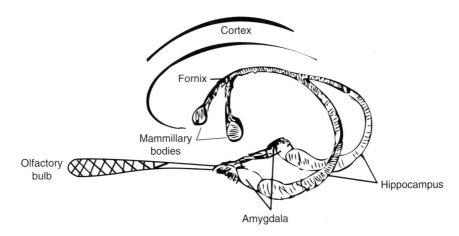

Fig. 2.7. A diagrammatic representation of the limbic system in the cerebrum, shown only to illustrate the complexity of this system. The overall integrity of its parts creates an elaborate system addressing and attempting general homeostasis in the animal.

The basal ganglia play an important role in the initiation and control of movement. Many neurons of the basal ganglia change their activity during movement of a specific body part. These neurons are typically clustered close together, forming a somatotopic representation of the body. Neurons whose activity relate to movements of the forelimbs are found ventral to those whose activity relate to hind leg movements. Characteristically, the changes in activity of these neurons take place before the movement of the body, indicating that they play a role in the initiation of movement. The presumptive basis of some pathological motor patterns, for example anomalous actions, is the dopaminergic projection from the substantia nigra to basal ganglia. Dopamine constitutes about one-half of the catecholamine in the brain, 80% of which is localized in the basal ganglia.

Hypothalamus

It is at the level of the hypothalamus that patterns of nervous activities become integrated and regulated so as to establish the adaptive reactions of the animal. Even behaviour that is largely dependent upon experience and learning in the animal is seldom, if ever, completely free of control by the primitive mechanisms established in the hypothalamus and in the subcortex generally. The neural links involving the subcortex, and the links between the hypothalamus and the surrounding brain in particular, remain the principal integrators of most behavioural patterns.

The working units of the hypothalamus are neurons, which are grouped into 'nuclei'. These nuclei operate together with a high degree of coordination. The information from various levels of the brain is received and processed by these nuclei before signals are subsequently reissued to more specialized parts of the body, which are geared to function under the control of the hypothalamus. Much of the influence of hypothalamic activity is directed at the production of hormones in the subjacent pituitary gland. The pituitary is the principal endocrine gland in the body, and its hormonal production is all-important in the maintenance of the bulk of the body's activities, including behaviour. Even the all-important central hypothalamus is responsive to some of the endocrine activity for which it is initially responsible. It has become clear that there is a considerable amount of hormonal control over the hypothalamus. The receipt of afferent stimulation provides the hypothalamus the role of maintaining and regulating the activity of the pituitary gland. The hypothalamus is characterized by its glandular appendage – the pituitary. It is also, of course, continuous, in the forward direction, with the limbic system.

Autonomic system

In the autonomic circuitry, fibres passing without interruption from the hypothalamus to the autonomic motor neurons of the spinal cord's grey matter constitute a small minority of the outgoing hypothalamic fibres. The hypothalamus appears in large measure to project no further than the midbrain, where neurons of the reticular formation take over. The pathways descending to autonomic motor neurons are interrupted at numerous levels. At each eruption further instructions enter the descending lines. The convergence of information on motor neurons is a characteristic of the autonomic nervous system.

Most sympathetic nerve endings release the neurotransmitter substance norepinephrine (or noradrenaline), which is chemically very similar to epinephrine (adrenaline), produced by the medulla of the adrenal gland. The nerve fibres creating such chemistry are therefore termed adrenergic. Thus, the adrenal medulla resembles a ganglion of the sympathetic system in its roles. The release of norepinephrine at the adrenergic nerve fibre terminations prepares the subject for actions. Notably there is an increased blood supply to the voluntary muscles. Most parasympathetic nerve endings release acetylcholine at synapses and nerve endings. They are therefore termed cholinergic in their chemistry of neurotransmission. After its synaptic release, acetylcholine duly spreads the parasympathetic effects. The effects of the two divisions typically tend to be opposite, and the two subsystems are therefore antagonistic. The antagonism is due to the chemistry of the two divisions. Parasympathetic stimulation produces the 'vegetating' effects of slower heart rate, lowered blood pressure, constriction of bronchi and increased activity of the gut for digestion.

The autonomic system acts as a behavioural integrator; its full role is in modulating the intensities of behavioural responses and in particular the emotional component of behaviour. The autonomic system affects and moulds all. It integrates glandular function and somatic behaviour. Since it is a moulder of reaction, it plays a part in determining the nature of behaviour and emotive states associated with behaviour. Through this system, conditioned reactions determine the nature of future responsiveness.

Autonomic conditioning may last for years and requires little reinforcement. Any reinforcement to this system is powerful and may even occur in anticipation of a set of circumstances without them necessarily occurring. The autonomic conditioned reactions are, in many cases, triggered by telereceptors and even in anticipation of what may occur. The reactions are very fast and precede somatic components of defence, alerting, fight or flight. Autonomic innervation improves the acuity of olfaction, taste, hearing, touch and proprioception. In equine life, the autonomic system is involved in agonistic reactions, self-determination, survival efforts, comfort-seeking and preparation for future circumstances. This supports an ancient and modern view that the autonomic system is the system by which modulations are dictated to behaviour, so that the subject meets the requirements of the environment and its society.

Spinal cord

The spinal cord and brain are extensions of each other. Specific tracts from the lumbar area of the spinal canal along the cord, to and from the brain, exemplify this scheme. The role of the spinal cord is sometimes autonomous, as in certain reflex mechanisms. Simple reflexes such as limb withdrawal in response to a local limited stimulus have cord organization. The scratch reflex is the outstanding example of coordinated cord reflex action. Spinal reflexes are quite numerous in equine behaviour. Reflex spinal arcs are by no means eliminated or replaced in evolution but, in horses for example, they are modified and controlled by superior reflex arcs involving the cerebrum. For example, a high order of control of defecation is seen in the elimination behaviour of horses, in which patterns of defecating behaviour are elaborate and specialized. At the same time, such patterns are not always operant; if the horse is being worked, for example. The demands of controlled work engage the cerebrum sufficiently to return the control of defecation to the appropriate spinal centres. As a result, the horse readily passes faeces during periods of restrained, enforced use. This example demonstrates that lower levels of CNS control are never eliminated or entirely replaced by higher ones.

Specific motor reflexes involve not only excitation of particular muscle groups but also inhibition of antagonistic muscles, as follows:

1. Stretch reflex involves excitation of extensor and inhibition of ipsilateral flexor muscles, as in pandiculation.
2. Flexor reflexes: painful stimulus to limb causes excitation of ipsilateral flexor muscles and inhibition of ipsilateral extensors.
3. Withdrawal reflexes are associated with extension of the limb of the opposite or contralateral side of the body. Inhibition of the flexors on that contralateral side also occurs.
4. Many neurons are common to all the above reflexes, i.e. ventral horn cells act as a final common path. These circuits are only part of more extensive circuits.
5. As well as allowing for many forms of integration, spinal interneurons allow a presynaptic input to be converted from excitation to inhibition or vice versa.

Complicated yet coordinated motor behaviour, such as occurs in equine locomotion, can be seen in terms of the above-mentioned mechanisms and reflex pathways. The nervous system is responsible for innumerable varieties of coordination, generating a continuum of behaviour that is directed at homeostasis. Disturbed physiology in the limbic, hormonal and neural autonomic network influences certain hormones and transmitter substances, such as adrenaline and dopamine, respectively. Severe or chronic imbalance in this elaborate network underpins stress and numerous equine behavioural anomalies. Many of the latter relate to excess dopamine activity (hyperdopaminergic). Stability in this network is of fundamental importance in the horse.

Chemical Operations

The nervous system and the endocrine system are cooperative. Contact between them is essential in their full function. The two systems cooperate with each other through the processes of neural secretion and the priming effects of hormones on the brain. Hormone secretion is subject to the influence of many forms of stimulation. An elaborate organization of interactions exists between the external stimuli received and the internal physiological state (Oliver and Lorenz, 1993).

Three factors – behaviour, environment and internal state – can alter to cause a change in motivation.

This can create complex situations of chemical activity in neuropeptides, hormones and pheromones. These are active in chemical communication within the body and between bodies. Such communication advises and instructs the animal's parts on the physiological status and requirements of the whole. This very active chemistry provides a powerful basis for bodily activity. An outline of the system of chemical messengers is therefore essential to an appreciation of behavioural motivation.

Endocrine system

Motivation is neuro-hormonally dependent. Hormones act on nerve tissue within the nerve system specifically to energize the production of output in those neural systems that are programmed to function in the presence of the chemistry of the particular hormone. Many 'new role' circumstances operate through the production of hormones, mainly from endocrine glands. The purpose of such hormones is to activate neural systems that are not involved in routine behaviour. Although hormone production is the role of the endocrine system, hormone release requires stimulation. The hypothalamus is responsible for controlling the secretions of both anterior and posterior pituitary lobes. It is also responsible for releasing and inhibiting factors, for feedback mechanisms, for the control of cyclic phenomena and ultimately for sexual behaviour.

Pituitary secretion is promoted by the output of releasers from the hypothalamus. Gonadotropin-releasing hormone acts on the anterior pituitary gland, causing it to produce and release dual hormones: luteinizing hormone (LH) and follicle-stimulating hormone (FSH). The gonadotropins have the sex glands of either gender as their target. Here they promote the physiology of the gonads. The gonads produce their gametes and their own hormones. Gonadotropic output is cyclical in the female.

Prolactin is a further hormone concerned with reproductive function. It is produced by the anterior pituitary and is considered to be the hormone that motivates the initial maternal behaviour. This latter activity does not entirely depend on prolactin, however, since it is also governed by the ratio of progesterone to oestrogen, typically occurring in the postpartum period. Prolactin also motivates grooming behaviour.

The notable hormones produced by the posterior pituitary are oxytocin and vasopressin. In terms of reproductive action, oxytocin is commonly known as the 'let-down' hormone – the hormone that encourages the free outflow of milk at the appropriate times. It also appears to be involved in male ejaculation. Vasopressin is associated with the increased blood pressure of arousal (Brownstein et al., 1980). Vasopressin contributes, unfortunately, to the problem of nasal bleeding in racing horses.

The two gonadotropic hormones from the anterior pituitary are essential to reproductive function. The two are produced in concert with one another in both sexes. The levels vary in the female. This creates cyclic ovarian activity and related behaviour in breeding mares. The production of gonadotropins in the male appears to be steady and continuous. The sex hormones of the gonads, in their behavioural roles, are androgenic and oestrogenic, respectively, in the male and female. High levels of either androgens or oestrogens can inhibit the secretion of both FSH and LH by feedback effect through the hypothalamus.

Corticotropin-releasing hormone (CRH) is another of the releasing substances. Through its action, there is output of adrenocorticotropic hormone (ACTH). ACTH secretion is involved in sugar metabolism (glycogenolysis) and stress. ACTH also controls some other endocrine glands. In particular it causes the adrenal cortex to enlarge and produce a variety of corticosteroids, typified by cortisol. Blood levels of cortisol, which rise in states of stress, are the result of increased ACTH activity. Sometimes the cortisol output in horses can be erratic as a result of major husbandry disturbances. ACTH is essentially the adaptive hormone for unusual circumstances. It has an increased secretion during any attempt at adaptation to an environmental or husbandry problem (Nelson, 2000).

Steroids are produced in the adrenal cortex as hormonal substances. The adrenal cortical hormones can generate glycogenesis by glucocorticoids and male activity by androgens. All of the adrenal cortical hormones are termed corticoids, among which cortisol is most active. This hormone quickly activates carbohydrate metabolism so as to increase blood sugar for the needs of sudden energy and to deal with stressful events.

The adrenal medulla is under the close control of the limbic system, and of the hypothalamus in particular. The hormonal product of the adrenal medulla is epinephrine; it is biologically similar to norepinephrine. Epinephrine prepares the horse for gross physical activity in situations of emergency. It is particularly responsible for temporary increase in blood pressure in response to stressful stimulation. Increases in epinephrine output are associated with agonistic events and alarm responses (Schulkin, 1999).

The small pineal gland, located in the centre of the brain, produces melatonin. The output of this hormone is influenced by the light–dark photoperiod and is basic to the operation of seasonal phenomena in horses. Melatonin influences their diurnal and cyclic behaviour. Testosterone motivates masculine behaviour; it is produced by the testicles of the adult stallion under the influence of LH from the anterior pituitary. In the stallion there is some seasonal fluctuation in testosterone output in high northern latitudes as a result of the photoperiodic influence of melatonin (Smolensky, 2001).

Physical activities depend on the thyroid gland for its secretion of thyroxine. This hormone influences energetic behaviour by affecting the metabolic pool of nitrogen and available energy. Thyroxine influences the activity of the gonads as well. Deficiencies and excesses of this hormone occur. Both hypothyroid and hyperthyroid females are sometimes found to have lengthened, irregular or arrested oestrous cycles.

In the mare's breeding season the ovary produces two hormones. As the ovarian follicle matures during pro-oestrus, its output of oestrogen increases. At the critical level of oestrogen output, the mare's behaviour exhibits the signs of oestrus. Some preovulatory progesterone is needed to synergize with oestrogen to produce all of the features of oestrus. Oestrous behaviour is strongly motivated while the follicle is at the peak of its development. When the follicle ruptures there is a sharp drop in oestrogen. A day or two later the disappearance of oestrogen in the general circulation is responsible for the termination of oestrous behaviour in the mare. This temporary motivation of sexual behaviour in the mare contrasts with stallion motivation, which is maintained by the continued output of testosterone by permanent interstitial cells in the testis (Mair et al., 1998).

In pregnancy, the placenta synthesizes the steroids progesterone and oestrogen. The placenta also contains a very high concentration of β-endorphin. During parturition it is now believed that the release of β-endorphin from the placenta permits its uptake by the maternal circulation, causing a mild opioid state to block some of the pain of parturition.

Pheromonal system

A pheromone is a substance secreted to the outside of the body by an individual animal and detectable through the odour-detecting system of another individual of the same species, motivating a special reaction in the recipient animal. Horses and many other animals communicate by pheromonal substances conveyed through their secretions and excretions. The pheromonal system includes the nasal apparatus as the receptor, the rhinencephalon of the brain as an integrator, and the olfactory region of the cortex as the executor. Stimulation through these steps is affected by the pheromone after its binding with the olfactory mucosa (Vandenbergh, 1983; Wyatt, 2003).

Horses possess specialized gland complexes located in the skin. These glands induce temperature control, excretion and lubrication. In each individual these products combine to create a specific body odour. In horses the convoluted type of skin glands have apocrine excretions. This volatile substance on the skin's surface is mixed into a product that contains the odorous substance. Special odours relate to certain functions and have specific motivating capacity. Some pheromones act as 'external hormones', affecting the internal endocrine state of other individuals. Other pheromones can be classified according to territorial marking, ranking, tracing, recognition, alerting and sexual stimulation. The perineal skin of the foal appears to be the source of a pheromone of identity for the mare.

Other pheromonal sources include faeces and urine. Exhaled breath and oral odours appear to have a similar function. Saliva can be involved in chemical communication (Block et al., 1981), and behavioural evidence of this is notable in social events in the horse. Nosing closely at the muzzle of another horse is seen as having some purpose when a bond or social tolerance is being negotiated. It is also a notable exchange between a foal and an adult.

The odorous substances of horses contain several pheromones at one time; such pheromones are secreted not only through their skin organs but also through the urine and other secretions. Releaser pheromones, such as sexual pheromones, can produce a latent but longer response, such as bonding. It is assumed that a pheromone feedback mechanism stimulates sexual activity in the male. The urine of stallions apparently contains 'indicator' pheromones relating to the concentration of

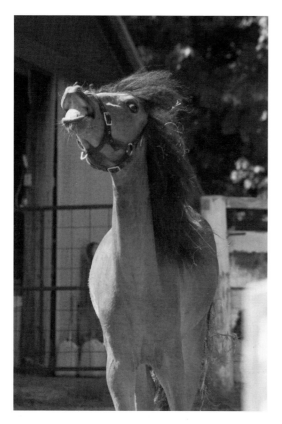

Fig. 2.8. The flehman posture. Photo: A.F. Fraser.

sex pheromone. Equine pheromone detection depends on the horse's macrosmatic ability, i.e. the possession of a highly developed sense of smell. As aforementioned, the horse possesses the vomeronasal, or Jacobson's, organ. The full operation of this olfactory receptor is dependent on the horse drawing in a fine aerosol in an olfactory reflex act known as flehmen (Schneider, 1930). In flehmen, the horse elevates and extends its head, its lip curled up, its mouth slightly open and its nostrils constricted. Pheromones detected via flehmen can signal the oestrous state of the mare to the stallion

(Fig. 2.8). This contributes significantly to sexual motivation.

Welfare Addendum

The equine eyeball loses some of its globular shape with advancing age, becoming slightly more contracted from front to back. This has some effect on vision. The conflicting accounts over the existence of a 'ramp retina' may have been the result of differing ages in the specimens examined. The excusable and simple fact of age causing poor eyesight has to be borne in mind when poorer responses or performances are found in an older horse.

When a horse is blind it usually keeps its ears in constant motion and, while walking, will lift its feet as though stepping over obstacles. The feet will then be put down with some uncertainty. If the animal is blind in only one eye, this typical gait will not be shown. Eyesight can deteriorate with ageing, and this reduction in sight can lead to instances of shying in older horses that did not show such behaviour previously. Total blindness in a horse calls for euthanasia because it inevitably establishes suffering, except in very special circumstances of intense care.

Very young foals are short-sighted, most especially in the early hours of life. This visual factor is not a handicap in outdoor habitats but is a serious defect in various domesticated situations. Young foals may run into structural obstacles around farm premises.

Many horses may 'spook' at minor, innocuous factors suddenly coming into their vision; horses are often reluctant to load into trailers that have 'unseen' interiors, for example. Adjustments to vision need quick changes of head position. To a very large extent a horse's vision is influenced by its prevailing attention and its sight can be affected by distractions. Good primitive reflexes to potential danger allow horses to be reactive to novel stimuli, but this may take the form of flight, such as bolting. Good training and experience, however, can restrain this reaction through habituation.

3 Neural Substrate

Introduction

The neuromechanism underlying behaviour is the intrinsic potential of the cells of the CNS. From each cell's substrate there is evidently an export system for its secretions to its terminus, contributing to neuronal excitation. Electrical impulses pass the length of the axon to hit the next cell's connection. The connection itself is a chemical exchange across the ultra-minute gap between the connecting of the linked neurons. By such a system, a 'live' network of signalling exists throughout a horse, determining its behaviour.

Studying the neural substrate of many finite features of behaviour, such as locomotion, requires an appreciation of the overall neural control of behaviour. The chemistry of transmission in the mammalian central nervous system has been studied to great effect with discoveries of biogenic amines and an increasing list of neuropeptides (Prosser, 1991).

Appreciation of the nervous system greatly improves the comprehension of the properties of the brain. Some awareness of brain anatomy helps to shed light on the major parts involved in the control of behaviour (see Fig. 3.1). In its entirety, the CNS deals with stimulation, sensory discrimination, motivation, learning, the inheritance of neural traits, and the release and control of action patterns. The neuron's main parts are its body, its main extension or axon and its additional extended processes or dendrites. Axons carry signals out and dendrites convey signals into the neuron. Neurons communicate with each other at the interface of the axon of one and the dendrite of another, via a synapse (Cunningham and Klein, 2007).

Neurons

Electrical messages are conducted from sensory organs, acting as receivers, to recipient aggregations and associations of neurons, acting as centres. These evoke additional electrical patterns, which mobilize the animal and establish conscious experience. Behaviour is founded on this electrical principle (Hockman and Bieger, 1976).

The brain's hypothalamic neurons have special secretory capabilities, relating to the production of releasing hormones. This additional attribute of neural tissue, namely production, draws attention to neuronal connectivity through use of axonal transportation. The neuron's endoplasmic reticulum has a cellular transport system, and the throughput system appears to originate in the lacunae within the Nissl bodies of the neuroplasm and terminate in the vesicles that accumulate in the axon end. The vesicles appear to be pinched-off portions of the neurotubule, which passes down the axon from its hillock in the cell body to its terminal bulbs. The vesicles migrate to the adjacent cell membrane and rupture into the synaptic space between associated neurons. In doing so, they liberate such substances as catecholamine and norepinephrine, and thereby communicate (see Fig. 3.2).

The Nissl body is the plant for polypeptide synthesis, which, in a sense, is the ultimate source of behaviour. Nissl bodies contain programmed ribosomes, which lie closely packed along the edges of the elongated lacunae, set out as a series of parallel spaces within the neuron body. The ribosomes are evidently marshalled there for a role of continuous production and exportation into the intraneuron transport system. In ethological terms, their basic product is behavioural potential. Behavioural information of genetically determined origin therefore resides, to some extent, in the Nissl substance, abundantly present in the cytoplasmic reticulum of the neuron (see Fig. 3.3).

The existence of two main classes of neurons is of basic importance in neuroethology. In the first class are cells called macroneurons, which have stable morphology. These are the large, principal neurons of the brain, whose long axons constitute the main nerve-fibre tracts. The second class consists of

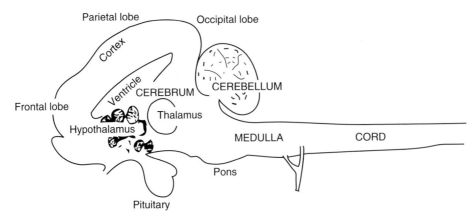

Fig. 3.1. Anatomy of the equine brain.

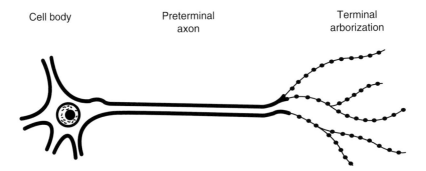

Fig. 3.2. Diagram of a complete neuron.

highly variable interneurons called microneurons. They are present in all parts of the nervous system, but are particularly prominent in areas of the brain known to be involved in modifiable behaviour, such as the cerebral cortex. These two classes of neurons differ not only in their morphology but also in their ontogeny.

The macroneurons with long axons are usually formed first in each part of the brain, and the small neurons with short axons are formed later. This generalization applies to all parts of the nervous system of vertebrates. The fact that these two classes of neurons arise at different times in development is evidence of a fundamental variance between them. The large neurons originate and complete their development at a time when the embryo is still protected from the variability of the extra-uterine environment. Macroneural development and differentiation therefore appear to be

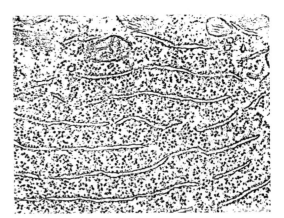

Fig. 3.3. Very high magnification of Nissl substance. The Nissl granules are packed along the edges of the lacunae. The latter are the start of the tubular system passing down the long axon to the synapse.

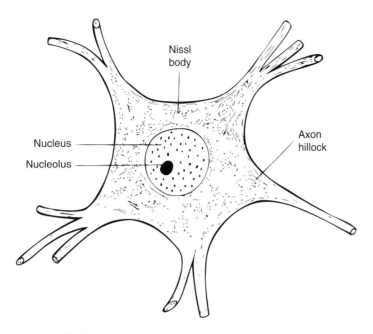

Fig. 3.4. Diagram of a nerve cell body.

largely completely controlled by intrinsic ontogenetic mechanisms. In contrast, the microneurons mainly originate and undergo their differentiation postnatally, when the animal is exposed to massive environmental discoveries and influences, including the discovery of a solid substrate, with which the foal must interact immediately. The small, variable interneuron cells are apparently responsive to environmental influences and are thus responsible for the plastic or modifiable aspects of neonatal and developing behaviour (see Fig. 3.4).

In the case of the large macroneurons, the axons grow along well-circumscribed routes or trajectories, which eventually constitute the nerve-fibre tracts that are among the most invariant features of neuroanatomy. Neuron processes terminate at characteristic positions in the nervous system and, in many instances, appear to make synaptic connections with selected cells. Neuronal circuits develop in this way by the formation of selective connections between different groups of neurons, or between neurons and sensory receptors or muscle fibres. The basic circuits, including the main input and output pathways, are thus laid down, to connect the different parts of the nervous system in the foal before birth (see Fig. 3.5).

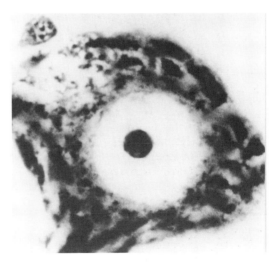

Fig. 3.5. Electromicroscopy of neuron nucleus. The dark masses are Nissl bodies.

Small groups of neurons from centres in the hindbrain, midbrain and boundaries of the forebrain send axons diffusely throughout the brain. The small focal origins and the wide diffusions of fibres suggest that this is a system issuing commands around the brain. All of these command systems have amine-containing fibres, so the transmitters in use are norepinephrine, dopamine and serotonin. For all of these amine-fibre systems the feature that stands out is that they have very small origins and very widespread influences. The norepinephrine, serotonin and dopamine systems are apparently a small triumvirate located deep in the brain, issuing command decisions to the whole brain (Prosser, 1991).

These systems link behavioural motivation to reward systems. The broadcast fibres of these systems form networks of terminals sufficiently diffuse to explain the relative lack of localization of the centres for motivation and reward. Items linked with such associated assemblies of cortical cells become alternative goals. This is apparently the neuroethological basis of 'redirected' phenomena in behaviour, such as displacement activities.

The axonal process must make appropriate connections once it reaches its predetermined target region, where the axon terminal undergoes extensive branching. Most of the branches will eventually disappear, leaving behind those which were able to establish permanent connections. This suggests that the axonal process makes tentative contact within its target area, maintaining only those branches and terminals that turn out to be functional, suitable and tenable. Firm and permanent connections become confirmed by the quality of activity generated in the developing nerve circuits. This can allow external factors, coming from the animal's interaction with its environment, to be involved in the selection (Oliver and Lorenz, 1993).

The neuronal interconnections that persist are those which best serve the functional requirements of the animal. An interesting aspect of this lies in the kinetic actions of the neonatal foal. The prominence of these in a neonate, which could otherwise be restful, indicates that kinetic functions are apparently having their postnatal neuronal pathways secured. A notable example of special neonatal kinesis exists in the form of saltation – sudden and spontaneous acts of jumping, dancing, kicking and running. The phenomenon of equine neonatal saltation will be considered in a later chapter in more detail, as it has not been reported previously in equine science.

This provisional coupling of certain neurons is the means of using information from the external environment to optimize the animal's ability to function within that environment. This validation of tentative connections must occur at the appropriate stage of epigenesis. It is governed by an appropriate and genetically controlled timetable. Selection of the appropriate connections from among the excess that have been created embryologically is delayed until the animal's first response to the external environment. One would therefore expect environmental factors to have their effect on the developing nervous system during the postnatal 'critical period', such as the first day or two of the foal's life.

The dendritic processes must also develop and establish contact with the proper axonal terminals to complete the developing neuronal interconnections. Differentiation of dentritic processes also follows precise timetables. However, in the sequence in which dendrites mature in the different regions of the brain, the differentiation of dendrites of large macroneurons occurs before that of smaller microneurons. Furthermore, there is a tendency for nerve cells in the motor fields of the nervous system to develop their dendrites before those of cells located in sensory fields.

Significantly an operant capability is established before a sensory one. By this means the newborn foal can act out certain items of behaviour without the need for much critical sensory ability. In addition, the newborn foal does not exhibit a keen sense of pain. One value of this is that the falls that occur in the first rising attempts are not painful enough to inhibit these attempts. One disadvantage is that the neonatal foal, without sensitization to trauma, can inflict injury on itself by walking or running into objects in an environment that has not been properly prepared for it.

Sensory stimulation plays an active role in the final differentiation of neurons and is necessary for the normal development of neuronal organization. Although the information necessary for tracts to connect with the appropriate part of the brain is supplied by intrinsic developmental programmes rather than by the animal's experience, such experience, or exposure history, during early postnatal development exerts a powerful influence on neuronal capability in the cortex. These effects are long-lasting since they can persist after years of overlying experience. Environmental conditions introduce variability into the developing nervous system. By this rule, it is evident that good standards of welfare in the management of the neonatal foal can have long-lasting benefits in physical functions.

Transmission

Neurons are distinguished from other cells by their molecular properties. Their characteristic properties are responsible for their signalling activities. Such activities include:

1. Responding to specific chemical transmitter substances by altering membrane permeability to common ions (Na^+, Cl^-, K^+, Ca^{2+}).
2. Conducting electrical impulses.
3. Communicating with other postsynaptic cells by the process of synaptic transmission.

Basic to each of these three physiological functions is the neuron's specific responsiveness to certain substances resulting from various intrinsic membrane proteins called receptors. Membranes of different neurons contain different receptors and this creates neuronal diversity (Prosser, 1991).

The release of transmitter substances from presynaptic axon terminals is another physiological function that is composed of many biochemical processes, some of which are characteristic of specific neuron cells, whereas others relate to pathways of numerous cells. Chemical transmission can be divided into four steps:

1. Synthesis of transmitter substance.
2. Storage and release of the transmitter.
3. Interaction of the transmitter with a receptor in the postsynaptic membrane.
4. Removal of the transmitter from the synaptic cleft.

Even though synaptic transmission occurs at nerve terminals, other parts of a neuron contribute significantly to the process. The terminal is dependent upon the cell body for the supply of components needed for transmission. These components are rapidly exported after being synthesized in the cell body and move along the axon to its terminal by either fast or slow axonal transportation. Some transmissions are obviously more urgent than others (Palmer, 1976).

In the horse, situational reactions, such as flight, are more urgent than seasonal responses, such as reproduction. In horse behaviour, some transmissions must be in constant operation to produce specific features of behaviour, but others may not be in regular operation if the transmitter substance is not in use or demand. For example, the anoestrous mare and the gelding do not use the transmissions innervating maintenance behaviour. The outstanding slow transmitters are the catecholamines, norepinephrine and dopamine. Acetylcholine is the well-known fast chemical messenger (Hockman and Bieger, 1976).

Each transmitter has the following four essential characteristics:

1. It is synthesized in the neuron.
2. It is present in the presynaptic terminal and is released into the synaptic space in order to exert its action on the receptive neuron or effector organ.
3. It mimics exactly the biological action of the endogenous transmitter when applied exogenously, as in a drug given to the horse.
4. It has a specific mechanism for removing it from the synaptic cleft, its site of action.

Nerve cells have been characterized according to their transmitter biochemistry, and the important generalization has emerged that a mature neuron makes use of the same transmitter substance at all of its synapses. The majority of neurons use only one transmitter substance – this is 'neuronal specificity'. A specific set of biosynthetic enzymes in a neuron determines this specificity. An enzymatic step exists in all transmitter pathways where the overall synthesis of the transmitter is regulated. This enzyme step is characteristic of the neuron and therefore endows it with the property of being cholinergic, norepinephrinergic (noradrenergic), dopaminergic, serotonergic, etc. Transmitters are substances that are released synaptically by neurons and affect other neurons or effector organs in a specific manner. Several substances clearly function as transmitters, but there are many other chemical substances with similar functions. The four types of transmitter substances are as follows:

1. Acetylcholine.
2. Biogenic amines, including dopamine, norepinephrine, serotonin and histamine.
3. Amino acids: γ-aminobutyric acid (GABA), glycine, glutamate.
4. Neuropeptides.

These four are considered below:

1. **Acetylcholine.** Acetylcholine (ACh) is the transmitter used heavily by the motor system and operates, therefore, at the junctions of nerves and skeletal muscles. ACh is diffusely localized throughout the brain but is highly concentrated in neurons of the basal ganglia. It is the transmitter for the parasympathetic nervous system.
2. **Biogenic amine transmitters.** Dopamine and norepinephrine (NE) are two important transmitter substances, which are synthesized in common pathways. In the central nervous system, NE-containing

nerve cell bodies are prominent in the locus ceruleus, a nucleus of the brainstem concerned with arousal. These neurons project diffusely throughout the cortex, cerebellum and spinal cord. In the peripheral nervous system, NE is the transmitter for the sympathetic nervous system (Axelrod, 1984).

Dopamine-containing cells are located in three regions: the substantia nigra, the midbrain and the hypothalamus. Serotonergic cell bodies are found in the brainstem. These cells (like the NE cells of the locus ceruleus) send fibres throughout the brain and spinal cord. Histamine is concentrated in the hypothalamus. NE and dopamine are catecholamines and serotonin is an indoleamine. Catecholamines, indoleamines and histamine are all referred to as 'biogenic amines'.

3. Amino acid transmitters. A number of amino acids exist, both as neurotransmitters and as universal cellular constituents. Glycine and glutamate are two of the 20 common amino acids that are incorporated into the proteins of all cells; glutamate and GABA also serve as substrates of intermediary metabolism. Glutamate is a transmitter in the cerebellum and the spinal cord. Glycine is an inhibitory transmitter in spinal cord interneurons. GABA is present in neurons in the basal ganglia, which project to the substantia nigra; cells of the cerebellum are GABA-minergic, as are certain inhibitory interneurons in the spinal cord.

4. Neuroactive peptides. About 25 short peptides have been found to be localized in neurons and to be pharmacologically very active, causing inhibition, excitation, or both. Some of these peptides were previously identified as hormones with known targets outside the brain (for example, angiotensin) or as products of neurosecretion (for example, oxytocin, vasopressin, somatostatin, LH and thyrotrophin-releasing hormone (TRH)). In addition to being hormones in some tissues, these peptides may act as neurotransmitters in other tissues. These neuroactive peptides are localized in regions of the brain that are involved in the perception of pain, pleasure and emotion.

Two classes of peptides possess opiate-like actions – the endorphins and the enkephalins. These opioid peptides are involved in a variety of functions, including the modulation of pain. Three pharmacologically active endorphins exist: alpha, beta and gamma. The most active is β-endorphin, which is synthesized in the hypothalamus and in the pituitary. The enkephalins are synthesized only

in neurons and in the adrenal gland. The precursor is synthesized in cell body ribosomes and transported within secretory vesicles to nerve terminals. Enkephalin molecules are produced during this transportation. Unlike β-endorphin, the enkephalins are widely distributed in the brain. The distribution matches that of the opiate receptors. It is now believed that forms of abnormal behaviour in horses, such as crib-biting and weaving, are associated with endorphin release.

Substance P is a peptide concentrated in certain neurons of the dorsal root ganglia, basal ganglia, hypothalamus and cerebral cortex. It is assumed to be the transmitter for sensory fibres involved in mediating pain.

The synthesis of the transmitter is only one aspect of the biochemistry of synaptic transmission. The transmitter within a neuron is packaged in storage granules or synaptic vesicles, which are concentrated at nerve endings. These vesicles are required to store the transmitter and mediate the synaptic release of the transmitters by the process of exocytosis. Supply of transmitter is an important factor in regulating synaptic transmission. Vesicular stores constitute a large reserve of transmitter substance protected from intracellular degradation, since the transmitter in vesicles is safe from intracellular enzymes. By this means, a reserve of potential behaviour is maintained.

Synaptic vesicles are directly involved at the site in the synaptic membrane at which transmitter molecules are released from the neuron by exocytosis. This vesicular rupture is the method by which transmitter is released into the synaptic cleft. Once released, a transmitter molecule is effective only if it interacts with a receptor. A given transmitter, however, does not always bring about the same biochemical change in every postsynaptic neuron. For example, ACh can excite some synapses, inhibit others, and do both simultaneously in others. Catecholamines (e.g. NE) may excite some synapses but not others. It is the receptor that determines whether a synapse will be excitatory or inhibitory.

All receptors for transmitters are proteins that have active sites that bind transmitter substance and have two common biochemical features:

1. The receptor location is in the membrane facing outward; this is important for their interaction with the transmitter arriving from across the synaptic cleft.

2. Receptors change membrane permeability to bring about exchanges affecting intracellular metabolism.

The method of disposal of transmitter to end the signal is critical to synaptic transmission; if a released transmitter substance persisted for a very long time, a new signal could not get through. Three mechanisms exist by which a neuron may dispose of soluble or unbound transmitter substance:

1. **Diffusion.** Diffusion will remove some transmitter substances; it is an important means by which the synaptic cleft gets rid of transmitter.

2. **Degradation.** Enzymatic degradation of transmitter substances is used primarily by the cholinergic system. This makes possible the retrieval of the choline fraction, which is readily taken up by the neuron from the extracellular space.

3. **Re-uptake.** Re-uptake of the whole transmitter substance from the cleft is probably the most widely used mechanism for inactivation of transmitter substance. Synaptic junctions have high-affinity uptake mechanisms for released transmitter, e.g. uptake of choline. Biogenic amines are also taken up into the presynaptic terminal by specific concentrating mechanisms. Amino acid transmitters are also taken up from the synaptic cleft by glial cells, as well as by neurons, in the central nervous system.

The systems by which neurons interact synaptically are important for an understanding of how information is processed into behaviour by the nervous system. A given neuron may have any number of receptors for a wide variety of transmitter substances. Thus, although a neuron's output is essentially unique, it can be influenced by many different inputs. For explanation, the various features of neuronal operation give abundant support for concepts relating to behavioural reserves, potential behaviour, actions patterns and critical periods that feature in ethological concepts (Lehner, 1996).

Motivation

Motivation affects the complex phenomena collectively termed emotionality. In displays of emotional behaviour, vast experimental evidence points to the involvement of the brain's limbic system. The limbic system is that interconnected group of brain structures within the cerebrum, including portions of the frontal lobe cortex, temporal lobe, thalamus and hypothalamus, together with linking neural pathways connecting all of these parts. The parts of the limbic system therefore have many connections with each other and with other parts of the central nervous system, so it is likely that information from all the different afferent routes influences the limbic system. Activity of the limbic system results in a wide variety of autonomic responses and body actions constituting behaviour of numerous forms.

Three distinct neural systems mediate the various emotional behaviours controlled by the limbic system. Following experimental stimulation of one area, the animal actively approaches a situation in a positive, exploratory manner. Stimulation of a second area causes the animal to stop any behaviour it is performing. Stimulation of a third physiological area of the limbic system causes the animal to show marked aggressive change, either from a quiet state to savageness or from the latter to docility. Alterations in stimulation of the different areas of the limbic system are therefore the foundation of emotionally motivated behaviour. Equine saltation may be an example of emotional motivation, to be discussed later.

Although physiological and endocrinological studies have shown that the hypothalamus is an integrating region, some neurophysiological activities are diverse in the organized control of their motivation. It becomes necessary to recognize that, in the ethogram of the horse, there are two main categories of behavioural production:

1. **Phasic motivation of maintenance behaviour.** This vegetative–expressive motivation supports the bulk of the behaviour of horses and is the behaviour concerned with such activities as ingestion, locomotion and social activities. Certain physiological needs, such as resting, body care and thermoregulation, are also featured in the motivation of equine maintenance.

2. **Occasional forms of motivation occur.** These are the motivations that are needed for dealing with occasional, specific and often critical circumstances. These instances include such matters as the new role of a mare with a foal, the new role of a colt post-puberty and the new role of stallions following the start of the breeding season.

It will be seen that most of these examples of occasional motivated states relate to 'new roles'. This would seem to be an important feature to recognize, since many 'new role' circumstances operate through the production of hormones. The major purpose of such hormones is to activate neural systems that are not involved in routine maintenance behaviour. These new roles, and emergency roles of behaviour, must nevertheless be established in the neuromechanism of the individual animal, to be called upon only when circumstances require their activation. In some circumstances their activation may never occur in the entire life of the horse if the appropriate motivation is not coordinated. An example is the absence of sexual behaviour in a gelding.

The neural circuits are laid down in embryonic stages of development and these remain in all individuals of both sexes. For this reason the sex hormones will activate only those neural circuits appropriate to their chemistry. Neural circuits for the alternative sexual behaviour exist, but are not normally called into play in the domesticated lifetime of the animal. However, when abnormal circumstances occur, e.g. the presence of an ovarian tumour, the alternative neural system of sexual behaviour may then be motivated. This will result in the manifestations of behaviour characteristics of the opposite sex. For example, mares with ovarian tumours often exhibit the typical prancing behaviour of stallions, including the masculine arching of the neck. The neuronal circuit for sexual behaviour of the opposite gender evidently does not lose potential merely because it is never called into play by the key hormone in the lifetime of the animal. It must be remembered that the lifetime of the neuron equals the lifetime of the individual animal.

In relation to this neurological fact and returning to the example of neural links being formed in the newborn foal through saltation, it follows, as a theorem, that such saltatory linkages remain. While many of the individual component items of saltatory innervations serve various locomotor activities into adulthood, the neural schemes for the behavioural patterns that were formed in the original spontaneous displays will also remain and should be capable of reproduction in the adult. They are certainly reproduced in juvenile play in some instances. Through this theorem, a question arises about the possibility of actions of neonatal origin intruding spontaneously into motiveless adult equine behaviour in unusual or peculiar fashion, such as so-called 'shadow jumping' (where there is no shadow). In fact, other saltatory behaviour is occasionally demonstrated in adult horses. Further

consideration should be given to the phenomenon of equine saltation and its wider significance.

Self-stimulation behaviour is characterized by automatic and repetitive compulsion. Experimentally, the administration of amphetamine, which is one of the drugs used to liberate amines, often causes such repetition of behaviour in animals, even though the stimulation no longer has a directly rewarding effect. Herein lies the neuroethological basis of stereotypes. A feature of significance of amine fibres is that they can proliferate. By this means, disruption to the reward system can find alternative routing and create stereotyped activity, which can also lead to consolidation and fixation of stereotyped behaviour. This fits ethological findings on anomalous behaviour and explains their obvious characteristics.

Neurophysiological research has pointed out that motivational mechanisms of the brain may be mainly peptide events. Changes in the chemical state of the brain can bias neuronal processes (Kandel and Schwartz, 1981). Catecholamines are involved in controlling hormonal states. Catecholamine actions modulate the various steps in sequential step-by-step procedures, such as in so-called fixed action patterns of the more extended type, seen notably in reproduction. Catecholamines help trigger hormone events, and then the hormone process continues the motivation. The catecholamine transmitters are set off by normal action patterns and they can carry the reward message returning from them.

The biogenic amine system is the basis of the behavioural changes that facilitate the animal's achievement of homeostasis. At the same time this system can redirect behaviour in seemingly anomalous forms of activity, which are capable of being strengthened in their neuronal substrate. The manner in which the terminals infiltrate the cerebral cortex, mainly in its upper layers, shows its pervasive influence in voluntary behaviour.

Control over motivation can be seen under certain typical circumstances of season and husbandry. In a free state, horses aggregate in groups of their own kind. Through systems of social organizations, harmony is a prominent feature of collective behaviour. Phenomenal features of group behaviour are synchrony and conformity of motives in the group, leading to social facilitation. The discipline of synchronous conformity is imposed on the maintenance behaviours of a group. The discipline shows in the way that a herd of horses will feed together, move together, react together, associate together, utilize territory together, shelter and rest together. Group behaviour shows cohesion, which often appears in a state of higher motivation than would normally be observed in the behaviour of the solitary individual. Examples are seen in feeding, kinesis, body care, territorialism and resting. Reproductive behaviours also appear to be influenced by group or population dictates called social facilitation, which amplifies mass motivation.

Neuroethology has shown that some motivational hormones are controlled by the catecholamine system (Schulkin, 1999). The catecholamines involved are norepinephrine and dopamine. Fibres containing these catecholamines pervade the critical brain areas and course through them to many other parts of the brain. Changeability in the outlets of centres, throughout the limbic system, may be the basis of certain ethological phenomena in horses, such as redirected drives, displacement activities and some anomalous behaviour.

The substantia nigra, where one dopamine bundle has its main origin, controls motivation-rewarded behaviour and voluntary performances aimed at avoiding noxious stimulation. The dopamine pathway can carry incentive messages. The norepinephrine pathway can carry motivation-reducing messages of satiety. Reward is implicit in both of these arrangements. Rewards both start and stop actions, depending on whether they are incentive rewards or terminal consummatory rewards. Incentive rewards, such as the smell of food, utilize the dopamine pathways. Final rewards, such as the ingestion of food, act through the norepinephrine pathways.

Relationships between physiological, neural and hormonal factors in motivation are coordinated in specialized areas of the hypothalamus. Organizations for both feeding and drinking behaviour, including the searching and appetitive components, are finally located in areas of the hypothalamus. Stimulation of certain hypothalamic areas of limbic structures elicits behaviour with a very strong 'emotional' component. The medial hypothalamus exerts inhibition on the circuits, producing the fight-or-flight response. Clearly, emotional behaviour is the result of limbic stimulation. The main structures involved in the control of emotional behaviour are predominantly located throughout the limbic system. The main units for consummatory behaviour are located within the hypothalamus, although they come under other controls also.

Programmes of motivation in the animal are modified or directed by exogenous environmental stimulation, such as temperature, light intensity, day length, social factors and social circumstances. Endogenous stimuli such as hormones and the chemical status of the animal also influence motivations. These have sequential components. Initially a period of appetitive behaviour occurs – a period of seeking out a specific goal, such as food, or any other goal associated with the homeostasis of the subject. This behaviour is specific searching, directed towards an appropriate goal. The subsequent component period emerges when the animal is presented with the appropriate goal and begins consummatory acts designed to satisfy the motivation. The behavioural classes of self-maintenance are all examples of consummatory behavioural processes, which can be regarded as expressions of emotive states such as hunger, thirst, pain (or discomfort), fear and anger (Spruijt et al., 2001).

It may be necessary to reflect on the subdivision of behaviour into that which is motivated by the normally extant chemistry of the body, and other action patterns that are only motivated by the presence of short-lived chemical agents in the form of hormones. The principal chemical messengers are neuropeptides and hormones – most of these have phases of production. Phasic motivation characterizes many homeostatic activities of horses. Principal motives can be recognized, and feeding is a most obvious example. Other major types of motivation relate to aggression, avoidance and reproduction. In addition to these, there are a number of others, such as the reproductive activities of copulation, suckling and care-giving, which have high priority. By contrast, play and exploration motivations are subordinate in priority to most others in the pursuit of homeostasis.

4 Behavioural Homeostasis

General Concept

The bedrock of well-being is homeostasis, or balanced maintenance. Homeostasis is a physiological balancing arrangement, which is seen at many levels of operation. Cellular homeostatic phenomena occur, and homeostasis also takes place at the level of organs, whole systems and multiple systems (Heidemann, 2007).

The great Harvard physiologist Walter Cannon first developed and named the concept of homeostasis. This was initially viewed as the condition of stability, or steady-state, in cellular chemistry, in tissues and in fluids. Cannon saw that body homeostasis was supported by a 'cerebral defence system', which could deal with challenges to general homeostasis. Cannon's attention progressively shifted to the autonomic and endocrine systems, which regulated bodily function. He explored the controlling forces of these in the brain, including the cerebral cortex, and this duly led to recognition of the role of emotion in bodily function. Such function extends into self-maintenance and even into species maintenance through reproduction via emotional motivations.

Behavioural homeostasis is an obvious extension of Cannon's concepts (Cannon, 1953). It is very clear that motivated behavioural processes are used to attain general physiological stability, whole-body homeostasis and social balances. Furthermore, these behavioural processes can be perceived to be under the control of Cannon's cerebral defence system, which is in essence the limbic system. The view is taken here that the animal's limbic system and the autonomic and endocrine systems vitally and collectively support comprehensive well-being. This view is considered to be totally consistent with Cannon's concepts.

The ramification of the three systems named creates a vast network of influential forces. From the frontal and prefrontal cortex, through all its numerous parts, to the hypothalamus, the limbic system has roles of profound importance in sustaining life and controlling physiological activities. The autonomic nervous system ensures bodily operations without conscious input and has a self-balancing capability in its two opposing subdivisions. The endocrine system, from the brain's pituitary gland, through the thyroid gland to other endocrine parts such as the adrenals, secretes hormones into the circulation, carrying chemical messages of instruction throughout the entire body. This ensures the animal's balanced maintenance with appropriate activities, notably in a maternal role. Priorities of activity are determined by means of a motivational time-sharing arrangement in the prefrontal cortex. By this means, priorities of activity can be efficiently determined in favour of the animal's defence, its general social existence and its general maintenance (Robinson, 2007).

Maintenance is seen as a major category of behaviour. Much of the behaviour of horses is concerned with self-maintenance. Highly successful self-maintenance is the basis of an animal's health. Activities involved in such maintenance can be divided into primary generic systems, which interlock. These are basically of innate origin and include much instinctive behaviour. In general, the needs of animals relate to the maintenance systems of reaction, ingestion, body care, motion, rest, association, exploration and territorialism. These are reviewed in Table 4.1.

Reaction

The principal generic class of activities utilized by animals to maintain themselves in harmony with their environment and to adjust themselves to sudden environmental changes that are harmful or potentially so is reactive behaviour. Aggressive activity, in general, can be recognized as falling within this broad category. Other reactive states included learned responses, simple reflexes and vocalizations (see Fig. 4.1).

Table 4.1. Equine forms of maintenance behaviours directed at general homeostasis.

Category	Varied features	Function	Usual priority
1. Reaction	Reflexes, responses in general, fight or flight	Defence	xxxxxxxxxx
2. Ingestion	Grazing, drinking, chewing, browsing	Nutrition	xxxxxxxxx
3. Body care	Rubbing, rolling, scratching, nibbling	Hygiene	xxxxx
4. Motion	Natural gaits, play, comfort shifts	Exercise	xxxxx
5. Rest	Drowsing, idling, lying, sleeping	Restoration	xxxxx
6. Association	Affiliation, bonding, herd unity	Companionship	xxxxx
7. Exploration	Attention, curiosity, wandering	Learning	xxxx
8. Territorialism	Affinity for home base and home range	Security	xxx

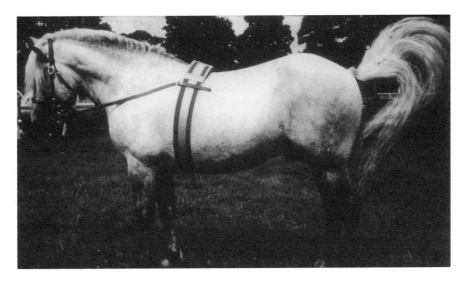

Fig. 4.1. Tail thrashing by stallion. Display of emotional reactivity. Photo: A.F. Fraser.

The phenomenon of 'language' is quite remarkable. On studying the means whereby horses communicate vocally, it is found that each horse has its own individual 'language', using sounds to convey various meanings. Anyone knowing a particular horse becomes able to understand these messages. The horse uses 11 distinct notes to convey a message by sound; sounds vary from a low snuffle to a scream of rage, fear or pain.

Many reactions among horses are vocal expressions (Kiley-Worthington, 1999). The production of vocal sound is a major feature of reactivity, which is typical of a given horse during most circumstances. Many vocalizations are incorporated into responses concerned with alarm and threat. Vocal sounds also occur according to the sex and age of the horse and the particular type of stimulus

that has caused the vocal expression. The neigh is the loudest sound emitted by the horse. It is often given when a horse is curious about events happening outside of its range of vision or when it is seeking to communicate with other horses some distance away. Grunting and threat noises are various; the most frequent is the type expressed at feeding time, when a mixture of hunger and excitement seems to be the stimulating force for this vocal expression. The crying or squealing sound varies in volume a great deal from one set of circumstances to another. It is usually heard during short, sharp aggressive encounters between horses, when one horse attacks another unexpectedly. Additional forms of vocal expressions of horses include the trumpeting of the stallion in a state of sexual arousal and gurgling throaty sounds, which are common in both sexes of all ages, but deeper in stallions. These sounds are produced in circumstances that indicate that the horse is expressing general satisfaction, as, for example, when it has been fully fed or when it greets the arrival of a person or another horse of which it approves. One interesting form used by horses is the wicker. A low wicker is frequently used as a message of welcome or an invitation to 'come here'. By raising the note of the wicker, the horse can make the communication more emphatic. This welcoming call has several different tones, which vary the intensity of the greeting call.

Most aggressive reactions in horses are shown when they are mixed in their own company. Much of the restless activities that are exercised socially relate to the status of each horse in the group. In a typical encounter between two horses of different social status in the one group, one horse will act aggressively, reaching out to snap at the skin around the shoulders and neck of the adversary. If the adversary then recognizes itself as subordinate in the social hierarchy to the animal attacking it, its response will be one of quick submission. At this point the aggressive exchange between the two animals ceases because its purpose has been fulfilled. A lot of minor aggressive acts are shown when one horse's 'individual space' has been violated by the sudden intrusion of another horse. Horses also use physical reactions, body language or displays as forms of expression, which advertise their presence, status and hypothetical intention. These are important forms of communication between horses so as to provide others with a clear understanding of the individual's motive state.

A first line of defence in the individual is behaviour in reflex form. Reflexes require the integrity and full function of the central nervous system and rely on the peripheral nervous system with its specialized sensory transducers, the sense organs, conveying sensory input. Reflex responses are typically prompt and brief. Their suddenness makes behaviour of this kind important to animal handlers, but their predictability is high, making preventive measures possible if the handler has experience. When disturbed, associated horses first join and then run away together.

Ingestion

Feeding and drinking are addressed in Chapter 5, but their behavioural characters are presented here as basic homeostasis. Ingestive behaviour among horses represents the primary category of behaviour involved in their maintenance. The various forms that ingestion takes vary according to the nature of the material being consumed, the age of the animal and its individual preferences. Horses graze by shearing and grinding after using their strong muscular lips to gather enough to bite. They prefer to crop young grass that is short, cutting away such grass to ground level. Oats and concentrates are taken up by the lips and moved by the tongue to the molars for grinding. Root crops and apples, when provided, are bitten into pieces by the incisors before being quickly conveyed to the molars for shearing and grinding.

Free-ranging horses spend much of their time grazing. Perhaps about 12 h or more per day is usually given over to this chief activity. Where grazing is poor, horses will travel considerable distances each day in order to select preferred grasses, but they will not use an area greater than that which contains a fresh supply of water within reasonable walking distance.

More than any of the other farm animals, horses suffer from various mouthing and eating problems: wood eating is one. Other examples of depraved appetites include the consumption of bedding, dirt, sand, tail hairs and their own faeces. Some horses develop the various bad habits of swallowing air, bolting their food and drinking water excessively. Most of these bad ingestive habits can be considered as ethological disorders. They are potentially dangerous to the horse since they can cause serious types of colic.

The normal ingestive habits of horses are regular. If fed only in its stall, the horse eats for about 3 h each day. About 15 min daily are spent drinking; the average horse taking about 22–38 l (6–10 gal) of water each day. The drinking of abundant water is a great ingestive need for horses. Most horses take only two or three drinks per day. Some only drink once daily. When drinking, they consume very large quantities of water, taking up to 15–20 swallows. At the time of its main drink the horse has to have some freedom of movement and, if watered at a trough, it usually raises its head at least once during its drink. If they have a choice, horses show a preference for soft water over hard water. Horses also enjoy ingesting salt: they can spend up to half an hour each day licking at an available salt block; while they do not require this amount of salt for their systems, there appears to be a special fondness for it as well as a basic need.

Emotional tensions in horses can affect their digestion (Herdt, 2007). Some, under difficulty in adapting to their circumstances or the type of work, become so emotionally affected that their digestive processes become noticeably impaired. The texture of their dung changes and is evacuated much more quickly after consumption; the digestive upset causes food to pass out of the body before it is properly digested. When the horse becomes relaxed and accepts its condition its digestion can return to normal.

Body care

This category is best recognized as grooming, but grooming itself is complex. Among horses outdoors, grooming occurs as nibbling, rubbing, rolling and scratching. Both sheltering and bed selection are included in this category. These behaviours may be undertaken individually or mutually with others. Although maintenance behaviours generally cease on illness, with those of lowest priority ceasing first, it is often the cessation of body care that is first noticed as a sign of illness. The arrest of other maintenance behaviours of higher priority occurs in sickness at a severe clinical level.

In general, body care deals with skin hygiene, thermoregulation and comfort seeking. Horses seek to preserve their physical comfort to the best of their ability under the circumstances in which they find themselves. The motivation they show in the pursuit of these activities clearly indicates a high level of priority relating to body care. The activities produced by this objective relate mainly to the active seeking of physical comfort for themselves, the continuous attempts to maintain satisfactory thermal harmony with the environment, and periodic but intensive activities relating to skin hygiene, such as grooming, scratching and rubbing (see Figs 4.2 and 4.3).

Physical comfort activities are evident in the way in which horses select sites on which to bed themselves and the way in which many of them will evacuate in locations not used for feeding or resting. The common activity of mutual grooming, although relating to skin hygiene, is practised in a precise manner over certain dorsal sites on the trunk. The manner of this behaviour indicates that physical comfort is derived from this activity. The search for physical comfort indicates this as a basic need in horses. Mares and their foals will often groom each other. At pasture, pairs of horses may

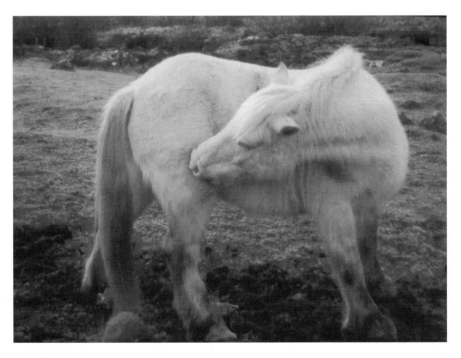

Fig. 4.2. Gelding grooming its winter coat. Photo: A.F. Fraser.

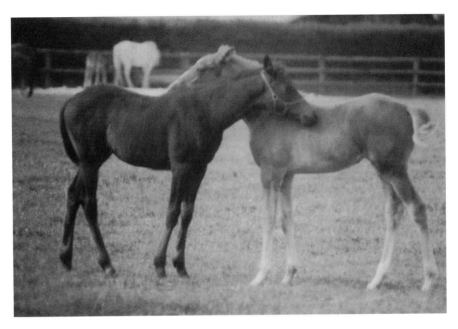

Fig. 4.3. Mutual grooming. Photo: H. Hastie.

spend quite lengthy periods in mutual grooming. This form of grooming is shown in all age groups, though the pairs formed by individuals are usually matched for age and size. In the normal grooming arrangement, two horses face each other and one extends its head past the other's neck and nibbles vigorously over its back, while the other horse responds in like fashion. Presently both animals vigorously nibble over their back regions simultaneously. Some horses will even groom other animals with which they have some social affiliation, such as goats or dogs (see Fig. 4.4).

Horses also spend some time grooming their own bodies. Their own hips and flanks are reached by turning their head around as far as possible and snapping at the skin of these parts. They may also groom their limbs, both the forefeet and hind, in the same manner. Occasionally they will clean their nostrils and faces by rubbing them up and down the inside of one foreleg and then the other.

Horses at pasture have another form of grooming, which they practise fairly frequently. This is the routine of rolling themselves on to their backs and working the back region into the ground. They will usually select a patch of ground that is bare of grass. In this activity, a horse lies down in the normal fashion and

then proceeds to kick itself over on to its back. It then rubs its back vigorously into the ground while keeping its feet in the air. After several rubs and rolls the horse rises to its feet and shakes all the skin of its body in a manner called the 'wet dog shake'. With this movement the entire body shakes and the skin ripples in a wave from head to hind legs, while dust particles are thrown out from the coat.

Motion

Horses may be genetically programmed to travel considerable distances daily, foraging for suitable food. Even when travelling is not required of them in order to obtain food, it is found that there is still a basic need for an expression of a kinetic urge, which motivates them to walk, to exercise their natural gaits and to seek radical changes of location. When stationary, there are certain characteristics of movement, in the form of stretching of the limbs, back, head and neck. Kinesis, therefore, can also be recognized as a basic behavioural need in horses.

Certain patterns of action and movement apparently require regular expression. The horse in full health has much greater kinetic output than other

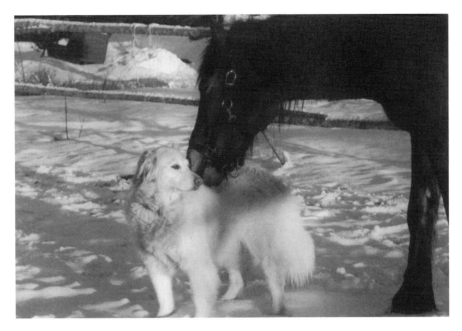

Fig. 4.4. Grooming an alien friend. Photo: D. Critch.

livestock. An output of the gaits of the walk, trot and canter are essentially the equine kinetic need. Various kinetic activities are tied to other specific behaviours: perambulation in grazing, for example. Patterns of kinetic activity become mixed in equine playful activities, which are also included in this system of gross motor activity. The typical intense playing in young foals and their output of the natural gaits show a need for kinetic output from the start of equine life, as illustrated in Fig. 4.5 (McDonnell, 2002).

Play is pure kinesis, even though it can serve other purposes. Racing at the gallop is a notable form of play in groups of horses, both young and adult. One partner biting or nipping the crest of the other often initiates play in pairs of all age groups. The thing the horse does best, the thing it has the greatest need to do, is performance of movement. The need for movement is essential for a horse's physical and mental well-being. A horse also desires variations in its circumstances. The more fit the horse, the greater its need for exercise or work, and constant activity is needed to preserve fitness. In distant history the horse was vulnerable to predators, and nature ensured that it was provided with a means of defence and survival by the ability to travel a great distance without rest.

Rest

General features of rest will be addressed in Chapter 9, but some of its characteristics are given here because of its significance in homeostasis. Horses rest in various ways. Some rests are acquired in a state of drowsing, while standing or lying. Even in a conscious state, horses in static postures can acquire some degree of rest for periods of time. Resting stances or resting recumbency can be used for true sleep, but deep sleep, in the form known as rapid-eye-movement (REM) sleep, involves such muscular relaxation of the neck that head support is needed by such surfaces as the floor or ground. Deep sleep in a standing position with muscular relaxation of the neck can sometimes be accomplished, however, by older horses using tactics they have learned. They may use a location outdoors where they can stand downhill and allow the head and neck to droop. In a stall they can hang back on the halter rope to support the head and neck. With the head extended in either position breathing is not embarrassed.

Horses require significant quantities of true sleep. Mostly, this sleep is acquired at night, when sleep episodes are punctuated by periods when the horse is wakeful. The sleep patterns of horses in tune with their environments are fairly fixed.

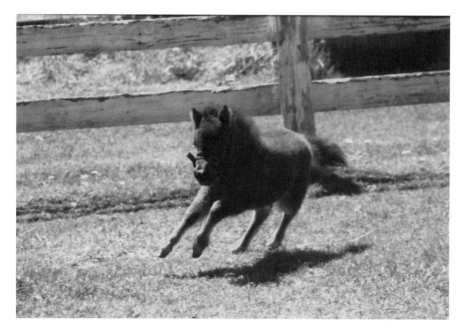

Fig. 4.5. Rotary gallop in young foal. Photo: Melanie MacDonald.

Adequate rations of sleep on a daily basis are necessary for horses to thrive and maintain fitness. When their circumstances are disturbed, as for example when they are relocated or subjected to excessive crowding, sleep patterns become disrupted and sleep can cease entirely for extended periods of time, such as several days. Resting and sleep are forms of physical conservation and restoration, which may occupy a third of a horse's life. It occupies a great deal of time in the young foal and much of this is in the form of deep sleep (see Fig. 4.6). Continuing homeostasis is dependent on this. Regular periods of deep sleep are the norm in foals. They conserve energy and grow during these periods (Home, 1977).

Association

A most pronounced feature in equine behaviour is the active way in which individuals associate with each other. An assembly of horses soon becomes an integrated herd. General association does not always satisfy the need for association and close pairings are often formed. The force that maintains social cohesion among horses is considerable. It is through social actions that the living strategies of horses are implemented. Affiliations

are basic to the equine nature and for the transmission of learning. The group effect (social facilitation) influences communal activities. The intimate association of individuals permits the organization of numbers of animals into breeding groups and herds. The discipline that the social force brings to the component individuals of animal assemblies ensures the common pursuit of tactics required for living. Such social stability safeguards their immune systems (Schorr and Arnason, 1999).

Horses are very gregarious animals and enjoy the company of each other. Small groups will tend to become closely compacted and move around a grazing area together, while still maintaining a certain amount of individual space around them. Many horses show a marked preference for certain other individual horses. Two horses encountering each other for the first time show keen, mutual examination. This involves an investigation of each other's head, body and hindquarters by smelling. Bonds of friendship can become quickly formed between pairs of horses that are allowed to associate with each other outdoors. When they have the opportunity to associate with each other at pasture, closeness is featured prominently in their daily activities (see Fig. 4.7).

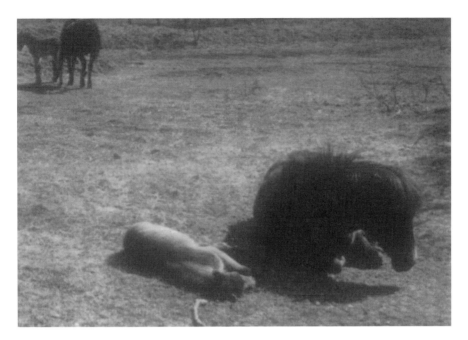

Fig. 4.6. Foal in deep sleep beside mare. Photo: A.F. Fraser.

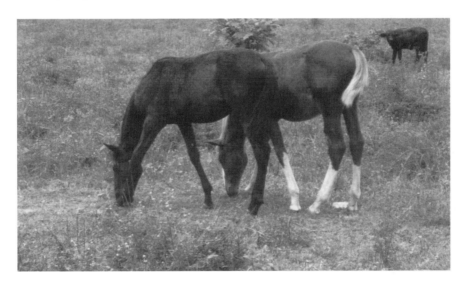

Fig. 4.7. A close partnership. Photo: A.F. Fraser.

Like many of the other highly developed animals, horses show a form of social order when they live in the company of their own kind. In the hierarchy that becomes formed, the older and larger animals are usually found to be high in rank. Stallions do not necessarily dominate geldings or mares, however. A dominant individual horse often dictates the movement of the herd throughout the grazing area, serving to act as a leader in the grazing movements. Such a horse will, with evident jealousy, sometimes break up close encounters among other horses. Socially dominant horses are sometimes found to have much more aggressive temperaments than others in the group. If a group of horses of mixed sex contains a number of geldings, these males are very likely to separate to the edge, forming a close-knit bachelor group.

When horses have been living in a group and the group moves from place to place throughout the pasture, it is generally observed that the same horses lead the way each time, while others tend to repeatedly lie to the back of the group. In the way some horses assume full leadership and others assume the role of followers, there is a remarkable consistency. The role of dominance in horse groups is very real. Some horses will persistently find their way into a position of leadership in a group, while others seem quite ready to accept a position low in the ranking order, even in a small herd. Removed from one group and placed in a new one, horses usually attain for themselves a similar position in the hierarchy that they held previously. A phenomenon in horses at pasture in a group is the emergence of one that always investigates any new developments in the vicinity. The horse has an inbuilt need to be assertive much of the time. No doubt this is an additional part of its natural equipment for survival. Without this, horses low in the 'pecking order' or the social structure of the group might become deprived of nourishment by being driven away from the best grazing. Existence could be in jeopardy in these cases, but even horses at the bottom of a social hierarchy will retain some capacity for self-assertion. Some dominant horses adopt a 'preferred associate', which benefits in society (see Fig. 4.8).

Social interaction with people varies considerably from horse to horse, depending on the rearing system, its nature and whether the animal has received a traumatic human association. This form of special relationship involving the positive association of the animal with man is termed socialization. Interspecies affiliations can occur in remarkable forms. These demonstrate the equine need for close companionship.

Established groups of horses have a social hierarchy with a dominant individual at the top of the pecking order. It is a common and almost traditional belief that dominance, by itself, establishes and operates social hierarchy. However, there is an avoidance system in social behaviour, which operates with the dominance system. It is the vital component of group association and it effectively generates social stabilization. Subordinate horses deliberately avoid moving too close to dominant animals. Avoidance serves to reduce contests between individuals in most other circumstances of association. However, this avoidance tactic does not work well in all situations. Social dominance is

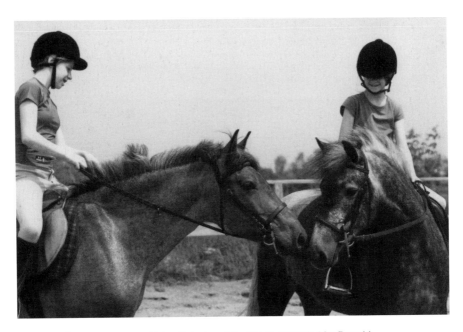

Fig. 4.8. Friends greeting, nose to nose. Note dilated nostrils. Photo: Melanie MacDonald.

exhibited in competition for supplementary feed, and dominant animals will frequently threaten subordinates while eating. A lack of feeders can mean that dominant animals command resources at the expense of subordinate animals, unless they are 'preferred associates'. The latter ultimately do not suffer from food deprivation.

In clearly established hierarchies there is maximal group bonding and minimal aggression, creating the social stability that is a vital requirement in good animal husbandry. A social hierarchy is merely the state of settled-out relationships between individuals. Partnerships and friendship pairs are formed, and these involve mutual tolerance. The function and durability of the hierarchy is dependent upon component relationships and upon ongoing, operative avoidance tactics within these. 'Dominance hierarchy' may be a misconception for a social relationship based on a mixture of social arrangements. It seems that horses have organized tactics of stable social living, which involve their own pacts and systems of pacts that create social understanding.

Pair bonds are a very notable feature of associative behaviour in horses. Within herds, it is often found that discrete pairing through mutual selection of each other's company is a common social strategy, which operates to the advantage of both, particularly in aggressive situations involving other dominant animals. When they form pairs with great understanding, they seem able to read each other's intentions and to function almost as one bonded unit. Pairs of horses in states of intimate understanding have been termed 'empathic pairs'. Very specialized forms of close association occur in some pairs of horses that have become closely bonded to each other. To put this fact in simple terms, horses enjoy friendships, particularly when their emotional characteristics are satisfied (see Fig. 4.9). These characteristics are very real and give the horse its individuality or 'personality'.

The use of the term personality, in regard to describing regular dispositions in horses, has been favoured in some recent reports in the scientific journal *Applied Animal Behaviour Science*. McGrogan *et al.* (2008) reported three differing horse personality traits: (i) a human agreeableness factor, with obedience, kindness, sociality and non-aggressiveness; (ii) human extroversion, with intellect and curiosity; and (iii) neuroticism and emotionality. These authors suggest that the agreeableness factor may dominate from millennia of domestication and thereby infer that this is a heritable trait manipulated by selection. In some agreement with these findings is the report by

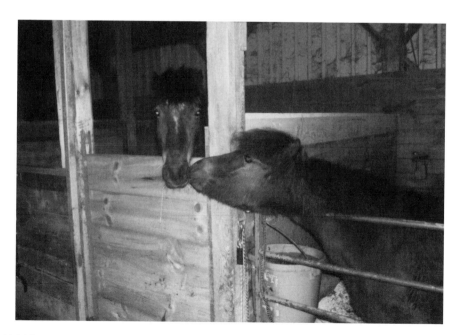

Fig. 4.9. Neighbours greeting. Photo: J. Scanlan.

Lloyd *et al.* (2008), which recognizes six components of horse personality: dominance, anxiousness, excitability, protection, sociality and inquisitiveness. In this latter study, the authors found differences between horse breeds with regard to the most common personalities observed. They noted that the personalities within breeds were in accord with popular opinions.

Exploration

As with the other generic classes of maintenance behaviour, exploratory behaviour, which is essentially investigative in purpose, is motivated by its own forces. In general it facilitates natural learning in horses. Exploratory activities take many forms according to the age of the horse, its previous experience, its environment and, in particular, novelties within the latter. It can take the form of directed attention and of simple curiosity. In the continuing presence of an environment that is sterile in regard to a variety of features, the investigative thrust of most horses can become intensively directed to close environmental fixtures. The motivation behind exploratory actions appears to be quite strong in many horses and is notable in foals. Very young foals will direct their intentions to features or persons in their immediate environment to which their mare shows no evident interest. A horse's harmony with its environment is partially dependent on adequate exploratory activities. However, equine exploratory behaviour is featured in all age groups, allowing learned behaviours to be acquired throughout life. A lack of curiosity is not a healthy sign. Curiosity is one of the norms of well-being in horses.

Territoriality

The affinity for a home range and the bond for a home site feature prominently in the motivation for most horses. Spatial arrangements vary in a large herd of horses. Although there may be closeness in the general herd, subgroups of two to four are often formed. These have their own intimacy and keep slightly apart from others. Although they group, horses require extensive territorial facilities for the total herd strategy. When similar herd densities are used in domestication without adequate territory, crowding develops, which is particularly stressful for horses. Without the provision of significant territorial variation, alternate territory or expansive territory, spatial density simply becomes a state of concentration. In horses, the stressfulness in this arrangement is considerable. Social density among horses without territorial adequacy is responsible for much agonistic behaviour, fight-or-flight responses, threat displays, bullying and much avoidance behaviour.

The periphery of the herd in adequate territory is the escape zone for subordinate horses. Even in a moving harem of mares, constantly herded by a stallion, there will be frequent changing of neighbours and movement to the herd periphery for avoidance. A stallion's own position is well outside the harem periphery and he does not counter herd movement, only territorial dispersal (see Fig. 4.10). The spatial need of a horse is yet another natural need. A foaling mare needs a spacious box and is more restful in one to which she is accustomed. Nevertheless, it is best for a mare to foal outdoors in suitable weather on familiar territory.

In their territorial habits, horses soon become proprietors of certain areas and they will frequently become aggressive in defence of these. In quarrels over space they fight with one another with their own offensive and defensive tactics. They bite, kick out with their hind feet and strike with their forefeet. In a territorial defending situation, a horse will establish its defence by kicking out with its hind feet when its flight distance is violated. The flight distance is the perimeter of area that the horse views as the outer limit of its individual space and that which it will defend when encroached upon by another alien or unacceptable animal. Both hind feet are usually involved in this kicking. This double kick is delivered directly to the rear without particular aim. Kicking out defensively with one hindlimb is usually directed more maliciously, and is usually aimed very specifically at an intruder whose presence is unwelcome. Since horses have a great need for action and exercise, they use territory as a facility for running. This running behaviour is usually a group activity, with one of the group setting off and generating a mood in the others to follow.

Maintenance Priorities

Of the eight primary categories of maintenance behaviour given above, the first two, namely reaction and ingestion, are probably the most fundamental in terms of survival. The vital business of fending for itself is taken care of by each animal through feeding, fighting and fleeing. This is then

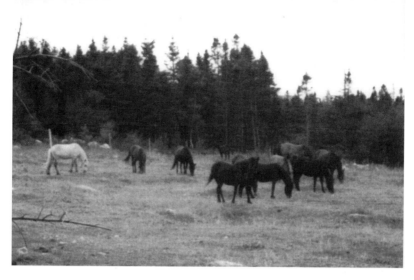

(a)

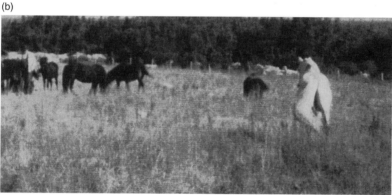

(b)

Fig. 4.10. (a) Grey stallion patrolling on perimeter of harem of mares. (b) Stallion herding harem. Photos: A.F. Fraser.

first-order behaviour of maintenance in motivational time-sharing.

The agenda of maintenance continues into other items of behaviour, which relate to a 'second-order' level of behaviour homeostasis in motivational time-sharing. These consist of six generic classes of behaviour, which have fundamental importance to the animal but do not usually have the motivational priority typically shown in reaction and ingestion. They are as follows: body care, rest, motion, association, exploration and territorialism. Their relative priorities are probably close to the rough order in which they are presented here.

Welfare Addendum

The forms of behaviour that address physiological needs feature in continuity and support well-being in the individual horse, and they are more than those most basic activities such as feeding, watering and sheltering. It can be concluded that behaviour that effects maintenance is the means of general homeostasis. They should therefore be facilitated via good welfare for any horse and in particular for a breeding mare and her progeny. It is a fundamental fact that any form of suffering suppresses maintenance behaviours. Evidence of these behaviours can therefore serve as indicating norms of health and freedom from suffering.

5 Eating, Drinking and Ingestive Welfare

A great deal of a horse's well-being has its source in the gut. Proper nutrition is clearly a vital factor in the welfare of this animal. The proper feeding of horses in their various circumstances requires that a standard textbook on animal nutrition be consulted and followed. Basic factors in equine feeding and watering are considered here to underline the fact that food and water are principal elements in equine welfare. The feeding and drinking habits of horses need to be appreciated for their proper management (Stafford and Oliver, 1991).

Motivation

A centre involving the motivation and regulation of hunger is located in the hypothalamus. Cortical and limbic contributions add to a comprehensive ingestive organization, although physiological factors alone do not explain all aspects of ingestive activity. Feeding behaviour is strongly influenced by reinforcement, both positive and negative, from food palatability and by the environmental and social associations of feeding (Giraldeau and Caraco, 2000). Young foals learn much about grazing from their mothers, for example. It is necessary for the concepts of motivation, learning and reinforcement to be incorporated into any comprehensive view of food intake (Toates, 2002; Hogan, 2005). Feeding may occur frequently and in modest amounts because the horse anticipates the pleasures of ingestion (see Fig. 5.1).

Homeostatic mechanisms do not exist to stimulate consumption of specific and essential nutrients in proportion to their need by the body. The answer appears to be in two parts. First, regulatory systems exist for water and sodium, creating thirst and a salt appetite (Pilliner and Davies, 2004). Secondly, nutritional deficiencies in general do not have specific homeostatic methods of self-correction, although some can affect behaviour through creation of depraved appetite, which may or may not address the deficiency. The ability of the horse to correct a specific mineral deficiency, even when given free access to the necessary mineral, is poor.

Horses have a marked desire to ingest salt. For this reason, freely available salt licks are put to full use. They provide one way of supplying trace elements that might not be ingested even if made equally freely available in another mixture. At times a salt appetite in horses can be very acute and can lead them into active searches, travelling considerable distances to known salt lick locations. Grazing horses with access to the seashore can be seen foraging on the shore below the high tide line, where they will frequently ingest seaweeds (and occasionally seawater); they may also lick and chew other salted material present. This is evidence of the pleasure quality of a salt appetite.

General Feeding

The quality of food needed is not only dependent on the environment of the horse but also on its size, use, age and special state, such as pregnancy, lactation and convalescence. Idle horses can be maintained chiefly on roughage in the form of good-quality hay, such as white clover, lucerne or a mixture of grasses, but they also require supplements. As a general rule, about 340 g (0.75 lb) of grain or concentrates and 900 g (2 lb) of good hay can be fed to a horse daily per 45 kg (100 lb) of body weight, provided that the horse is not working hard in sport or labour. Precise amounts should be tailored to the individual horse. This amount of hay is virtually *ad libitum* feeding of roughage (see Fig. 5.2). Good-quality hay (e.g. lucerne and timothy) remains an essential and major food, which provides not only energy, vitamins and minerals, but also the intestinal bulk that is required. The large intestine of the horse must have a critical mass of content in order to function properly (Canadian Agri-Food Research Council, 1998; Herdt, 2007).

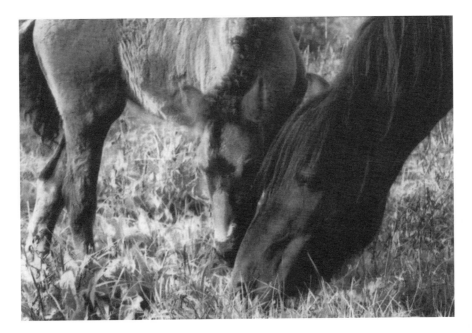

Fig. 5.1. Foal eating with its mother. Photo: R. Butler.

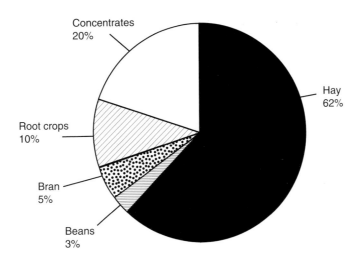

Fig. 5.2. Approximate proportions by weight of the main constituents of the daily food ration for a horse in light use.

It is imperative to provide hay of good quality to a horse. Poor-quality hay is often dusty or damp, mouldy, smells abnormally or appears dead-looking. Horses will refuse to eat such hay, even if they are hungry. Good-quality hay has a fresh appearance with recognizable grass heads. It has a fresh odour and is dry without dust. The stems are firm and can be teased out easily when flakes are set out for eating.

Grazing

While grazing, horses select short young growth of plants and often show a preference for the more fibrous grasses. They also graze the higher-carbo-hydrate grasses in a mixed pasture. The preference of horses for different plants and seed mixtures is evident in the way they prefer grazing a clover-rich seed-mixture pasture (Cunha, 1991).

The areas grazed by horses in a limited area do not include soiled grass. They do not encroach on excretory sites, and the grass over such sites is therefore allowed to grow in height and become coarse in nature. Since the horse closely crops the grass during grazing, these coarse spots eventually stand out as 'roughs'. By contrast, the favoured grazing areas tend to resemble lawns. In a limited area of grazing land, the sharp divisions between very smooth 'lawns' and tufted 'roughs' become very conspicuous through severe overgrazing (Francis-Smith, 1979). This is a danger signal. Horses will refuse to eat grass that has grown out from a faecal deposit. Such outgrowths can increase in number and size; they can create a false impression of the available grazing matter remaining to be eaten (Odberg and Francis-Smith, 1976). A horse in such a situation has its well-being at risk from helminth infestation and poor nutrition from the lack of grain and restricted grazing (Freire et al., 2009).

Food quality and availability influence the duration of grazing time. Although they graze for as long as 8 h/day, horses have some diurnal patterns in their grazing behaviour. Grazing periods are correlated with daylight, but some night grazing is also performed. The onset of active grazing is closely related to the time of sunrise, and continuation of grazing activity is largely confined to daytime. Most of the daylight hours are occupied with grazing periods. These periods usually add up to more than half of the total daylight time, longer if pasture management is poor (Singer et al., 1999).

The ratio of day to night grazing is affected by hot weather. Heat and fly attacks can adversely affect summer grazing activity. More frequent night grazing occurs in summer than other seasons, while cold and wet spells of winter weather can reduce grazing activity. Both of these circumstances demand a change to body care activities in seeking shade and shelter instead of grazing.

Horses graze by cropping the pasture close to the roots with their incisors. They cover large areas and seldom take more than two or three mouthfuls before moving at least one step further, avoiding grass patches containing excreta. They maintain some distance between each other when grazing in groups; however, bonded pairs usually eat in close proximity to each other.

Grazing is, of course, the horse's natural manner of feeding. A great advantage in grazing for a horse with an airway problem is that the head-down position facilitates drainage from the lungs and the major respiratory tracts. Apart from lower airway disease, horses can have their respiratory systems contaminated with dust and blood while racing. Long transportation after racing causes accumulation of airway debris. After racing, a horse should be turned out to graze for several hours daily for 3 days. Alternatively, it could be fed from a container at ground level to facilitate airway drainage.

In a stabled environment, the feeding behaviour of horses is influenced by their diet. If fed exclusively on hay, they spend 40% of their day eating. If fed chiefly on concentrates, they spend one-tenth of that time eating. Horses eat about ten meals a day of pelleted feed. Each meal averages 40 min in length, during which each horse eats 0.5 kg of feed, on average (NRC, 1989).

Summer grazing on good-quality pasture can be adequate feeding, but the staple diet of the horse when stabled or out-wintered is hay and grain or concentrates. Compounded, concentrated food is now generally used in place of grain. It is provided in the form of pellets, nuts, cubes, nuggets or other compacted forms. These rations are now technically composed of all the various nutrients required for equine health. Out-wintered horses not only need the same nutrition as stabled animals, but also need a greater supply of heat-giving, energy-rich food. Winter grass has poor nutritional value. For this reason, a weatherproof feeding station should be given to out-wintered horses, although they still enjoy eating fibrous matter that is available (see Fig. 5.3). In a study of out-wintered horses in Iceland, it was found that those with the highest social rank ate better than the others and came through the winter in good physical condition, while the others ultimately lost condition (Ingolfsdottir and Sigurjonsdottir, 2008).

Horses and ponies, in particular, show some preferential selection of very fibrous matter in their diet. They can eat hedges, dead nettles and fallen leaves, particularly in autumn and winter (see Fig. 5.4). They also eat bark off of trees, sometimes to the point of 'ringing' the trunk. Frequently, the bark of trees is eaten in restricted areas of grazing. Trees can be de-barked to a height of 2 m (6 ft) or more, although bark-eating

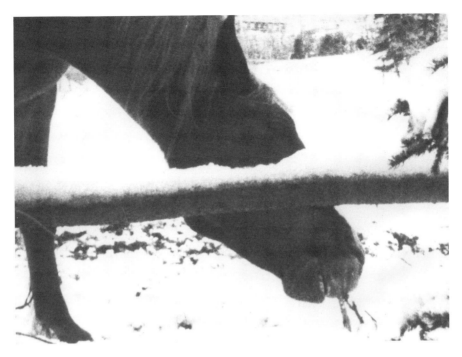

Fig. 5.3. Fibre is appreciated in winter. Photo: A.F. Fraser.

will always commence at the lower levels of a tree trunk. The bark of some trees is chosen in preference to others, with poplar a principal choice. Ash, oak and rowan are also favoured for their bark. Occasionally, horses will nibble off small branches of trees. In cases when horses nibble pieces of the yew tree (*Taxus baccatta*), sudden death through poisoning can occur.

Concentrates

The ease of rationing and dispensing concentrates allows good control of the feeding regimen that has been determined for the individual horse, bearing all of its requirements in mind. As they are already prepared with their proper proportions of ingredients, they are a very convenient food, which can be given in two, three or more feeds per day. It should always be remembered that a horse's stomach is comparatively small and has a limited capacity. It also empties in a short time. Regularity in feeding time is very important. Watering should always precede the feeding of grain or concentrates so that the fluid can readily pass through to the large intestine. Since horses take in large quantities of water at a time, this aids the flow through the stomach

and small intestine to the caecum. Water should not be forced to compete with a bulk of solid food as it washes its way through the gut. For this reason, and others, it is better to give water before any concentrated feed. Furthermore, the addition of a large amount of water to grain or concentrates already in the stomach will cause such material to swell up and create a digestive crisis.

Rationing

It is advisable to give one-quarter of the hay in the early morning, one-quarter at midday and the remaining half of the daily ration between afternoon and evening. The grain or concentrate ration can also be subdivided into a mid-morning, afternoon and evening feeding. Root crops such as carrots or turnips can be used carefully to supplement the diet. Some slight variety of foods can guard against deficiency in the diet, but any significant food changes must be made very gradually.

Traditional Food Items

Apart from general nutrition, some traditional food items have their own features in equine welfare

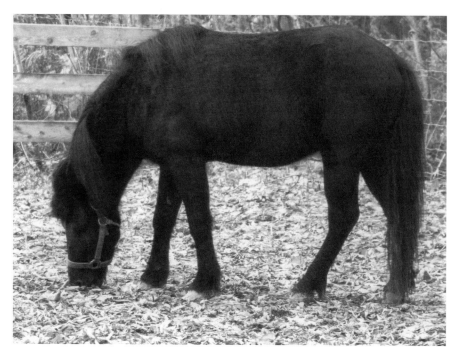

Fig. 5.4. Healthy horse enjoying fallen leaves. Photo: J. Scanlan.

(Rollin, 1995; Goodwin *et al.*, 2005). These can provide desirable variety to the horse's diet.

- Processed barley is very useful for a horse in convalescence or in need of improved nutrition. A few pounds per day can be fed. It is usually prepared by boiling and cooling before being offered. Barley contains vitamin B complex and carbohydrates. If uncrushed barley is used, it should first be soaked for 12 h and then boiled until the grains can be squeezed easily.
- Bran is a good basic ingredient in horse food and can be added to any diet including a ration of concentrates. In addition, a bran mash is a traditional feed for laxative purposes in horses. It is made by putting about 1.36 kg (3 lb) of bran into a bucket and mixing with boiling water while stirring, until the mixture is thoroughly wet. Two tablespoons of salt are then added. The bucket is then covered until cool. When this mash is fed to the horse, it may be sprinkled over with crushed oats in order to tempt the animal to consume it. The laxative effect occurs some hours later.
- Molasses, as a high-energy food that is extremely palatable, is a good additive that may improve

appetite. After it has been reduced with water, it can be spread over any other food.
- Bean substance, notably soybean meal, has high digestible protein content. This can be used as an additive to the main diet if it is not considered adequate in digestible protein for the particular needs of the animal (some proteins are non-digestible). A suitable quantity of bean meal would be about 454 g (1 lb)/day to a large horse of average activity. This amount could be increased to 900 g–1.36 kg (2–3 lb)/day for a working animal of one of the very heavy breeds. On a day of rest, a workhorse should never receive a full ration of its regular food, except hay. This is a vital rule of feeding.
- Shelled maize may be used as an alternative to oats in a similar quantity. Since it has a low protein content, maize should be supplemented with nitrogenous food such as bean meal and should be crushed or given as cooked flakes to assist digestibility. Maize needs time to be digested, and a horse fed on it must not be allowed water within 3 h of the feed due to a risk of sudden swelling in the stomach or small intestine, causing colic. Since maize is denser

than oats, it can provide a high amount of digestibility by volume.

- Oatmeal gruel is an old and traditional preparation of food intended to provide an increase in the nutritional value. It is made more digestible by prior cooking. About 3.78 l (1 gal) of milk and water is boiled while 225 g (0.5 lb) of coarse oatmeal is gradually added with a tablespoon of salt. The mixture is simmered for an hour or so and fed when cool. It must only be fed to the animal when freshly made. Some horses are keener than others for this special dish. It is undoubtedly nutritious and can be fed often to a horse in convalescence.
- Certain root crops, such as carrot, turnip or beet (as pulp), can serve as additives to a horse's basic diet. In general, they are rich in iron, vitamins and other minerals. All of the material should be cut into portions of a size that can be easily swallowed. Dicing is a good method, as is slicing. If carrots are to be fed, they should be cut into lengths rather than circular sections. Vegetable pieces in limited quantity are enjoyed by most horses, as are apples. All of these materials must be fresh and clean. They should not be used to economize on proper horse food.
- Horses cannot easily digest starch; potato pieces are therefore unsuitable as horse food. Excess starch fermenting in the large intestine of the horse leads to the production of D-lactic acid. This increases the level of acidity in the intestine, causing a condition of 'hindgut acidosis'. This results in the passage of soft, moist manure with a paste-like consistency and a sour odour. These faeces are often termed 'cow-pat' droppings.

Hindgut acidosis limits subsequent fermentation of food. It particularly hinders the digestion of fibrous matter. This condition has been linked to a variety of equine dysfunctions. It can cause sore feet, a scratching style of gait with an uneven foot fall, a low-grade laminitis, loss of appetite, dehydration and nervous behaviour. It has also been linked to a greater incidence of the 'tying-up syndrome'. Dietary alteration is needed to deal with hindgut acidosis. In particular, starch overload must be eliminated.

Special Food Items

Some modern techniques in the feeding of horses include use of the following items:

- Lupins and sunflower seeds. Cracked lupins and sunflower seeds do not contain starch. The energy value within them is provided by vegetable oil. They can reduce the volume of food being given to a performance horse. The volume of lupins must be limited to a quarter of the grain ration. For sunflower seeds, the limit is one-fifth of the total grain fed. Young horses in training for racing can benefit from a few cups of sunflower seeds daily.
- Cooked grains. The extrusion process is a form of pressure cooking for maize and barley. It improves the digestibility of the starch content by making the starch granules expand for the benefit of the enzymes in the digestive system. Extrusion also improves the digestibility of the protein content of the grains. The palatability of such material is good. Using a food with an extruded base of these grains reduces the risk of hindgut acidosis. A step-by-step introduction of such food over a period of 2 weeks is needed.
- Vegetable oils. As a source of fat for energy, some vegetable oils are now used in the feeding of performance horses in the midst of training. Horses can use such fats to increase their muscle glycogen and conserve this for metabolism during racing or fast performance. It takes some time, however, for the horse to adapt to such a constituent of feed. It may take up to 3 months for complete adaptation. Ideally, the vegetable oil is added slowly to the diet when training for racing begins. Eventually about one full cup of oil can be added to the feed in the morning and evening for a horse of Standardbred size, for example.

Maize oil, sunflower oil, canola oil and blended cooking oils are used as energy-dense substances to substitute partially for high-starch food matter in the horse's diet. Replacing a portion of the raw grain with vegetable oil has certain advantages for some racing horses, for example. One cup of vegetable oil has the same amount of energy as three cups of oats, rolled barley or cracked maize. The oil is digested in the small intestine. This evidently reduces the hyperactive behaviour caused by starch overload in the hindgut. The reduction in hindgut weight can be as much as 5 kg. This is of benefit to a horse running a mile or more in a race.

Excess oil in the diet has an adverse effect. More than two cups per day can reduce hindgut fermentation and result in the passage of poorly digested, oily droppings. Cold-pressed canola oil is slightly more palatable than some other oils and is less likely to go rancid in storage. It is advised that large quantities of vegetable oils be stored in a refrigerator and only added to the food at time of eating. It requires thorough mixing with the feed to prevent clumps from forming. This also dampens the feed and prevents inhalation of dust from the feed. The inhalation of food dust contributes significantly to long-term lower airway disease, while hay dust is the most common source of allergenic mould particles.

- Minerals. For a high-performance horse, some traditional equine diets can be deficient in minerals such as calcium, iron, copper, manganese and selenium. For example, grains contain up to 20 times more phosphorus than calcium. For bone metabolism, the ratio of calcium to phosphorus has to be 3:4. Calcium deficiency can cause lameness and spinal bone problems. A daily food supplement of 6 g of calcium can reduce the incidence of spinal problems in racehorses. Calcium is lost in sweat and it follows that a calcium supplement would be advisable for any horse sweating frequently. Some racehorse trainers provide 600 mg of iron to their horse daily.
- Vitamin D. A vitamin D supplement aids calcium metabolism. A restricted amount of time in outdoor sunlight could limit a horse's capability for natural synthesis of vitamin D. Although good-quality lucerne hay should provide its vitamin D requirements, there are times when hay may deteriorate or be cut back in the diet. This may be a misguided attempt to cut back on abdominal bulk. In such cases a vitamin D supplement could be needed. About 3000 international units (IU) of vitamin D daily is the required dose for treatment of a medium-size horse.
- Vitamin E. The American guidelines for a working horse recommend that 1000 IU of vitamin E are provided daily in the animal's food. A low level of vitamin E can occur in grains after they have been in storage for a while. Racing horses may require up to 1800 IU of vitamin E daily in order to provide normal levels of this vitamin in the various tissues requiring it for health.
- Vitamin A. Doses of 50,000 IU daily have been found to reduce the incidence of tendon weakness and breakdown in racing Thoroughbreds. Again, the long-term storage of grain can result in great vitamin A loss. Horses under the stress of training require vitamin A supplementation (Meyer, 1987).

- B-group vitamins. These are necessary for energy production and blood formation. Horses working on grain-based rations usually benefit from B-group vitamin supplementation daily. It has been found that extra B-group vitamins help to maintain a good appetite in the performance horse. For this purpose, a daily supplement of 1000–2000 mg of vitamin B12 in the feed has been found to be useful.
- Electrolytes. Horses readily lose body salts or electrolytes when working hard or racing. Sweat loss under these circumstances can often be up to 15 l/day. Electrolytes such as potassium and sodium chloride are leached from the horse's body in an outpouring of sweat. In addition to fluid, there is a need of electrolytes to prevent dehydration.

If electrolyte loss is excessive, a clinical state of 'alkalosis' can develop in the horse due to chloride depletion. In this state there are elevated blood alkaline levels. This alkalosis eventually leads to a condition of heavy blowing during and following fast work. Prolonged blowing after exercise is typical. Severely affected cases of this alkalosis can become very 'spooky' and may 'shadow jump'. Daily supplementation with an electrolyte mixture of potassium chloride and sodium chloride will correct the problem. About 3 tablespoons of common salt daily in food would provide enough electrolytes for a normally active horse. An athletic horse could require more electrolytes in potassium and chloride supplements. Travelling over a distance, a horse can become dehydrated. In such a case, a rehydration fluid can be given over the tongue for prompt restoration of electrolytes. It is essential to provide adequate drinking water to a horse receiving electrolyte treatment or supplementation, to help the horse cope with the thirst that will develop.

Feeding Welfare Addendum

As has been previously described in this chapter, horses in pastures with trees often spend time vigorously de-barking the trunks. The reason for this apparently aberrant form of eating behaviour is unknown. It is possible that some wood-eating is normal and might be considered vestigial browsing behaviour. In support of this idea is the common observation of horses browsing occasionally, eating very small trees, branches and leaves, given free range in brush land. Bark-eating is likely to be adopted by each horse in an enclosed group with tree access. This can lead to trees being debarked and 'ringed' from the root level up to the height of the highest reach of the horse. In wild or deprived natural circumstances, browsing may serve a horse beneficially as auxiliary feeding. In a good domesticated enclosure with good-quality grazing, the consumption of wooden fences or gates, for example, is abnormal and not particularly healthy. An adequate supply of a good supplement is the answer (see Fig. 5.5).

Various abnormal eating behaviours occur in some ill-managed horses. These disorders include gulping air and eating dung, hair, soil and sand. Horses cannot detect poisonous plants and trees as a rule and have to be protected from encountering them. Such eating disorders are addressed in Chapter 15.

A horse has the capacity for overeating when it is not properly rationed. Overeating is dangerous, particularly in ponies; it can cause very debilitating laminitis. A horse's natural greed has to be controlled. A good supply of hay can serve such a purpose for any idle horse, in the interest of its own well-being. Intestinal accidents resulting from improper ingestion, such as impaction and spasm, can be fatal. A bowel twist condition can occur as a true accident, causing severe colic and death.

A horse is only as good as its nutrition. A hungry horse can be an angry horse, and a disturbed temperament does not go with proper well-being. The general state of good health that all good horse keepers want their horses to possess and display is dependent mostly on good nutrition. Fat and fibre-based diets (FF) have lately been found to be very satisfying to horses (Hothersall and Nicol, 2009).

Nicol *et al.* (2005) conducted a study on the effects of foal feeding on behaviour and well-being using two diets. Twelve foals aged 2–40 weeks were fed either starch and sugar (SS) or FF diets in paddocks or barns. Barn-weaned foals were more stressed than paddock-weaned. FF foals cantered less at weaning and appeared more settled. Foals are inclined to consume their mare's faeces, or others' faeces, so the foal's enclosure should be regularly cleaned out (see Fig. 5.6).

Drinking

Water is clearly essential to health and well-being. Its need is signalled by thirst, which is created when body fluid volume is diminished. Dryness of the mouth and throat is a means to direct thirst. Oral and pharyngeal moistness appears to be capable of metering water intake. Water adequacy is signalled even before the ingested water has time to be absorbed from the gastrointestinal tract. In the horse, uniquely, the caecum is the main site of water absorption, with the colon a secondary site for water uptake and holding. In other words, the horse uses its large bowel as its water reservoir.

Every horse needs an adequate supply of good clean water on a daily basis (Houpt *et al.*, 2000). Depending on size and other conditions, any equine subject will need from 26 to 60 l (7–16 gal) of water daily. Flat water is not good for a horse's digestion. Stale, old or stagnant water is quite unsuitable. Clear running water is best for a horse, and so constant access to a spring, stream or river is ideal. Water in a trough or bucket should be fresh and aerated. The mixing of air with still water can be accomplished by stirring with a clean stick. Water in buckets in the stable should be changed often, at least once daily.

When they drink from water at outdoor ground level, horses like to step into the water. For this reason, the site of access to the water should be sloped and not muddy. A flow of good-quality water is the best standard for the drinking needs of outdoor horses and ponies. Frozen water must be well broken. Regular daily checking is needed to ensure proper maintenance of the water supply all year round.

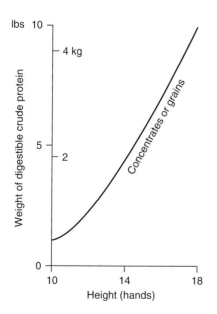

Fig. 5.5. General guide to daily requirement of solid (non-hay) food supplement for stabled horses.

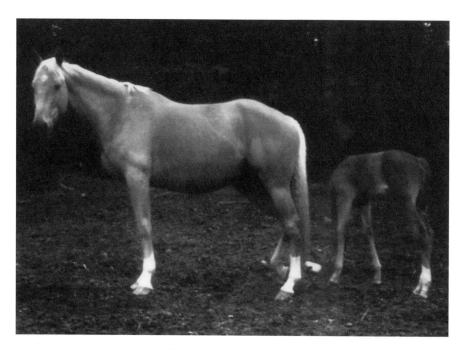

Fig. 5.6. Foal eating mare's fresh droppings. Photo: A.F. Fraser.

Horses do not drink very frequently in a 24-h period. Commonly, they only drink two or three times per day. Some horses drink only once daily. When they do drink, they typically consume very large quantities, taking 15–20 swallows of water. At the time of its main drink, the horse has to have some freedom of movement. If watered by hand at a trough, stream or carried bucket, it usually raises its head at least once during its drink. It should not therefore be taken from the trough when it first ceases to drink. About 5 min should be allowed for a drink under such a controlled condition. The last water of the day should be given as late as possible to a stabled horse that has no automatic water supply. The modern automatic watering system operated by the horse is best of all, while an outdoor paddock for several horses requires a large trough with running water.

Size also influences water intake. A medium-size horse requires an average of 30–40 l (8–10 gal)/day, but this varies according to the season. In hot weather, a large, heavy horse will drink up to 56.5 l (15 gal). Mares drink more when nursing a foal, to replace the extra fluid given out as milk. Most Thoroughbred horses take 30 l (8 gal)/day. A typical pony will swallow, on average, 20–25 l (4.5–6.5 gal) of water daily (see Fig. 5.7).

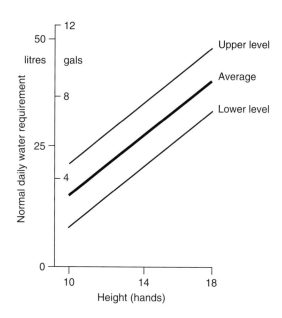

Fig. 5.7. Daily water requirements.

Whenever possible, drinking should be monitored to verify that all is well with this vital process. It is perfectly normal for some water to run out of the horse's mouth when it stops drinking. Excessive drinking is not normal and may indicate a behavioural disorder termed 'polydypsia nervosa'. Horses with this condition can drink 55–75 l (15–20 gal) daily. This abnormal drinking interferes with digestion. Polydypsia sometimes occurs in horses that are permanently confined. Proper management and water restriction are required to control this condition, which is more fully described in Chapter 15.

Water Welfare Concept

The horse is a uniquely strong and mobile domestic animal. Its generous muscling ensures its powerful mobility. Perhaps its musculature can be regarded, figuratively, as a great hydraulic system, so that this animal's need of fluid might be better understood and appreciated by horse caretakers in general (Friend, 2000).

6 Body Care and Evacuation

Before human society took care of them, horses cared for themselves over millions of years. Undoubtedly they did so by the behavioural means that they still possess in domestication today. The evident goals of the behavioural class of body care are physical comfort, hygiene and thermoregulation. Together, these play a role in well-being (McDonnell, 2002) and homeostasis (Robinson, 2007).

General

Through self-grooming, systematic stretching, particular evacuation and the practice of comfort seeking, care of the body is an ongoing system of self-maintenance in horses. Many acts of body care, such as rubbing, scratching, shaking, biting and licking, are usually brief and varied in form. As a result, they are not conspicuous as a system. However, these acts are numerous and important. Their total occurrences per day constitute a significant proportion of overall activity in many cases. A feature of this behaviour is the flexibility of its display, allowing it to intrude into other activities such as feeding or resting (Waring, 2003).

In addition to the many behavioural acts collectively grouped under the general term 'grooming', horses also tend their bodies by selective evacuation, sheltering from strong wind, shading from sunshine and repulsion of flies (Keiper and Berger, 1982). Friction on integumental areas activates body surface sensors in satisfying ways (see Fig. 6.1). With a pair in mutual grooming, sessions are usually extended, probably for the satisfying feedback in both horses. Such equine acts of mutual care indicate a degree of social sentience and behavioural organization (Toates, 2002). Many horses can scratch parts of their bodies with a hind foot. All of this expresses the horse's natural care of its entire integumental surface, including its hide, mane, face, legs, dock and tail. Integumental self-care is a sign of its well-being; it ceases in poor health.

During use, such as work, the horse evacuates its bowel or bladder without any evident discipline. It can defecate while walking, but for urination it must be stationary, when it adopts the male or female urinary stance. At pasture, the horse tends to excrete at selected spots (Odberg and Francis-Smith, 1976). Stallions are most particular in excreting at fixed locations. They typically defecate regularly at a given site, and when faeces build up they back up to the faecal mound to defecate on it. They also tend to urinate at selected places.

Another feature of body care is a particular form of stretching in which the movements are performed symmetrically to regional parts and to paired limbs. It is a phenomenon occurring in quadrupeds and man, and sometimes involves the whole body. In medical terminology it is called pandiculation. In horses, its incidence is highest in foals, but it occurs in all ages (see Fig. 6.2). It obviously serves to maintain orthopaedic functions, occurring usually after a period of inaction or at the approach of sleep. This is another item of behaviour that ceases in poor health. Pandiculation is an action pattern; once started, it leads on to conclusion.

In the behaviour of rolling, the horse lies down on one side, then rotates its trunk with a lateral push-off to attain a supine position. It holds this fixed position while it performs one or two slight rubs of its back on the chosen substrate. By laterally swinging its legs, it then falls back on its original side. This procedure is quickly repeated a small number of times until the horse falls to the other side. From that side it performs further rolling actions. When the rolling repetitions cease, the horse rises, stands squarely, then performs the 'wet dog shake'. In this, a wave of rippling skin passes from the head to the hindquarters, the legs and tail, dislodging matter from the hide and hair. The vigour in the shake is such that the limbs quiver down to the hooves. The entire process represents a classic 'fixed action pattern', as recognized in pure ethology.

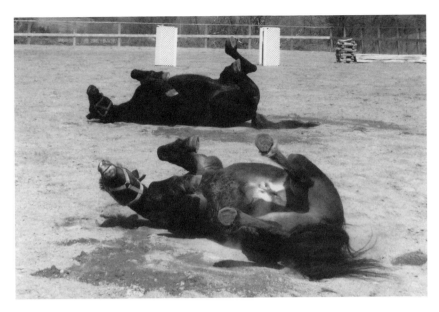

Fig. 6.1. Rolling on sand. Photo: Melanie MacDonald.

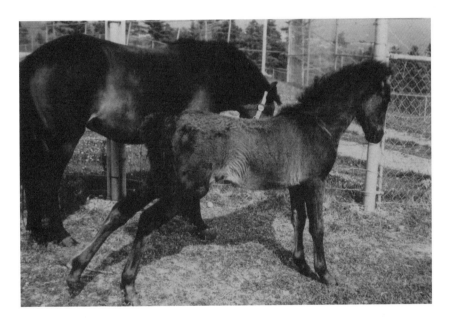

Fig. 6.2. Overall pandiculation in a foal. Photo: P. Barker.

Grooming

Horses groom their own bodies regularly, especially around the hip and flank. This auto-grooming is done by turning the neck, extending the head and nibbling repeatedly at the skin in these regions. They may occasionally also groom their limbs, both fore and hind, by nibbling or snapping. Horses groom their crests by rubbing them to and fro beneath a manger or tree branch, for example.

Horses do not use their tongues to clean out their nostrils as do cattle; instead they snort to do so. Nasal secretion in the horse can be considerable. In severely cold weather these secretions can freeze and become very prominent on the horse's muzzle. Abnormal nasal discharges may also accumulate in some illnesses. This is due somewhat to their excessive production and partly because surface body care activities are suppressed in most illnesses (Fraser, 1995).

Another peculiarly equine form of grooming is scrubbing of the buttocks. This is another region that cannot be attended to by nipping or rolling. A swaying action of the rump is used against a convenient structure such as a post, tree, building, gate or fence. Special scrubbing places become adopted, and fences can be broken down by such continual use. While this behaviour can be a sign of parasitism in the horse, it is also normal grooming and has no clinical relevance unless the incidence of the action becomes significantly excessive. The effect of rump grooming is twofold. It scrubs the skin of the buttocks and the outer face of the tail head, removing scurf. It also causes the tail to be pressed into and across the skin of the perineum, wiping this hairless region, which can accumulate skin scales, salt from sweat, sebaceous grease and small faecal accumulations. Some grooming acts make use of items in the environment (see Fig. 6.3).

Climatic Body Care

In severe cold, horses group closely together to afford mutual shelter and to conserve body heat. As an example of such a tactic, horses often gallop in snow (see Fig. 6.4). This generates energy to boost body temperatures. In the absence of wind or moisture, they tolerate temperatures down to −20°C (even to −40°C if provided shelter), but horses are most comfortable in mild temperatures in the range 10–20°C. Shade from direct sunlight is normally sought in temperatures over 25°C if there

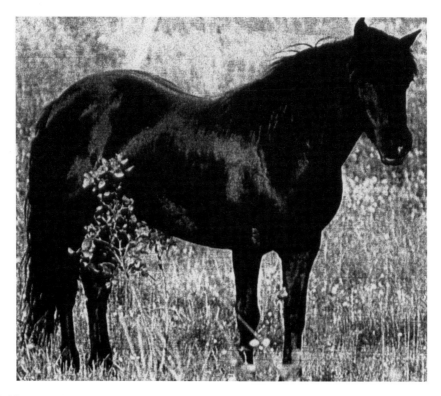

Fig. 6.3. Gelding grooming its belly on a well-used bush. Photo: J. Woodman.

is no air movement. Sheltering from rain or snow by outdoor horses is particularly noticeable when the precipitation is severe (Robinson, 2007).

In severe, stormy weather a horse will cease to graze. The tail will be held close in to the dock, allowing it to be blown between its hind legs. The tail hair then shields all of that hairless area of its perineum, its inguinal region and the inner thighs. By this means it spares itself some loss of heat and energy. The density of the winter coat and the direction the hair lies, especially over the hindquarters and back, provide an outer periphery to the body, which acts as a weather shield, so efficient that ice may form on top of it without transmitting chill to the skin. Rolling on top of the snow, therefore, does not chill a horse (see Fig. 6.5).

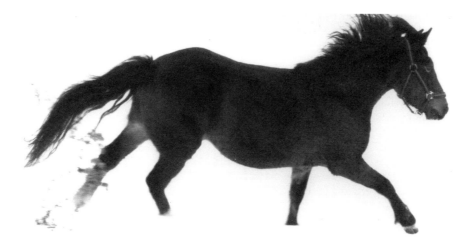

Fig. 6.4. Galloping in snow. Photo: Melanie MacDonald.

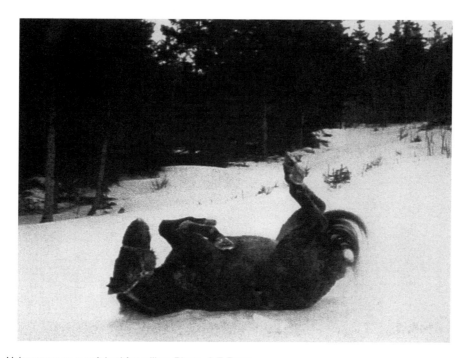

Fig. 6.5. Using snow as a soft bed for rolling. Photo: A.F. Fraser.

A combination of cold and wind, especially combined with rain or snow, can inflict great stress upon a horse. The effects of frost in severely cold weather can be worst in a saturated horse. A quantity of hair over the head can be both waterproof and a watershed, to ensure that ears and eyes are not subject to weathering. A full mane with natural length and density can act as a waterproof screen for the head, jowls, throat and neck. When left uncombed, numerous long, ropey segments become formed throughout the mane of mountain and moorland ponies, for example. In a strong wind, horses usually graze with the wind at their backs. In hot, sunny weather, horses spend their lounging time in any shaded or partly shaded area that is available. They put their heads, rather than hindquarters, into limited shade. In like manner, they direct their hindquarters into strong, inclement wind if no windbreak exists in the pasturage (see Figs 6.6 and 6.7).

Shelter from flies is often difficult for grazing horses to achieve, unless they can find an area receiving air currents where they can stand. If they are in a social group, horses may gather closely together and, with tail switching, they can set up a fairly proficient fly screen for themselves. In addition, agitation of the head and ears helps in fly defence. Whisking the tail is a good fly repellent. Horses usually shake manes and forelocks as an additional means of creating air movement and fly disturbance.

Horses can adapt well to climatic extremes. By no coincidence, the heavy cold-blooded types and northern ponies can deal well with cold, while the hot-blooded and warm-blooded breeds cope well with very warm climates. Of the heavy horse breeds, the Percheron copes best with warm weather, including tropical climates.

Pandiculation

Pandiculation is a somatic form of body care. It is defined as the extension of the legs, the raising and stretching of the arms and the throwing back of the head and trunk, as occurring before and after

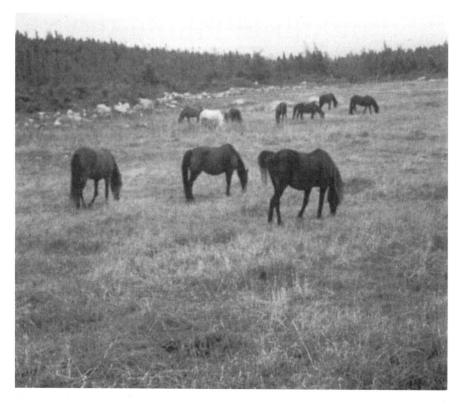

Fig. 6.6. Grazing with the wind. Photo: A.F. Fraser.

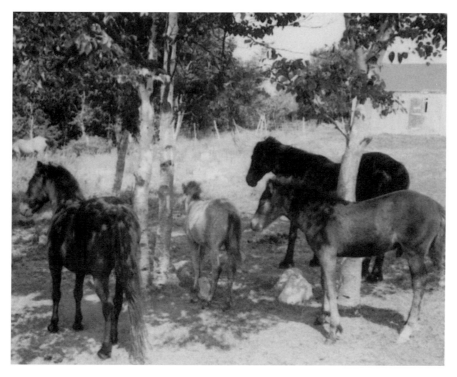

Fig. 6.7. A group in shade together on a hot day. Photo: A.F. Fraser.

sleeping (SOED). The general manner in which horses stretch themselves in a stationary position shows that the specifics of such equine stretching actions have much consistency. In its variable forms, pandiculation appears to function as an expression of well-being, especially in foals, in which it is very commonly observed. Healthy foals average about 40–50 pandiculations per day in various forms and in recumbent or upright positions. Being the uniquely kinetic domesticated animal, the young horse presents itself as a suitable subject in which to note this remarkably neglected feature of behaviour, serving as both body care and movement. The stimulus to pandiculation can be assumed to be feedback from stiffness. In addition, the phenomenon at times may be in response to a period of asymmetry in position.

Pandiculation as a comparative phenomenon has a core of common characteristics from time to time and from subject to subject. These characteristics are:

1. Extending the forelimbs.
2. Extending the hindlimbs.

3. Extending the head and neck upwards or forward.
4. Flexing the vertebral column by depressing it or arching it regionally.
5. Stiffening the trunk.
6. Periodic yawning.

The above features in horse pandiculation have a high degree of constancy. Among them can be variations such as absence of yawning or exertion at only one pole of the body, i.e. anterior or posterior. Equine pandiculation can have symmetry in simultaneous or alternating extension of limb pairs. Obviously, all four limbs cannot be easily fully extended simultaneously in the standing subject, although they are typically involved in simultaneous extension in pandiculation when the animal is lying in lateral recumbency. In this latter situation the tensile form of the phenomenon is most evident.

Other notable characteristics of pandiculation in horses include those given below:

1. Polarity. Although the action pattern is not directed in relation to the environment, it has direction in relation to its body base. It can therefore be recognized as being variously outstretched, upraised, anterior or posterior.

2. Position. Pandiculation can occur in the two basic positions of upright stance or lateral recumbency.

3. Totality. The whole pattern of pandiculation may occur in a given manifestation, or recognizable portions of it may be produced. It can therefore be complete or partial.

4. Periodicity. Many occurrences of pandiculation are in perisomnolent circumstances, e.g. when the animal is arousing from sleep or as sleep is being initiated. It also often occurs at the end of a period of flexed sternal recumbency. Occurrences are most common when voluntary action is being initiated after inactivity. Pandiculations may recur as a series of events in close succession.

5. Illness. Pandiculation is remarkably absent in all forms of general illness. Equally notable is its return to behaviour when the animal is progressing in convalescence and returning to a state of health.

6. Diagnosis. It is of prognostic value in appraising a recovery to health. Equally it is of some diagnostic value in ascertaining a state of well-being, particularly in young horses.

7. Age. The complete forms of pandiculation appear to be shown with greater frequency in young animals than in older ones. In the latter, incomplete manifestations are more common, such as yawning.

8. Confinement. Whereas it appears that release from confinement or change of locus often induces pandiculation, it is noted that the full pattern cannot be reproduced by the animal until it has sufficient space for the vigorous bodily extensions that are the main feature.

9. Comfort. Clinical subjectivity affirms that the phenomenon is associated with evident satisfaction. In the animal's bodily and behavioural conditions, an element of comfort attainment can be assumed.

Although the impression is of musculature being stretched, many of the above actions clearly involve joints. The atlanto-occipital joint is subject to considerable articulation in some of the above actions. Other major joints that are notably involved in fully extended articulations are shoulder, elbow, carpus, stifle and tarsus. Stretching also stiffens the extremities and trunk. In such patterns of stretching, the musculature, tendons and articulations involved are, in general, used in equine kinetics.

Yawning may occur with body-stretching episodes or it may occur alone. Its form is slow and displays maximal extension of the temporomandibular joints. If eating is important for life, it follows that the only chewing joints – the temporomandibulars – must be maintained permanently functional.

An interesting minor feature in this stretching is eye closure during the activity. It may be that the eyes are closed for saccadic suppression, to allow the exercise to be performed without opposing visual signals, which could interrupt the process. Slow movement also overcomes any influence from optomotor feedback, which would be aimed at correcting the body's position. The centre of gravity changes and body angles are changed during bodily stretching. Finally, the body-based (somatic) character of pandiculation emphasizes the need for primary space for basic kinetic output and for general comfort in the interest of the horse's welfare.

Evacuation

Stallions and geldings straddle while urinating. The mare, when urinating, does not show the same marked straddling posture as is shown by the stallion; nevertheless, the posture is similar, in that the hind legs are abducted from each other. Following urination by the mare, the vulva contracts. More elaborate patterns of urination are shown by brood mares with young foals and by mares in oestrus. Mares in oestrus urinate limited quantities frequently. They straddle and eject mucoid urine in an oestrous display, which includes tail arching and touching the ground with the toe of one hind foot as that leg is abducted significantly. Each ejection causes a splashing of clear fluid behind the mare. This eliminative behaviour continues for the period of oestrus, which commonly ranges from 4 to 10 days in duration. Pregnant mares periodically straddle and strain and pass small quantities of urine in the first stage of labour.

The stallion and the gelding adopt a characteristic stance while urinating; the hind legs are abducted and extended so that the back becomes hollowed. Urination takes place with the penis released from the sheath. Following urination, the stallion usually smells around the area before walking away. Normally urination occurs about three to six times per day. Most urine is passed during rest periods in the hours of darkness. For purposes of urine sampling, horses can usually be induced to urinate when they are led into a stall deeply bedded in fresh straw.

On average, a horse defecates about 6–12 times per day, depending on the nature of the feedstuff consumed. A common output is 9 l (2 gal)/24-h period. Faeces are passed without posturing, apart from tail elevation, and no straining occurs. In normal health, the faecal material is passed in the form of substantial accumulations of compacted balls that are mid-brown to olive green in colour, according to the material eaten. The faecal mass has a dry nature and breaks up when it falls to the ground. In health, the odour is not particularly offensive in nature. Fluid faeces are a serious indication of an alimentary disorder.

Stallions show careful and deliberate selection of the spot where defecation is to occur. As is performed following urination, a stallion turns and smells the spot where defecation has taken place. In the case of both the stallion and the mare, the muscles of the perineum contract following defecation and the tail is lashed downwards several times. The faecal deposits of geldings have been found to be random in long grass.

Breeding stallions grazing with a herd of mares create mounds of manure in a few specific locations. These mounds can build up to the height of the horse's belly with repeated use throughout a season. Controlled eliminative behaviour avoids soiling of resting areas and favoured grazing places. Horses do not normally lie down where they have excreted; they often choose the perimeter of a grazing area to urinate.

A Body Care Organization

Methods employed in general body care are practised with remarkable precision with regard to position, posture (even awkward posturing), group density and duration. Neural organization is evident in all of this, and it is apparent that specific motivation governs grooming and other forms of body care. Prolactin induces grooming, and the dopamine system supports grooming, and all comfort behaviour is opiate-related. Prolactin stimulates dopaminergic turnover in some brain areas, notably the nigrostriatal system. It is known that opiate-induced and sustained grooming behaviour is dependent on the catecholamine system. The mechanism of excessive grooming involves the dopaminergic system. It is known that striatal dopamine can be involved in stress-induced excessive grooming. Excessive self-grooming can escalate to self-mutilation in horses.

Individual grooming activities depend on the reverberation in the tactile sensorimotor circuits of the nervous system. In comfort-seeking, the tactility of extensive skin areas is a determining factor for horses. They often show clear preference for the tactile nature of the substrate on which they will more readily stand or lie, if given opportunity of choice. A great deal of physical comfort seems to emanate from cutaneous attentions, and these make up most of the actions that can be grouped in the general category of body care behaviour.

Varying with the health and well-being of the animal, a physical comfort system obviously functions as a caretaker organization. In general ill-health, body care diminishes and grooming activities become reduced or arrested. In many illnesses the coats of affected horses lose their normal clean and orderly appearance. Such coats become dirty or 'harsh' in appearance as they lack the effects of friction from rubbing, moisturizing from licking, and removal of debris from scratching and brisk shaking. Sick horses have reduced body care motivation and do not discriminate in choice of resting place or time and place of evacuation. In illness they are recumbent more than usual and their coats become heavily soiled as a result. Similar soiling can be the result of dirty or insufficient bedding when welfare is poor.

Welfare Addendum

Under the common controls of domestication, horses are not always able to let their body care organization function. For this reason, there is a welfare need and an ethical demand to supply comprehensive body care to any horse confined in a stable or premises with limited space. Hand grooming is the way to meet that need and fulfil humane ethics for the animal's satisfaction and its general well-being. A horse's skin is, after all, an organ of the body with critical functions. It is vulnerable to infestation, infection and trauma. This calls for regular skin inspection. Hand grooming facilitates such inspection while the integument is being cleaned and massaged (Marlborough and Knottenbelt, 2001).

Hand grooming

Horses kept in stables need to have their body surfaces cleaned off regularly and their long hair brushed or combed. The equine hoof is like a scoop and it needs to be cleared out frequently. These requirements are met by routines of grooming. The type of grooming should relate to the horse's circumstances as much as to a prescribed schedule or grooming drill. Certain traditional routines in grooming need to be recognized, but these can be modified by common sense and the need of the individual horse and its use. The objectives in grooming are hygienic, physiological and aesthetic, in addition to the probable provision of some sensory satisfaction to the horse.

During the grooming process the five specific aims are as follows:

1. To massage the animal (specifically the muscular areas – see Fig. 6.8).
2. To stimulate cutaneous circulation.
3. To remove skin debris, loose hairs, old sweat and skin secretions.
4. To monitor the need for treatment of any skin damage, infection or parasitic infestation.
5. To improve the appearance of the animal.

The removal of the old winter coat can be a major objective of grooming in the spring. When the horse has produced sweat, the removal of this is important when it dries. Old sweat becomes part of the dander in the horse's coat, and removal of dander is a basic objective in routine grooming. Proper grooming takes time. Hurried grooming

cannot be very effective in addressing the five specific aims listed above. Other interests should not affect the style of caring for a horse. When it is a recreation, horse keeping should not be undertaken as an attempt at a profitable commercial enterprise. In this it does not differ from other recreations. Notable exceptions, of course, are the horse racing, breeding or riding industries. With this matter accepted, grooming can be given its necessary time. Large horses require more time, while tall horses might need a stand for the groom. The elements of grooming are as follows:

- **Quartering.** The body of the horse is regarded as having four quarters. Quartering is the term for the cleaning of a horse's fore and hindquarters after a night in a stable stall. Urine staining in particular is dealt with appropriately. For example, it can be dusted with sawdust and then brushed off as often as is necessary. Urine staining and wetting is a greater problem with male horses kept in stalls, and this demands more grooming time and work. Since their urine falls under them in the centre of the stall, male horses often become urine soiled on the lower surfaces of their bellies. This area, which is not very accessible, must also be attended in quartering. The use of a damp sponge or moist cloth in this work can be useful. It should be realized that such items can serve as fomites (physical agents of transmissible infections, or infestations by ectoparasites). They should, therefore, be limited to use on one animal only. They can be sanitized later. Brushing is needed to complete the quartering.
- **Wiping orifices.** The horse's eyes, nostrils and dock area need to be cleaned, in that order, by wiping off these sites with a small, dampened towel kept thoroughly clean but not soapy. This should also be regarded as a potential fomite, as mentioned above.
- **Dandy brushing.** A dandy brush is one with stiff, long bristles, made of a variety of materials. It is a large hand brush to be used with vigorous, sweeping actions to dislodge debris from the coat and clean off adherent particles of dried-on foreign matter, such as faeces, bedding, etc. In this form of brushing the groom faces the rear of the horse and uses the hand closest to the horse. A start is made on the upper neck region with brisk light strokes of the dandy brush, going in the direction of the coat hair.

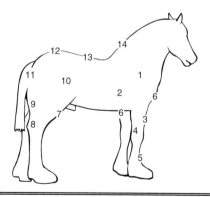

1. Prescapular	8. Lateral digital extensor
2. Triceps	9. Gastrocnemius
3. Radial carpal extensor	10. Quadriceps femoris
4. Common digital extensor	11. Semitendinosus
5. Common digital extensor tendon	12. Gluteal
6. Pectoral	13. Longissimus dorsi
7. Long digital extensor	14. Trapezius

Fig. 6.8. The main muscular areas to massage in the course of grooming an active horse.

This brushing is continued over the body and down the leg. Areas to be dealt with cautiously include the inner thighs and belly floor. Some horses are very ticklish in the flank region and may give a reflex action when touched there. A regular groom soon learns any idiosyncrasies of the horse in its reactions to grooming. Strokes with the dandy brush should be short and end in an outward flick. Reverse strokes may be needed to dislodge stubborn matting of a coat. This would be followed by strokes flowing along the normal lie of the hair.

- **Body brushing.** The body brush is a grooming item with soft, short bristles or rubber teeth. It is often oval in shape, with a broad band across the back to fit over the groom's hand for security of grip. It is used in conjunction with a curry-comb, on which it is periodically wiped. A currycomb is a broad metal scraper with several ridges of teeth over its open side. It has a handle and sometimes it also has a metal comb on its reverse side. Projections from the sides allow it to be cleaned by knocking it sideways on the ground. This is done from time to time, as it accumulates material from the body brush. The body brush is designed to be used as it is named, to go over the horse's body with a heavy massaging action. Its use is to massage the neck, forequarters, trunk and hindquarters. The body is gone over, small area by small area. Circular actions are used over fleshly parts but the final direction is with the natural flow of the hair. After a few strokes the body brush is cleaned off by scraping it over the face of the currycomb. The groom should not attempt to press the body brush heavily over sensitive areas or body prominences. Although they are available, mechanical grooming machines are not the best, chiefly because of their noise and the failure to use them with variable pressure.

- **Combing.** Ponies kept in a natural condition outdoors do not benefit from severe combing, but when the mane and tail need to be untangled a strong metal comb with teeth wide apart can be used. Riding horses are generally combed regularly, chiefly for good appearance. To enhance the horse's appearance further, the mane and upper part of the tail may be plaited. A wide variety of styles of plaiting and ribboning are utilized as decorative features. These are very time-consuming attentions to the horse and are not part of any formal grooming regimen. They are extras, which some grooms like to perform for a particular event.

- **Hoof picking.** The tool for cleaning out the sole of the hoof is a small metal pick with a handle at right angles to the head of the pick. It is held with the point of the pick away from the groom. To clean the sole, the foot is lifted and the fetlock flexed to put the sole on view. While the foot is held in this position with one hand, the groom uses the point of the pick to clean out the sole on both sides of the frog, around the bars at the heel and between the sole and the shoe. The direction of picking is away from the heels. Some picks have a wire brush attachment to brush off the sole at the conclusion of picking. In hoof care there may be rasping of the edges of an unshod hoof with a file. The wall of the hoof should never be rasped, except around its lower margin. The wall is sometimes painted with grease to preserve its covering of periople. The periople is the transparent tissue that gives a waterproof surface to the wall of the hoof. Its integrity prevents the hoof wall from becoming dried out and brittle.

Although a grooming regimen will vary from person to person and from stable to stable, three forms can be characterized as being basic, routine and special. These are summarized in Table 6.1. Since stabled

Table 6.1. Grooming types for stabled horses.

Type of grooming	Procedure
Basic	Quartering; wiping face and dock.
Routine	Head to feet brushing; body massaging; wiping face and dock; rough combing of mane, tail and limbs; cleaning soles and hoof walls.
Special	As above, plus fine combing of all long hair; full body brushing; special attention to face, belly, thighs and lower limbs; hoof rasping as necessary.
Extra	Trimming mane and tail; clipping body and limbs; washing legs; painting hoof walls with protectant.

horses are groomed twice, or even three times per day, it would be in order for at least one of these to be basic. Special or extra grooming would not be involved as a daily practice, as a rule. Proper grooming of a stabled horse in use is an ethical requirement, for which the designated custodian of the animal must take, or delegate, the responsibility. It is a major constituent of horse welfare.

The grooming of horses is a chore of fundamental importance in their care when they are stabled. Sometimes attendant volunteers enjoy performing this work. For those who are limited in capability to perform other work, this type of occupation can be enjoyed and may provide some therapeutic benefit (Katcher and Wilkins, 2000). Horses often relate well to attendants with disabilities who are nevertheless diligent with their attentions.

A Note on Thermoregulatory Welfare

In outdoor conditions horses can find themselves in extremely variable states of weather, with which they have to cope. In doing so, they seek shade from hot solar radiation, often putting the head and forequarters into shade. As aforementioned, they seek a windbreak in driving rain or blowing snow; they turn their hindquarters into strong wind; and they seek refuge in their own close company from fly attacks. These are their tactics in body care thermoregulation. Without shelter, they are unable to avoid becoming thoroughly wet in conditions of rain, wind and cold; they then experience hypothermia, along with shivering, particularly of the pectoral muscles, followed by inactivity. In such a state they lose weight dramatically in a day or two – the weight loss being most notable between the shoulders, the breast area becoming narrower. Illnesses can develop in such circumstances. Horses can tolerate extreme cold if their coats are dry; similarly, they can tolerate dry, tropical heat and have well-being in either type of temperature. The proviso is that, unless they are free in an extensive, variable environment where they would be able to find natural shelter, outdoor horses in limited space must have access to structured shelter – otherwise they should be brought indoors during inclement weather.

7 Kinetic Behaviour and Racing

Among the principal features in equine behaviour are ambulation and running in their various forms. The horse is a kinetic animal above all else; its modes of locomotion need to be recognized as the animal's expression of its nature. Every one of its numerous gaits can be performed at variable rates, giving the animal great control of its ability to move actively and progressively. Flight was probably this animal's principal defence system in the ancient days of its wild life, when, it is believed, it had the role of being prey to carnivorous predators. Its power of flight is great, in both the speed and the distance over which it is able to run. The muscular mechanics of all of its gaits are very distinct. The gait is the way-of-going, in which the animal progresses by the moving order of its four limbs.

Muscularity

The muscular activity occurring in the forequarter and limbs of the horse during its fast forward movement is an exact system of coordination (Barry, 2001). While the forelimb is moving forward and back, certain neck and chest muscles are alternately contracting and relaxing. These are the muscles that form a sling in which the chest is supported between the forelegs. The forelimb, of course, has no bony or joint attachment with the forequarters. When the leg is moving forward, the very long muscle that extends down the side of the neck to the forearm contracts and relaxes rhythmically. As it contracts, it pulls the forelimb forward. Muscles of the breast also pass from the chest to the forearm to aid in its motion. This alternating strong contraction and relaxation of these muscles in pairs is known as reciprocal muscle action. It is this important muscle feature that gives such proficiency in equine striding (Pearson, 1997). The reciprocal muscle action, when carried out most proficiently, gives the animal not only strength but also an even, flowing gait when running (see Fig. 7.1). The hindquarters have

the reciprocal apparatus, linking stifle and hock in fibrous bands (Chapter 9).

In the role of absorbing impact is the rounded and prominent muscle mass above the elbow joint: the triceps muscle. One important function of this muscle, particularly in jumping, is that it acts as a shock-absorber. When considerable weight is put on the forelimb, it takes some of the impact. In jumping, most of the body weight of the animal, together with its load, is applied to the forelegs when the horse lands. The tendency of such impact will be to force the elbow joints into flexion, and this is resisted by the powerful mass of this triceps muscle as it contracts. Other forms of special apparatus take up impact; one is the suspensory ligament and the other is the check ligament (Dyce *et al.*, 1996). Both of these pass down the back of the lower leg, together with the flexor tendons' ligaments (Wentink, 1978). They serve critically to reinforce the limb when the foot is pressed on the ground.

The Gaits

The gaits can be distinguished by the sequences in which the hooves are lifted from the ground. They alter with acceleration. In each form of locomotion the limbs act synchronously in any one of a variety of patterns, each of which is termed a gait. Two forms of gait pattern exist: symmetrical and asymmetrical. In symmetrical gaits the movements of limbs on one side repeat those of the other side but half a stride later. In asymmetrical gaits the movements of limbs on one side do not repeat those of the other. Symmetrical gaits include the walk, the pace and the diagonal trot. Asymmetrical gaits include the various forms of the canter and gallop, including the lope and the rotary gallop. The gaits of the walk, trot and canter are basically similar in most quadrupeds but are best shown in the horse. In addition, the horse has the potential for jumping ability.

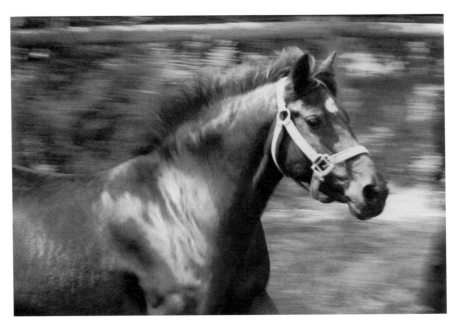

Fig. 7.1. Shoulder muscular action during impact. Photo: Melanie MacDonald.

The full cycle of movements of a leg during the support, propulsion and flight phases is termed a stride. A stride is a full cycle of movement of all limbs, while stride length is the distance covered between successive imprints of the same hoof. The sound produced when a hoof strikes the ground is the beat. If each limb strikes the ground separately, the gait will be a four-beat gait. If diagonal limb pairs are placed down simultaneously, as in the diagonal trot, the gait is two-beat, since only two beats will be heard per stride. The canter is a three-beat gait, resembling waltz-time. The lead leg is that leg which leaves the ground last during the canter or gallop. The gallop, of course, resembles the canter, but since it has more propulsion, it has an extra-long 'floating phase' at the end of each stride. The longer this phase, the greater will be the running horse's speed. Within every stride, each limb for a time acts in a support phase and in a non-supportive or swing phase. As a key factor in stability, the support phase is more critical in the forelegs, which are nearer the centre of gravity. Approximately 60% of the static weight is taken by the forelegs. The propulsive role has more investment in the hindlimbs (Hoyt and Taylor, 1981).

The gaits of the walk, the trot and the canter are the principal forms of action fundamentally involved in equine locomotion of any significant duration.

The full gallop can only be sustained for a limited time, such as a few minutes. In addition to muscular physiology, one reason for this is that respiratory action is tied to running, as is oxygen use. When running, the horse must breathe in rhythm with the gait. The oxygen consumption of a horse when running increases linearly with the speed. The full gallop presents most difficulty in breathing and the greatest oxygen cost. By contrast, the walking horse is an example of a most economical form of motion, since the metabolic cost of moving fast as opposed to not moving fast, which is the energetic cost of locomotion, is remarkably small in this animal (Hoyt and Taylor, 1981).

The walk

The walking gait can be very brisk, steady or slow. Its slowest form is when the animal is grazing. At this time, most of the duration of each stride is spent with all four feet on the ground simultaneously, each leg only moving singly forward during the remainder of the stride. The steady pace of the walk is at a rate of approximately 5 km/h (3 miles/h).

The walk has the least elevated action of all gaits. The walk is started by propulsion from the hindquarters, followed by the raising of a forefoot – either right or left. If the right forefoot lifts before the left, the stride is as follows. There are four movements. First that of the right foreleg, followed by the left hind leg to make the second movement. When the right foreleg is off the ground and moving forward, the left hind leg is raised and follows the movement of the foreleg. The third movement is that of the left foreleg, followed by the right hind leg in the fourth movement. Obviously the gait continues with the forward movement, alternating between each pair of diagonal legs. The walk is therefore a slow, steady, four-beat movement, and the four beats should be evenly separated from each other so that one four-beat movement blends in with the next one, creating equal time and emphasis with each individual beat.

In its slower walking stride, the horse always has three of its hooves in contact with the ground while one leg is advancing. For convenient identification, the legs and their hooves can be numbered as follows: 1, near hind; 2, near fore; 3, off hind; 4, off fore. If the near hind starts the walking stride, the footsteps in one stride of the walk will be in the order 1,2,3,4. With no. 1 advancing, no. 2 leg is flexing. With no. 2 advancing, leg 3 is flexing and so on. As a result, the three legs with their hooves on the ground are weight-bearing, while one leg is flexing. The energy used in this walk is therefore minimal, providing that the animal is not in heavy work as it walks.

At the faster rate of walking, the horse already has the flexing leg's hoof raised, as the advancing hoof hits the ground, while the next leg starts flexing. The animal's full weight is then borne for a moment by a diagonal pair, with the other pair in the motions of advancing and flexing. Although these two latter leg actions are not exactly simultaneous, they bear less weight than the other two, which have their hooves flat on the ground in the continuum of the stride.

The action of each limb in the walk (and other gaits) can be divided into two parts. These are the 'swing time' and the 'standing time'. The latter relates to the duration of time when the foot is on the ground, while the swing time is the remainder of time, when the foot is in flight. During the swing time the feet are normally raised well clear of the ground, with good flexion of the knee and the fetlock in the foreleg, and the hock and the fetlock in the hind leg. The foot is carried forward over the ground without the action being exaggerated or sluggish. A limb that moves in this fashion is set down on the ground firmly. Sluggish action ultimately leads to stumbling.

The amble is a specific type of walk; essentially it is accelerated walking. In the amble, the increase in walking speed is achieved by quicker swinging action. The following leg has started its flexion while the preceding leg is lifted. This is obviously a gait which is more demanding than the normal walk since only two legs are fully weight-bearing at one time. However, it permits a good breathing rhythm and it can be sustained for long periods.

The trot

The major difference between the walk and the trot is that the trot is more energetic, active and elevated in its manner and speed. The horse commonly trots by lifting two diagonally opposite legs at exactly the same time. Thus, the right foreleg moves with the left hind leg in synchrony. During the trot, there are only two supportive beats because the horse raises and sets down two diagonal feet at the same instant, giving the typical two-beat tempo of this gait.

In the trot the horse is solely supported by the alternating diagonal pairs of limbs. The suspension phase and support phase are of equal time in a steady trot, but if there is an extended period of time in the phase of suspension between the support phases, the gait is referred to as a flying trot. In this very fast trot there are two brief floating phases when all four feet are off the ground. If the support phase is longer, the trot is called a jog or dogtrot. In this slow trot there are two brief support phases when all four feet are on the ground.

The term 'dog-trot' may mean that the animal's position is oblique to the line of travel, with the hindquarters shifted to the left or right. The trot is also classified variously as ordinary trot, extended trot, collected trot and the pace. 'Extended' and 'collected' refer to the distance that the feet are carried forward in each swing of the diagonal limbs. Extended obviously implies maximal stretch forward of each limb, while collected indicates that the upper regions of the limbs are restrained in forward action. The collected trot is characterized by flexion and high carriage of the knees and hocks in a generally elevated way-of-going. In this trotting gait there can be two brief floating phases, one following the lift of one pair of supporting legs and another floating phase following the lift of the second pair. This gait is termed the flying trot and has a faster pace than the regular trot, but still has the two-beat pattern per stride. Figure 7.2 illustrates three distinctive trotting gaits.

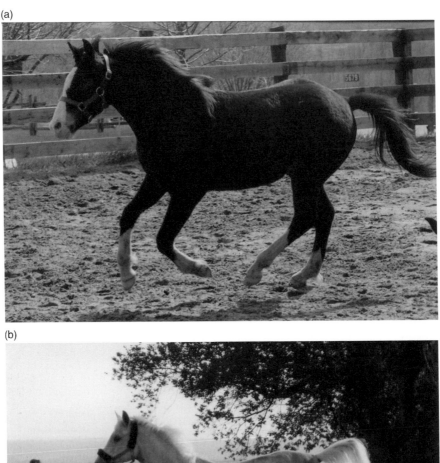

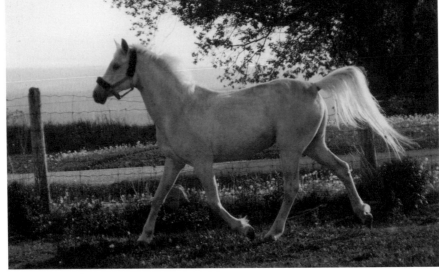

Fig. 7.2. (a) Slow trot. (b) Limb action in a perfect diagonal trot. Photos: Melanie MacDonald.

A form of trotting in which the paired legs are on the same side is called the pace. This gait allows slightly greater extension of the hindlimb since the paired forelimb (on the same side) is also extended at the same time. Some horses are born pacers, while others have pacing trained into them in the sport of harness racing. Pacers typically have longer swing time than support time in their gait. Pacing is symmetrical and permits full respiration at a fast rate. The pacer can slightly turn its body to the side of the extending pair of legs and away from the two supporting legs to increase its reach and speed. This

(c)

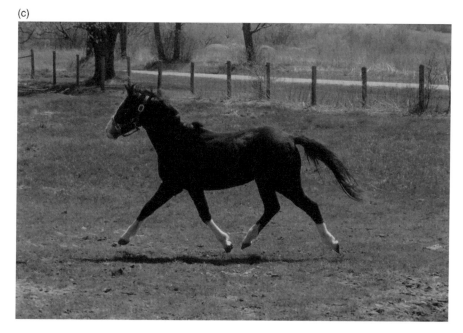

Fig. 7.2. *Continued.* (c) The flying trot. Photo: Melanie MacDonald.

slight side-to-side spinal swinging cannot be done in the diagonal trot since the paired limbs are on opposite sides of the spine in that gait.

The canter

In the cantering gait the horse has an asymmetrical style that permits a slight forward leap within each stride (see Fig. 7.3). In this form of running the horse has only one pair of limbs in synchrony, namely one foreleg and the opposite hind leg. The footfalls give a three-beat time as follows: 1, a hind leg by itself; 2, the other hind leg and its opposite foreleg together; 3, the remaining foreleg. This last forelimb, the lead leg, leaves the ground in each stride. It creates the slight forward leap before the originating hind leg lands to begin the next stride. The upward throw of the head and neck on the lead leg uses the musculature of the neck and forequarters.

A left-lead canter has the following sequence of leg movements.

1. The left foreleg throws the horse into a brief floating phase, with the aid of a muscular up-raising of the head and neck.
2. All four legs are gathered under the body, with the right hind leg extending forward to land on the ground.
3. The right hind takes the weight as the horse pitches forward to land on the left hind and right fore, almost simultaneously.
4. The left foreleg extends forward and takes the remainder of the impact of the stride.

During (1) there is a sharp inspiration. This is followed by an expiration during (4). A right-lead canter has the correspondingly opposite movements.

A left lead is suitable for taking a bend to the left and a right lead is necessary for the horse taking a curve to the right. In a straight run of significant length, such as half a mile, an efficient horse will change its lead in an action termed a flying change. In this, the horse brings its lead leg down on the ground quicker than the other foreleg, which then becomes the lead leg. The leading leg performs more muscular effort by stiffening the shoulder and the elbow, throwing the body upwards, and by taking the final impact of landing on a firmly fixed leg. The horse effectively vaults itself over this leg in this diagonal gait.

Changes of lead are helpful in giving some relief to a tired lead leg. This leg not only raises the horse for the leap, or the floating phase, but also takes the final impact of landing on to its support phase alone. In the training of a running horse, it is essential for

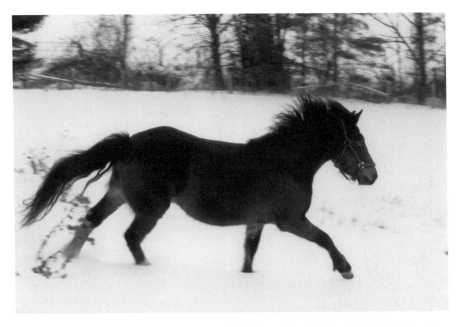

Fig. 7.3. Cantering in deep snow, providing absorbent underhoof conditions. Photo: Melanie MacDonald.

it to learn how to change its lead appropriately; going around a clockwise turn, a cantering or galloping horse should be on a right lead. Coming out of a turn, a change of lead can relieve the tiring foreleg.

The gallop

The gallop is a diagonal gait and is essentially the same as the canter except that it is the result of maximal effort (Fig. 7.4). The thrust of the lead leg is great and the resultant floating phase is also greater. This floating phase allows the fullest flexion at the croup and the fullest reach of the hind legs under the belly. Because of the extra effort and speed, the trunk has a more vigorous shunt forward with each stride. This causes greater respiratory difficulty, with the inevitable oxygen debt building up as the gallop continues. This gait can only be maintained for a relatively short time. Depending on the horse's fitness, a galloping period of a few minutes would be the limit of maximal speed of the gallop.

In the gallop, unlike the canter, the diagonal pair of legs does not hit the ground exactly simultaneously. As a result, there are no more than two legs bearing full weight at any time. The oxygen debt creates air hunger as exhaustion occurs. This is revealed by the horse extending its bobbing head and neck to the fullest extent while running. Horses breathe only through the nose, so the nostrils are now dilated to their limit. With fatigue, the forelegs develop a shorter reach in a chopping action. At this time, there is also a shorter floating phase.

The physiology of such fatigue shows that this running behaviour is associated with a decline in availability of adenosine triphosphate (ATP). The decline in ATP correlates significantly with the accumulation of muscle lactate. As muscle ATP content decreases, there is a loss in running speed. Some horses appear to tolerate a higher lactate load better than others, apparently for reasons of physiological idiosyncrasy. In normal circumstances of this fatigue, the running musculature accumulates a lactic acid burden, and the animal's physiological changes do not then tolerate full muscular activity. A further enforcement of running can cause serious muscle damage as myopathy.

The sprint

The fastest form of running in the horse is the sprint. Only a minority of horses have the ability to produce a full sprint, except among Quarter Horses, where this ability is a feature. In the full sprint, the

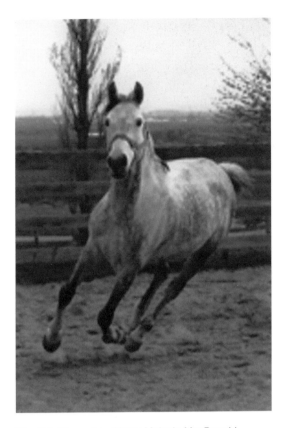

Fig. 7.4. The gallop. Photo: Melanie MacDonald.

since the sprinting posture involves raising the head and neck, with slight elevation of the forequarters.

The rotary gallop

A variation in the leg use in galloping sometimes occurs in a pattern called the rotary gallop (Fig. 7.5). This gallop is an asymmetrical gait of high speed, in which the horse's weight is more evenly distributed in the support phase. The feet are placed down in a circular order, e.g. right hind, left hind, left fore, right fore, as the horse lands from its floating phase. The rotary gallop is not employed by all horses. Some do not use it at all, while some use it only when they tire of a diagonal gallop, such as towards the end of a race, for example. Some use it when they are running in a long, straight direction. For some horses, the rotary gallop is not suitable while rounding bends. It is nevertheless an efficient and fast gait. Compared with the diagonal gallop, it permits better respiration, since the rotary movement modifies the force of the abdominal viscera pressing on the diaphragm. More pressure of viscera occurs when the direction of landing from the floating phase of a gallop is entirely in one forward direction against the diaphragm.

Other gaits

In addition to these natural gaits of the horse, some other ways-of-going exist, which are classed as 'unnatural' gaits, such as a very brisk 'stepping pace' or 'slow rack'. With such gaits there is no bouncing of the back and there is no bobbing of the head. This fast form appears to be related to other unnatural gaits, such as the 'paso' and the 'rack', which characterize the Latin American and Tennessee Walking horses, respectively. Other 'gaited horses' include the American Saddlebred and the Missouri Fox-Trotter, which, with the Paso breeds of South America, have the easy 'gliding' gaits.

These breeds have an innate aptitude for such special ambulatory gaits, in which the head is held very high and still; it must be noted that they are of Spanish origin. Such 'gaited' horses remain of special appeal in the Latin American culture and in many regions of the USA.

The Paso Fino gets gait characteristics from its ancestors: Berbers, Arabians and Andalusians. These breeds were crossed to produce the Spanish Jennet, a horse that displayed an exceptionally

horse surrenders its normal breathing rhythm and forcibly inflates its lungs before fixing its thorax in an expanded state. This permits the reciprocal apparatus of the forequarters to have free function. With the thorax held in a fixed state, the animal's trunk is also held in firm condition and this firmness helps the contractile function of the muscular pelvic region and the hindquarters. As a result, the running speed is improved for a limited time and distance.

A common sprinting distance is about 150 m (160 yd). Essentially, the horse is running anaerobically in the sprint, with regular breathing all but suspended. This fact soon results in deteriorated blood chemistry and depressed performance (Littlejohn, 1982, personal communication). At the end of its sprinting capacity, the horse can continue its momentum at a reducing speed but cannot produce a second sprint immediately. In a race, if a horse can be sprinted in the final length of a mile, it can finish the race strongly. In the stride of the sprint, the forelegs are thrown forward prominently,

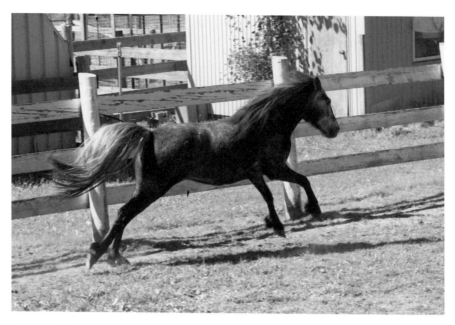

Fig. 7.5. The rotary gallop. Photo: Melanie MacDonald.

comfortable saddle gait. History has it that in 1492 Christopher Columbus left such horses in Santo Domingo in the Caribbean. Later, they were used as a foundation stock by the *conquistadores*. Known as *los caballos de paso fino* – 'the horses with the fine walk' – it was the *conquistadores* who established the Paso Fino throughout Central America in their centuries of rule there.

Paso Finos inherited their characteristic gait from ancestors that evolved in an Iberian environment, where short, quick steps were possibly an adaptation to the terrain there. This breed is unique with its natural four-beat gait. According to the breed's standards:

> Each foot contacts the ground independently in a regular sequence at precise intervals creating a rapid, unbroken rhythm. Executed perfectly, the four hoof-beats are absolutely even in both cadence and impact...In all speeds of the gait, the rider should appear virtually motionless in the saddle, and there should be no perceptible up-and-down motion of the horse's croup.

The 'unnatural' gaits employ a staccato rhythm of four-beat footfalls in a style that allows the horse to hold its back in a very stable state. The hindlimbs perform long steps in each stride and are placed in a forward position below the animal's trunk. The forelimbs have an elevated

action. All the footfalls are quick; the principal effect of this is that the 'gaited' horse is very easy to ride at a brisk speed, which approximates the rate of the trot.

Jumping

With training, horses are capable of effecting quite spectacular jumps, in both distance and height covered. Few horses readily jump until they are taught to do so. Untaught horses usually avoid obstacles only 60 cm high, rather than clear them by jumping. Normally horses avoid jumping over ditches and show a reluctance to jump over horizontal obstacles in general. Nevertheless, they possess great capability for jumping while running (Jones and Faure, 1984). This aptitude is best demonstrated in showjumping and steeplechasing.

Horses can pop over gaps in terrain in any normal gait; however, a significant jump can be considered as a special, upward, symmetrical stride. In sport jumping, the horse typically approaches the jump in a canter. Immediately before the obstacle the horse usually makes a short, strutting bound, bringing its hind legs under it to the take-off point in front of the jump. The horse throws up its forequarters and leaps with its hind legs together, about 2 m in front of the jump. At the same time, the knees are fully flexed, with the hooves coming close to the elbows. The lightened weight of the forequarters with the hindquarters under the body allows the forelegs to be fully flexed to clear the jump. The forearms are raised so that the knees lead over the jump. This latter posture is not a normal action and some horses have to be taught full knee flexion for high jumps. Since the horse enjoys this activity, it tends to learn quickly (Ferguson and Borgh, 2004). The horse goes over the jump in a horizontal position and extends its forelegs as it descends, the hind legs trailing over the jump (Leach and Ormrod, 1984). Some horses employ extreme sideways twisting of the hindquarters as an additional technique in jumping.

On landing from a jump, both forefeet hit the ground about the same time, with one slightly ahead of the other to become the lead leg when the canter is resumed. At the time of impact on the forefeet, the fetlocks go into hyperextension. On landing from a particularly high jump, the fetlock extension can be so extreme that the fetlock points hit the ground. It says much about the horse's great construct that such foot action can be tolerated repeatedly. Inevitably, of course, leg injuries can and do occur, requiring veterinary attention (Houpt and Wolski, 1982).

Saltation

A previously undescribed action pattern in neonatal foals usually first appears within 2 h after birth, in the form of an abrupt, jumping little dance. The behaviour is soon an established activity and recurs more frequently in subsequent days. Coupled with this action are sudden short runs, jumps and leaps of various types. Such forms of sudden and spontaneous bursts of activity are known in the human adult, termed 'saltation' (definition: 'leaping, bounding, jumping; a leap; a dance; an abrupt movement', *Shorter Oxford English Dictionary*) and 'saltatory' (definition: 'bounding; leaping; dancing; advancing in irregular spasms', *Penguin Concise English Dictionary*). The action in the foal is performed vigorously and is produced within very limited space. In the neonatal foal it has a strutting character, using the limbs firmly in a quick, downward-thrusting manner. If the foal has the necessary space, the activity soon progresses to sudden outbursts of running for further distances.

As the foal matures, frequencies of typical saltation diminish and instances of running increase, given sufficient space. The distances of these runs also increase as the foal's general activity blends into the common kinetic forms of foal behaviour. Nevertheless, saltatory characteristics continue to be apparent in the way that episodes of running and bucking play are often initiated and performed, either alone or with other foals. It is usual for an associating foal of similar age to reciprocate with the same activity. Within the young foal's saltatory actions, there appears to be some motivation to energize its locomotor anatomy (see Fig. 7.6).

Neonatal saltation may have facultative properties since the physical actions in it are not limited to one particular function. The experiential returns from saltatory actions are several, including stabilization, propulsion, gravitation, extension, flexion and elevation. These are essential items of self-knowledge for this kinetic novice that needs to use its limbs in numerous functions featuring mobility. Not only is this an imperative need in its neonatal stage but it also serves the animal throughout its entire existence. That the experiences of saltatory sessions would have fundamental value and permanent neurophysiological lodgement seems obvious. As a developmental factor in this physically competent animal, it represents a first lesson in variable kinesis.

Without this instruction on self-dynamics, the horse's particular ecological history could have been less than successful. Even today, some of the extraordinary performances of horses in dressage and in 'airs-above-the-ground', as shown by Lipizzaner stallions, may have parts that have a basis in early saltatory actions. These demonstrations contain certain special acts involving sudden leaps, kicks, rears, dancing steps and elevations. They are suspiciously similar to some juvenile saltatory actions. The question arises whether such staged capability is a by-product of saltatory experience and its 'hard-wiring' in the CNS.

Although equine saltation has no evident motivation, the manner of its expression in juvenile play indicates that it is linked to an emotional state of pleasure. This relationship could also exist in the successful neonate. Having recovered from the travail of becoming ambulatory and achieving satisfaction in suckling, the saltatory foal could be experiencing a degree of pleasure. Again, when an adult horse has been involved with regular containment in a stable, given demanding use over a period and then released on to pasture, a prompt saltatory display is common (see Fig. 7.7). It usually takes the form of kicking and running immediately after

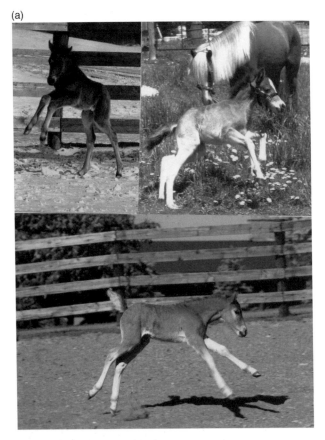
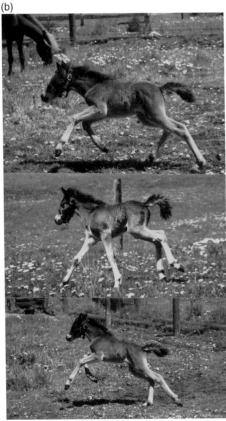

Fig. 7.6. (a) Foals in saltatory jumps. (b) Foals in saltatory runs. Photos: Melanie MacDonald.

release. It is reasonable to suppose that this is an expression of pleasure. In the horse, motivation for the sudden kinetic outburst of saltation would therefore appear to be from the equine version of mental enjoyment stemming from the limbic system (see Fig. 7.8).

Racing Behaviour

Racing

It is second nature for horses to run with each other and to put some effort into the run. In natural conditions, horses in a group readily run collectively in close association. Their circumstances in racing are therefore basically in accord with their inherent behaviour. In racing, the great differences lie in the fact that they are being ridden, that they are being forced to run at their rider's directions and that, at

some point, they are forced to run at maximum speed. They are commonly driven to a physiological limit in the race, either throughout it or at the final stage of it. Other differences between natural running and racing are that, for the latter, the horses are in their own age groups, are physically fit and have been conditioned by selection, training, feeding and general care. The racing horse is an athlete. Following a race, a horse is properly given a significant period of several weeks' rest. A degree of ethics exists in good racehorse management.

Horse racing is both a sport and an industry. It is controlled by its own authorized organizations, which establish rules and regulations for every aspect of racing. These exist to ensure that it operates properly, humanely, honestly and fairly in the interests of horses and race attendees. Since its events are under public observation, horse racing, as an acceptable activity, has the further guarantee of general scrutiny as a monitoring force. Individual horses that excel in this sport are of great commercial value and this underpins the industry. The gambling aspect draws massive public support. Some people are simply attracted to the sight of fine horses in motion. The sport is firmly established internationally.

The mobile functioning of the racing horse has not received very particular attention in general or technical literature, but this phenomenal item of equine behaviour deserves analysis for its full appreciation. To begin a dynamic examination of the racing horse, it must be recognized that the hindquarters serve as the main source of running power, propelling the trunk and foreparts forward. The connection between these two areas, i.e. the hindquarters and forward body, is the lumbo-sacral joint. This joint, recognized as the croup, is the vital coupling, or connection, between the source of power and the rest of the body. It is the hinge that determines the flexion capability of the spine when the hindlimbs are thrusting forward and backwards in the flat-out gallop.

The distance from the croup to the point of the buttocks is an indication of the amount of stretch forward under the trunk that the hindquarters can make at speed. If the line between these two points is a steep, downward-sloping one it suggests that the forward reach of the hindlimbs will be optimal. This forward reach is also facilitated by a tucked-up abdomen, which will not impede the forward movement of the legs' stifle joints. This forward projection of the hindlimbs is important since the thigh's femur does not increase its angle with the spine beyond 90° when the hindlimbs are being extended backwards. The femur's connection to the pelvis (i.e. the hip joint) permits much more flexion than extension.

In the diagonal gallop, the forward reach of the hind feet occurs during the 'floating phase' of the galloping stride. The hind hooves then strike the ground forcefully. One hoof (diagonally opposite the lead leg) is usually slightly ahead of the other, but they power in unison, with the non-lead leg projecting the horse forward on to the lead leg to complete the stride. A sharp breath is then exhaled through the wide-open nostrils. At this time, the back, from the croup forward, makes a minor upward extension, or elevation, as the animal's foreparts are slightly raised. This eases the weight on the lead leg, which is considerable.

In the rotary gallop, one front leg stretches forward (almost like a lead leg) and its hoof hits the ground before the partnering foreleg. The latter is the true lead leg and its vital forward reach is aided by the support from the other foreleg. The lead leg's reach is maximized by a vigorous forward throw, and this allows the leg to gain distance before it rigidly takes weight and 'pole-vaults' the horse into the floating phase. Both hind legs are then drawn under the body. The hind foot on the same side as the lead leg hits the ground slightly before the other and, with the pair of hind feet firmly planted, they push off together. The non-leading forefoot then hits the ground to complete the stride.

Fatigue, should it occur in the gallop, prevents the outreach of the lead leg occurring effectively, resulting in the two forelegs then simply chopping at the ground without gathering their greatest distance. Some horses, with energy in reserve and a capacity for sprinting, can elevate their forequarters coming out of the floating phase and throw their forelegs up and forward, giving them an extra burst of speed. Short sprints, as, for example, in American Quarter Horse

(a)

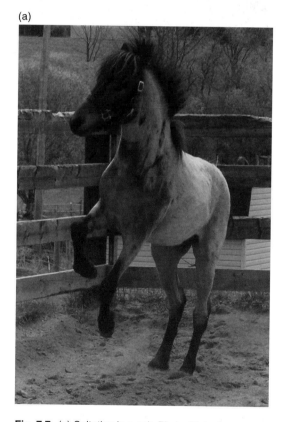

Fig. 7.7. (a) Saltation in a colt. Photo: Melanie MacDonald.

(b)

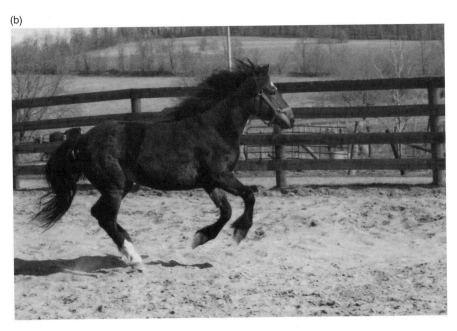

(c)

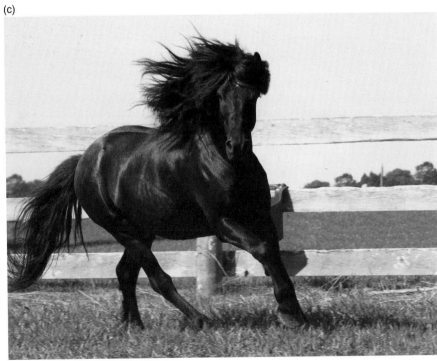

Fig. 7.7. *Continued.* (b) Forward leap in an adult. (c) An outburst of saltatory action in a pony stallion on release from stabling. Photos: Melanie MacDonald.

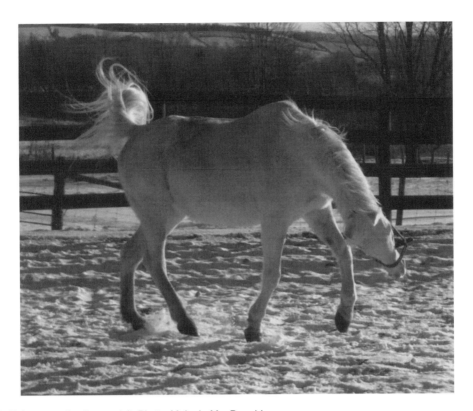

Chapter 7

Fig. 7.8. Saltatory action in an adult. Photo: Melanie MacDonald.

racing, can be performed virtually anaerobically. The oxygen debt from the short sprint can be corrected by panting when the run is complete.

When the lead leg duly takes the weight of the whole body, it is held straight. It then functions by 'pole-vaulting' the horse into the 'floating phase' of the stride. The vault briefly makes the horse airborne and this allows all legs to be drawn in under the horse. An inspiration of air can occur at this time. Coming out of the 'floating phase', the hind feet strike the ground and the muscular hindquarters propel the horse forward, beginning a new stride. These dynamics are the 'way-of-going' in Thoroughbred racing.

Standardbred horses race in harness and their form of running is limited to trotting. Their 'way-of-going' can be either the diagonal trot or the pace. In the pace, the pair of legs on the same side move in unison. Since this type of running permits some side-to-side bending of the spine, a slightly longer reach can be attained per stride in the pace than in the diagonal trot. Breathing is also slightly easier in pacing than in the diagonal trot. The latter style of trotting requires

the horse to keep its spine more rigid; however, the animal is in better balance in this diagonal mode.

Particularly in Thoroughbred racing, the horse's pulmonary aeration becomes increasingly compromised as the race progresses. In the period of the forward thrust and landing on the lead, the abdominal viscera are pushed against the diaphragm, preventing inhalation and enforcing exhalation. An intake of air can be made only during the floating phase of each stride. Breathing has therefore to take the form of short breaths. This is sometimes compromised by the sudden occurrence of epistaxis. Deep breathing cannot occur and, consequently, running at a full gallop causes physiological deteriorations to result and create exhaustion. The resulting oxygen debt and acidosis impair action severely. With the development of significant exhaustion, further enforcement of running would cause serious pathological repercussions in the animal, possibly resulting in death. However, full sessions of exercise in training can condition the racehorse for endurance and against early exhaustion.

Fear can add to exhaustion. To control fear, the use of blinkers on the bridle can be helpful. This cuts down on the horse's peripheral vision, which is its main alarm receptor. Some horses will always be timid and it can be helpful to restrict their vision with blinkers, visors, hoods, etc. An unblinkered, timid horse can move away in alarm from an aggressive competitor in the heat of racing. Any alarm is disturbing to the vital physiological functions of a running horse.

Use of the whip

While being ridden, some horses do not fully respond to the aids from a rider without a whip or crop. In racing, maximum effort is usually required of the horse at the concluding part of the race, and this is customarily conveyed to the animal with the whip. It serves as a signal of urgency. The horse, of course, does not know where the finish line is, so the jockey, or driver, must make it clear to the animal when a final effort is needed to conclude the run. Such whipping is done in various manners.

In recreational riding, a crop is sometimes carried by the rider and this, with its flat leather loop, can serve as a painless clapper to emphasize and aid. In Thoroughbred racing, the usual whip has a long, tapered end, and this can sting the horse and even cause welts if repeatedly applied vigorously to the animal's skin. The whip used in harness racing is much longer and very flexible, with a small flap on the end. Its lash can inflict a sharp pain, but it is usually applied to the side harness to urge the horse. Some harness racing tracks have introduced a 'no-whipping' rule.

In all circumstances, the use of the whip requires limitations for the horse's well-being. The latter concern is ethically and humanely of greater priority than the animal's achievement. Used tactically, the whip can provide a clear indication to the horse that a full effort is wanted from it. Improper whipping is punishment to the animal. In fact, painful whipping may produce a less positive reaction than an encouraging stimulus. The latter can help to inspire the horse to meet the needs of the moment. For improper use of the whip in racing, stewards have the responsibility and duty to impose disciplinary action on the offending jockey.

At the conclusion of the race, it is important for the jockey to keep the galloping horse running, while slowly and progressively reducing its speed. If the galloping horse is pulled up too quickly, the impact on the joints of the feet can be severe. The weight and great momentum of the galloping horse can create an exaggerated force being directed down the legs to fragile points if the feet are suddenly and firmly planted on the ground as a result of the horse being pulled up too quickly. When the horse has been brought to a walking pace, it should continue to walk for a while so that it can be progressively cooled and then covered to prevent chilling.

Swimming

As a rule, horses are not thought of as swimming animals. It is realized, of course, that a horse put in deep water is capable of swimming, even without previous experience. How competent they are as swimmers is a question which has never been seriously addressed. It is quite remarkable how pockets of free-living horses and ponies are to be found existing on so many remote islands around the world. Since many inhabit these islands as survivors of wrecks, they must be very competent swimmers.

The gait which the horse uses in swimming is simply the trot, the two-beat gait in which the diagonal pairs of legs move in unison almost in a mechanical way. If a horse can trot at speed for hours on land, he can swim steadily for hours at sea – at about a quarter of the land speed. It can be assumed that, if he can trot easily for about 100 km on good going, he could competently swim a 25-km distance in calm ocean. Indeed he might even swim for a longer time than he can trot, as a result of his good buoyancy in salt water. In swimming his legs bear no weight and the natural carriage of his head in trotting – elevated and extended, without bobbing – is another asset in water (see Fig. 7.9).

The horse is well built for swimming; each hoof can act like a scoop or paddle. His neck is long and he breathes through his nostrils, which can be held up easily and can also be expanded or closed. It is only at the canter or gallop that horses become tired quickly; during the trot they have almost endless endurance if they are fit. Trot-swimming appears to be effective. Either the diagonal trot or the lateral trot (the 'pace') allows high knee and hock action in the water and creates good swimming strokes.

Today, some convalescent horses are forced to swim in a few special veterinary clinics with circular canals, to hasten recovery from leg problems. More may be learned in the future about their swimming characteristics from scientific study.

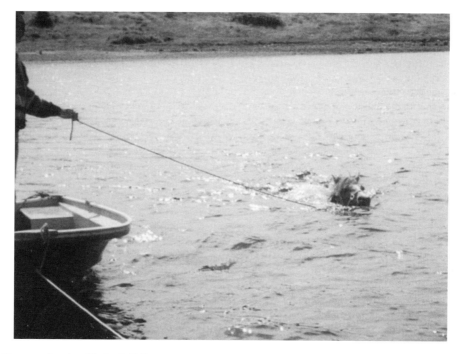

Fig. 7.9. Ocean swimming. Photo: A.F. Fraser.

Nevertheless, it can be stated that light horses can maintain a steady swimming speed of about 5 km/h, i.e. similar to a human walking speed of casual pace. At sea it could be anticipated that a fit and especially experienced horse could swim in calm water without difficulty for some hours.

Kinetic Need

Horses have an apparent desire for movement and the existence of a kinetic need is presumed (Collery, 1969). There is certainly a brain centre for such behaviour. The nucleus accumbens serves as a central location of cursive activity. It is located in the ventral forebrain region, where it organizes the continuity of locomotor limb movements. Many animals seem genetically programmed to travel certain distances in their 'time budgets'. Even when the need to travel has been removed, as in their domestic environment, horses are motivated to move. A kinetic need ensures a minimum level of activity to keep animals physically prepared for any necessary movement. This translates into a constant need for exercise in horses kept within any form of confinement. Regular exercise ensures proper activation of limbs and senses. Lack of activity causes sensory deficiencies through a

reduction in the animal's sensation of its own movement (Fagan, 1976).

The sense organs in the orthopaedic parts, such as tendons, joints and muscles, respond to mechanical action, movement, position and pressure. They obviously supply a major share of the horse's sensory input. The sensation of gravity is obviously less in a stationary horse than in a moving one. A sense of muscular effort also accompanies gross motion of the body. Seemingly, it is the general loss of such sensory input that is at the foundation of much anomalous behaviour in horses. A husbandry system that limits locomotor activity makes the environmental circumstances of chronic restriction impose two deficiencies in the physiology of sensation, i.e. hypostimulation (reduced stimulus input) and hypokinesthesia (diminished sensory receipt of body movement feedback). Evidently a sensory deficit adversely affects environmental homeostasis. The anomalous forms of behaviour resulting from this will be discussed in Chapter 15.

Exercise

Proper welfare includes regular exercise for the horse (Caanitz *et al.*, 1991). As a very kinetic creature, the healthy horse requires daily activity to preserve its well-being. While free at pasture, a horse can generate its own activity, but stabled horses require about 2 h of appropriate exercise each day. Athletic horses, even at pasture, require double this amount of steady activity on a daily basis to keep fit. Stallions need to be given a regular schedule of physical activity for their fitness and also to diminish their energetic behaviour while stabled. Horses can be exercised by being lunged, ridden, run or walked in a group. The form of activity must suit the subject. Stabled stallions are best exercised by a daily lungeing session. Enforced exercise can be given with a treadmill or a rotating pole with an overhead tether. Such exercise, however, provides no significant exteroceptive stimulation (Courouce, 2000).

Lungeing

For the lungeing of any horse, a lungeing head collar should be used with a lungeing line about 8–10 m (25–30 ft) in length. A cavesson with a ring on the noseband is preferred to a head collar. The horse should be lunged in a proper location. A smooth, sand-covered area or an indoor riding arena would be most suitable, but an area of pasture land can be converted for this use. With the aid of a driving whip, the horse is directed around a circular route. The person lungeing the horse occupies a central position and turns continuously to face the horse and urge it in its progress while holding the long lungeing rein.

The best gaits of the horse in lungeing are alternately the walk and the trot. The horse must be driven for equal amounts of exercise in both directions. At times, a lunged horse will engage in a canter. If cantering is included in the exercise, the horse must be directed in each direction long enough to adopt the proper lead for the direction. In the clockwise direction, the right foreleg should lead. In the counterclockwise direction, the exercise should continue until there is a left lead to prevent one-sidedness (McGreevy and Thomson, 2006).

Lead alteration helps a young horse to learn to change its lead easily. Such an ability allows a horse to vary its galloping gait to equalize muscular fatigue and also to gallop around bends efficiently. A running horse must be able to enter a bend on the correct lead. On moving from a curve to a straight course, horses often benefit in pace from a change in lead. Lungeing is also a method of examining a horse for soundness in respiration.

Riding

Horses can be exercised efficiently by being ridden. No ridden horse should be made to run long on a hard surface. Riding for an extended period of time at a very fast trot is not advisable as a form of exercise. A trotting speed of about 14.5 km/h (9 miles/h) is appropriate. Whenever possible, a rider should direct a horse on to soft going. Riding downhill puts extra weight on the forelegs, and a rider at that time should use the horse sensitively. The purpose in exercise is to afford the horse freedom for an appropriate quantity of activity without undue stress or strain (Clegg *et al.*, 2001).

For a horse to be ridden at a fast gait over an extended distance, it must maintain a good system of breathing, since its rate of respiration increases with increase of gait. The release of energy by the animal's body, in order to give it power to move musculature, is done with the production of heat within the body. Excessive heat accumulated by the animal readily leads to hyperthermia, which in the working horse is a serious physiological state if it cannot be relieved. Relief from hyperthermia in the running horse can only take place in two ways. One is to increase the output of heat from the body through expiration of its own warm air; this calls for respiratory efficiency in these features of conformation, such as a good clean throat and a wide muzzle. The latter is required to widen the nasal openings by the movement of the cartilaginous wings of the nostrils to make the nasal aperture as round and as open as possible. As previously mentioned, the horse only breathes through its nose.

The second and main thermoregulatory mechanism available to the horse that is becoming warm as a result of exercise is sweating. This facilitates radiation of heat over wide areas of the surface of the body. A degree of air movement over the surface of the body as a result of the animal's progression helps the loss of heat from the body as a whole. Sweating takes place over most of the horse's body when it is well heated from exercise.

One of the areas of the body that can lose heat very quickly and proficiently, when necessary, is the region beneath the tail, in the area of the dock and between the thighs. These are the same areas that require coverage by the tail when the animal is conserving its body heat in cold weather. This area can also act as a thermal vent when the animal is overheated. It is therefore a key part of the thermoregulatory system, together with conformation, breathing and sweating. When the animal becomes warm as a result of exercise, it promptly elevates the tail to allow the dock area to function as a thermal vent: a flue. For this reason, horses suitably warmed up by brisk exercise will raise and carry their tails out from the hindquarters. This style of the animal's carriage is to attempt cooling by improving the dissemination of increased body heat. Horses must never be cooled rapidly.

Under any sweated conditions, the rider should dismount and walk with the horse. If the rider chooses to remain on horseback uphill, the horse should be rested after the climb has been completed. The horse can then be walked slowly by the dismounted rider. By observing the respiration rate of the animal, it soon becomes evident when it has adequately ventilated itself. It is then ready to be ridden again.

Loose exercise

Grouping creates organization in dealing with a number of horses that are to be exercised simultaneously. They can be led around a circular track or put into a closed route with mounted riders leading

them and following up behind. The track should be at least 400 m (0.25 mile) long. The group should be moved at a walk until they have settled into the exercise. Once settled, they can be quickened gradually until they adopt a steady trot. Phases of walking and trotting should be alternated for a period of about 1 h. Shorter periods of walking are appropriate for mares with young foals (see Fig. 7.10).

Turning horses out of their stables into a large paddock can provide them with mild exercise and relief from tight enclosure if they are kept in stalls. In such circumstances, the released horses need several hours to move adequately. If this is a regular practice, a windbreak or shelter should be provided so the horses can deal with hot or cold weather during their release. The self-exercise period may need to be curtailed in very severe weather. Even in poor weather, installed horses need some release on a daily basis (Goodship and Birch, 2001). These are major welfare requirements.

Welfare Addendum

When a horse has sweated heavily, its coat becomes thoroughly wet. Again, a horse can become wet from rain or even swimming or washing. In all instances a wet horse should be dried off promptly. If the horse is also very warm from exertion, it should be cooled down progressively with a slow walk before being dried off. This controls further

(a)

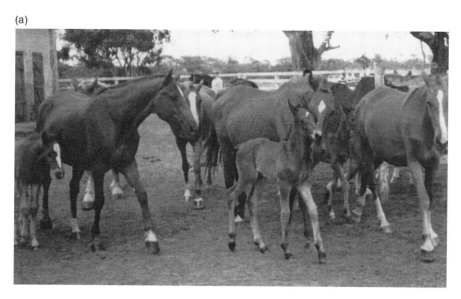

Fig. 7.10. (a) Mares and foals in loose exercise. Photo: A.F. Fraser.

(b)

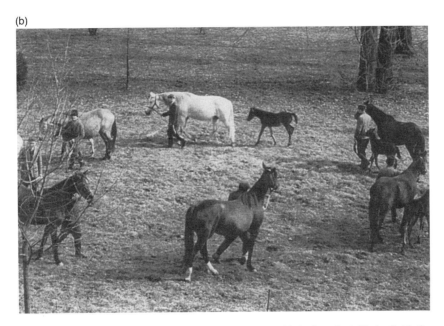

Fig. 7.10. *Continued.* (b) Exercising session for brood mares, some with foals at foot. Photo: S. Hlatky.

sweating. To control rapid heat loss, the horse can be draped with a light rug. No brushing should be started on a wet horse. As soon as the animal has been put into shelter and its tack is removed, it should have all of the moisture wiped off with a sweat-scraper. The scraper should take off as much surface moisture as possible, and for this reason the scraper should be taken over fleshy areas very firmly and repeatedly with slow downward actions. The scraper should, of course, be taken carefully over bony parts.

After the removal of moisture, rubbing down with thick wisp hay can dry off the coat of the horse further. The wisps are quickly discarded and replaced as this phase of drying progresses. The wisping phase can be sustained for 10–15 min. At the end of this time an armful of clean dry straw can be spread over the horse's body. A rug is then placed over this and secured with a surcingle. Drying will continue with the help of air circulation throughout the straw. The rug or blanket prevents cooling from being too rapid.

8 Spatial Factors

As a very large, energetic animal, the horse clearly uses space. As a grazer with a great hunger, it also has a natural lifestyle for feeding far and wide. Its daily energy output is balanced with rest, including sleep. An inherent scheme that combines two features, namely extravagant movement and self conservation, seems to be set in the horse's animal psyche. One feature requires territorial space while the other uses private or individual space. The composite scheme can basically be retained in the stable by day release of the horse into adequate outdoor space, on one hand, and provision of a freshly bedded box or stall at night, on the other hand.

Particularly in groups of horses, phases of spontaneous activity are counterbalanced with other and longer phases of lounging. The two are not usually connected by time, but they have their places in the diurnal time budget of healthy horses in spatial freedom. They give the animal routine episodes of exertion and lounging. These opposite habits, so commonly exhibited, reveal a marked dynamic bipolarity in the amplitude of equine behaviour. Positive action and negative inaction exist together as extreme contrasts in the manifold equine ethos. Figuratively, the equine performance of sharp, space-using activity is like a response to a green light for 'go', and the spells of lounging are due to a red light for 'stop'. This characteristic of bipolarity in their normal spontaneous dynamics is very equine. Displays of spontaneous activity are best seen in free-ranging groups of horses and more frequently among young animals in play. Available space evidently assists the motivation for such activity (Colgan, 1989).

Territoriality

Expressions of activity require a degree of space, particularly territory with which the animal is familiar. Horses soon acquire familiarity with allocated territory. Familiar territory is quickly adopted as the home base. Horses use eliminating behaviour to a large extent in defining their territory, and the home range becomes marked and mapped out by deposits of excreta. Three forms of territory can be recognized, according to usage:

- **Home range.** This is the area the horse, or horse group, habitually occupies and patrols. The horse acquires a close territorial bond with the home range. In some cases the home range may be the animal's total range, such as a pasture. An adequate home range would meet all spatial needs. Within it there will be other forms of actual territory. They exist where outdoor conditions are optimal.
- **Core area.** This usually becomes established within a home range. In an extensive area of pasture, one phase may become an area of regular use in idling, sheltering and sleeping, but not eating. The area becomes denuded of any grass that might have grown there previously. It is often located at a look-out point, a gateway, or by a clump of trees (see Fig. 8.1).
- **Basal territory.** This is the area a horse, or a group, uses regularly as the principal grazing area within a home range. A basal territory would be adequate to meet the needs of its occupants in feeding, watering and exercise. It would also provide shade in ideal circumstances.

Territorialism is a major determinant of agonistic behaviour, fight-or-flight responses, threat displays and herding behaviour. Territoriality entails proprietary behaviour in respect of all parts of the home range. The defence of this is directed primarily against members of the same species. In territorial aggression, horses fight with their own typical offensive and defensive means. They bite, kick out with their hind feet and strike with their forefeet. Both hind feet may be kicked out, for example after backing up to the intruder. This double kick is delivered directly to the rear without aim. Kicking out defensively, with one hindlimb, is sometimes used with more accuracy.

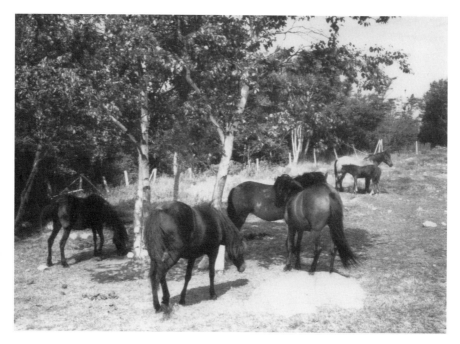

Fig. 8.1. Group idling in core area. Note that individual spacing is preserved. Photo: A.F. Fraser.

In order to minimize aggressive events among grouped horses, more extensive territories are best provided. Horses, like other livestock, react with set distances, e.g. the flight distance, the individual and 'critical' distance. When the periphery of these invisibly outlined areas is breached by an approaching individual, the distance between the animal and the advancing subject becomes so reduced that the approached animal must react. In the case of the 'critical distance', the animal will be more likely to attack than take flight. Individual distances are the finite areas of self-occupation preserved for purely social manoeuvres. These distances vary according to the typical reactivity of the animal, resulting from its inherent temperament, its experience, domesticated training, competition, housing and feeding (McDonnell, 1999).

Differences are recognized between horse breeds and types in regard to aggressiveness and speed of fight reaction when their space is invaded. Horses of oriental blood, i.e. hot- and warm-blooded horses, such as Arabs and Thoroughbreds, are more reactive than cold-blooded horses, such as draught breeds. Mares with young foals are particularly reactive to the approach of strange individuals into their infants' space.

Territorial exploration features in equine behaviour; horses will explore any new field they are put in and pay more initial attention to the field boundaries. They are likely to follow the boundary before exploring the interior of their enclosure. In small pastures that permit overall vision, a group disperses quickly and adopts the extensive spacing characteristics of grazing. In very large pastures, several days or weeks may elapse before each part of it has been explored by all the horses within it. Prior experience of similar terrain influences horses to explore extensively, while poor exploration is likely to be shown if they have not had previous experience of a similar environment. Horses raised on mountainous land and on ranges explore very actively if moved to different types of environments, such as fenced pastures.

One of the main features of exploratory behaviour in the horse is that it occurs only as long as the emotions of fear or apprehension are not present. The animal's curiosity is normally aroused when it sees an unfamiliar object or hears an unknown noise, but what may induce exploratory behaviour in one animal may very often be ignored by another. Such behaviour feeds their powers of learning (Forkman, 2002) and cognition (Roberts,

2000). Older animals, being more acquainted with the objects and sounds of their environment, are less curious than young animals. When curiosity is first aroused, the animal approaches with nostrils quivering and sniffing. The size and nature of the object in which the animal has become interested determines the speed of approach.

A great deal of exploratory behaviour is shown by very young and maturing individuals. This behaviour is directed towards the pasture, the ground and their boundaries, and other objects in the environment within its reach. In the course of this exploratory activity the foal may nibble and mouth unfamiliar objects. Within herds, very young foals learn the identities of their own mothers with the aid of trial-and-error exploration. Social relationships and hierarchies in all equine groups have been determined essentially through empirical activity. The support for such empirical behaviour is basically the motivation to explore. While this stems principally from associative and perceptive needs (Treves, 2000), it is also generated by other, even less tangible needs, such as determination of status (see Fig. 8.2).

Of clinical significance is the fact that exploratory behaviour becomes totally suppressed in many illnesses. Curiosity is a very healthy sign. The exploratory system in horse behaviour can be outlined simply as an organization of cycles of activities as follows:

1. A need in the animal for the perception of environmental factors that will feed its aroused senses.
2. Exploratory acts between the animal and its environment.
3. The receipt of sensory feedback from the environment to satisfy the original need.
4. The return of the cycle to a basal level of readiness with the lodgement of the prior events in either short-term or long-term memory (Fraser and Broom, 1990).

Spatiality

Horses have spatial needs and spatial factors influence their many activities. The horse's use of space meets its chief physical and behavioural needs (Mark and Whitney, 2003). Basic spacing for these animals falls into two general types:

- **Individual space.** Horses preserve private space through their behaviour. It includes the physical space that the animal requires for its basic movements of lying, rising, standing, stretching

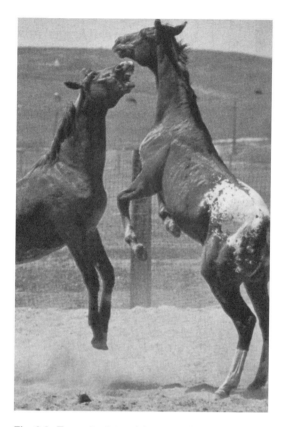

Fig. 8.2. Two colts determining status in their territorial space. Photo: V. Landell.

and scratching. This space is somewhat expanded in the head region in a radius of about a metre, for movement of the head in the course of ingestion, grooming, gesturing, looking-out and self-defence. This space is not maintained between foal and dam, between bonded pairs or between mutual groomers. Bonded pairs keep in close contact (see Fig. 8.3).

- **Social space.** This is additional to individual space. It is the minimal distance that a horse routinely keeps between itself and other horses that are not of 'preferred associate' status. Each horse in a group often has one associate and this animal is often contiguous or a very close neighbour. The second-nearest neighbour would be at a social distance of several metres during non-social activities, such as grazing. Social spacing is frequently altered. Should a group of horses include breeding females and a stallion, social arrangements can be disrupted (see Fig. 8.4).

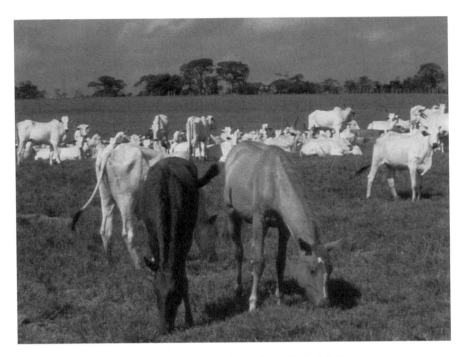

Fig. 8.3. A bonded pair sharing individual space in extensive territory. Photo: A.F. Fraser.

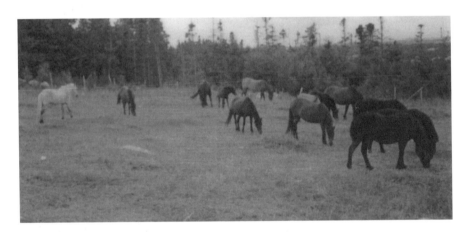

Fig. 8.4. A herd of horses held as one unit by a guarding stallion. Note: The grey stallion is closing in on a straggler. Photo: A.F. Fraser.

In any herd of horses, even those gathered together for a breeding or grazing season, the preservation of territorial space, as well as individual space, is important in the establishment of stability in social order. In particular, it is involved in acquiring preferential access to food, shelter, resting areas and close associates. In equine territorialism in general, many forms of space become integrated so as to provide a mixture of circumstances involving fairly continuous mediation of spatial needs such as defence of personal space and spatial surrender. Aggressive activities are common in equine territorialism in the form of biting and kicking. Territoriality can be seen to motivate aggression for defensive purposes to ensure access to physical provisions and to preserve bodily defence. Maintenance of territories by aggressive behaviour has been widely noted in various groups of free-living horses. Ways of territoriality are evidently fixed in equine behaviour; for example, they require abundant space for their natural excretory habits (Odberg and Francis-Smith, 1977).

1. Individual space. This exists as portable hoops of space seemingly carried about with the individual horse. An outer hoop meets the need for defence and territorial possession. An inner one is for individual protection. Both are important for social spacing within a group.

2. Actual territory. The given environment for the utilized horse is usually fixed by a physical boundary. This is its actual space for behavioural purposes. Such allocated space is used to meet various needs. In spatial behaviour, fairly precise rules of conduct determine the tenure of space and dominance privileges within it (Houpt, 1991). It is a determinant of resource use.

Spatial organizations are subject to dynamic change since individual horses adjust their close relationships continually. As a 'contact' species, horses allow very close physical proximity between each other, except in special circumstances related to sexual, maternal and aggressive behaviour. The distance they maintain between themselves and any potential foe is termed 'flight distance'. This, for example, is the space within which the horse may not remain if there is an approach by an unfamiliar person. The flight distance shortens with good husbandry and socialization. In socialized horses it may disappear, but most horses retain some flight distance. A more appropriate term would be the 'avoidance zone' for the majority of horses in common use that have a shy disposition.

Neighbour space

It is sometimes difficult to identify individual and social distances because it is not possible to know when they are affected by other factors. The individual distance in crowded areas may be simply inter-animal distance, and 'distance from nearest neighbour' on the periphery of grazing groups may indicate 'social distance', which is the radius of social space. A special type of spacing behaviour results when individuals with close bonds arrange themselves so that they establish a close 'distance to nearest neighbour'. Domestic horses, when grazing, maintain close contact with one and possibly more individuals, but the distance to the nearest neighbour varies much less than distances to other individuals in the group, for example the second-nearest neighbour. This gives a spatial structure of pairs of individuals within a group; the spatial relationship with a 'preferred associate' is stronger than any other type because the arrangement is basically friendship pairing. The distance to second-nearest neighbour can vary considerably, whereas the nearest-neighbour distance varies much less and sometimes may not be measurable owing to the physical proximity of the pair. In spite of the tendency to preserve space, a working group of horses can become preferred associates collectively. They can work closely in teams, very comfortably with each other (Fig. 8.5).

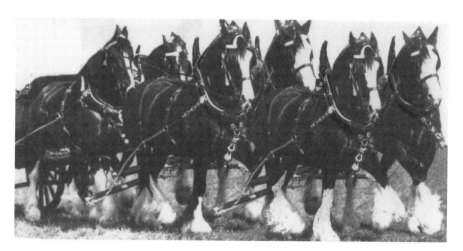

Fig. 8.5. A six-horse hitch of Clydesdales. Photo: W. Taylor.

Free-range space

In various parts of the world, indigenous or local ponies live in a state of comparative freedom. In some places the freedom is seasonal. In other places ponies live perennially in a wild state. In the free-living state they behave as naturally as if they were wildlife (Budiansky, 1997).

When ponies are free-living in a group and the group moves from place to place throughout its territory, it is usual for the same horses to lead the way each time, while others always follow at the back of the group. Remarkable consistency occurs in the way some assume full leadership and others assume the role of followers. A phenomenon in the behaviour of ponies free-ranging in a group is the emergence of subgroups that elect to occupy separate areas of a common territory (see Fig. 8.6).

Although they have preferred places, ponies have an urge to move from place to place. This urge becomes very evident when they are enclosed within a very limited territory. Ponies grazing on moorland areas have home ranges that are often shared or overlap considerably. Summer and winter ranges may overlap or be separate, but in general, different areas are used at varying intensities, according to the time of year and their ecological value to the animals.

Spatial Need

Space requirements were formerly viewed as those sufficient to contain the animal. Now it has been recognized that horses have a need for space, not only for containment but also to practise the social and maintenance patterns of behaviour embedded in their nature. This fact permits the recognition of three space provisions to meet the welfare standards of modern horse husbandry:

1. Primary space. This is the space needed for the physical containment and comfort of an individual animal. A horse stall of appropriate dimensions represents this space.

2. Secondary space. This is supplementary space that periodically allows the animal a change of direction, position or location. Secondary space also allows foaling or permits an appropriate companion to be accommodated. A large loose box represents this space.

3. Tertiary space. This is effectively free-range space. It would meet the cumulative needs of several individuals in a group. Where communal space is utilized for additional locomotion, it is evident that this potential space diminishes with increasing numbers, leading to crowding beyond welfare standards, e.g. in horse feedlots.

Welfare Addendum on Spacing

The outdoor custody of a horse calls for adequate standards of environmental welfare. When the horse is kept outdoors, its coat should be left in a 'natural' condition, although gross soiling should be removed promptly. Proper rotation of grazing areas is necessary, and sufficient land should be available to avoid

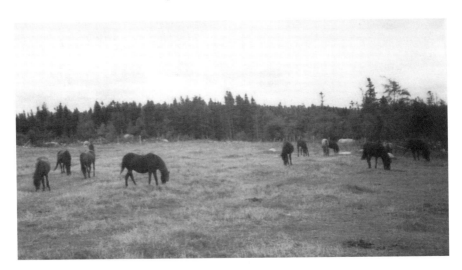

Fig. 8.6. Two subgroups in the same territory. Photo: A.F. Fraser.

overgrazing and the attendant risk of internal parasitism. Horses grazing on limited land should be wormed several times in the grazing season, perhaps monthly in some cases. To prevent clinical parasitism, a broad-spectrum anthelmintic programme can be instituted with veterinary direction. For their socio-behavioural need, horses require company, and an area for grazing or exercising sufficient for two horses is the minimal necessary outdoor space.

Horses grazing outdoors should have access to good shelter. Sometimes, good natural shelter, such as a wood, will be adequate. It is a humane and ethical obligation to provide a field shelter with an open doorway, hay rack, hay store, sound roof and dry floor. Many horses make strategic uses of such shelters without always going inside them; these shelters can also serve as windbreaks (see Fig. 8.7). The ground in a horse paddock should also be checked over regularly for any foreign items that need to be removed.

A horse is quickly chilled when exposed to cold, precipitation and high winds simultaneously. Chilled horses can lose weight rapidly and can become clinically ill from various conditions, including the possibility of carrying such conditions subclinically prior to the chilling episode. Cold, by itself, will not chill a horse with a natural coat. The additional components of wetness and/or air speed are needed for severe chilling.

Proper fencing is needed to contain grazing horses; electric fences, for example, are suitable (see Fig. 8.8). Barbed wire, however, should never be used for the purpose. Broad livestock netting about 1.5 m (5 ft) high can be used, as can wooden rails. Fence posts should be strong and properly sunk into holes 0.75 m (2.5 ft) deep, which are then fully filled with stone or concrete. Horses rub themselves against posts and fences using much of their full weight, and therefore only a well-built fence can tolerate this usage. The perimeter fence should frequently be checked out for weakness or breakage. Horses at pasture near an urban area will attract attention and visitors (see Fig. 8.9). The latter are capable of damaging fences and feeding horses inappropriately. Warnings should be signposted for visitors to be discouraged from inappropriate actions.

All housing for horses must be well ventilated, illuminated, rain- and draught-proof, equipped with fire extinguishers and well serviced with power, water and drainage. It should be sited appropriately and have good access and egress. As far as possible, it should have privacy and freedom from extraneous noise.

A stable should provide at least 350 m^3 (800 ft^3) of air space per horse. Natural light should be admitted by windows in the stable, about 1.5 m^2 (5 ft^2) per horse. Windows are best behind the horse's stall. The space for a horse kept nightly in a stable stall should allow the animal room to step forward or back, extend its head and neck, turn its head to its flank and, most importantly, to lie flat on its side. Horse stalls should be at least 1.5 m (5 ft) wide and 2.75 m (9 ft) long. To provide good-quality space, loose boxes are preferred to stalls. Closed box stalls should be about 68 m^2 (225 ft^2) or more. Two horses may be kept together if socially compatible. Stables should be rodent-free.

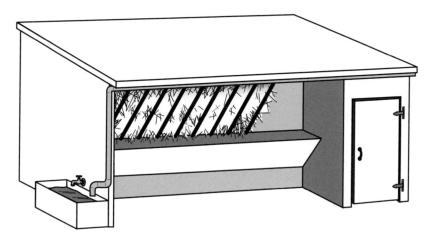

Fig. 8.7. Outdoor shelter and feeding station. Drawing by Stefanie Smith.

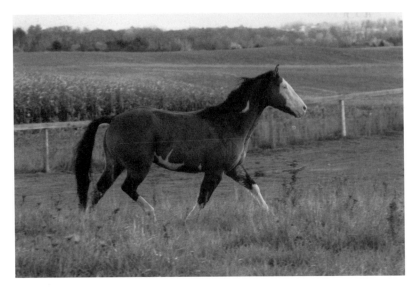

Fig. 8.8. Casual investigative canter around edge of a new pasture after release. Note: Good perimeter fence. Photo: Melanie MacDonald.

Horses should be fed in mangers, but these can be arranged to suit the situation. A high rack for hay is desirable, but a deep manger for hay is also useful. A separate grain box can be fitted in a corner by the manger or as part of it. Mangers should be about 1–1.5 m (3.5–4.5 ft) high, depending on whether they are for small or large horses. In the case of stalls, the passage behind the horse should be about 1.8–2.1 m (6–7 ft) wide. There should be no deep gutter. The gutter, from one end of the stable to the other, should slope about 2.5 cm/15 m (1 in/50 ft) and be suitable for shovelling.

(a)

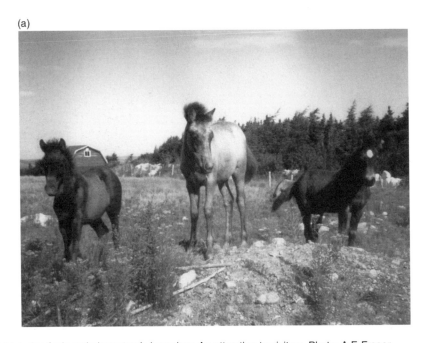

Fig. 8.9. (a) Maturing foals at their pasture's boundary. An attraction to visitors. Photo: A.F. Fraser.

(b)

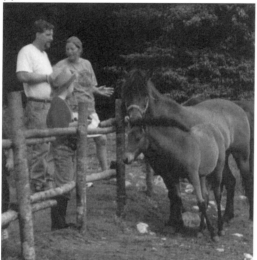

Fig. 8.9. *Continued.* (b) Ponies attracting attention. Photo: Anonymous.

To prevent fighting between neighbours, stall partitions should be of solid board and be 1.5 m (5 ft) high behind and 2.1 m (7 ft) high in front. If the stable is floored with concrete, the floor of the stalls should be covered by horse matting. The passageways should have a rough surface to prevent slipping. Doorways leading to the outside from the passageway should be at least 1.5 m (5 ft) wide.

Straw is the best bedding and should be liberally supplied. Depending on local availability, other forms of bedding can be used, including peat moss litter, wood shavings, sawdust or even shredded paper. A small drain in the centre of a stall can be helpful for male horses, but this can be difficult to service and keep unclogged. Drainage away from a stable should be enclosed and efficient. Manure heaps should be at a considerable distance from the building and enclosed by fencing.

Old stables should be given periodic renovation to maintain standards of space, hygiene and good order. At such times, repairs to surfaces can be done and drain traps and gutters cleaned out and disinfected. No paint should be applied to any surface where a horse can chew or lick. There should be no projections within stables that horses might encounter. Wheelbarrows should never be left in any section of the stable where horses are kept.

It is a common maxim that charity begins at home. Similarly it can be axiomatic that welfare for the horse begins in the stable. Indoor space is where the majority of horses spend most of their lives. Even outdoors they need space and company (see Fig. 8.10). This fact has long been common knowledge among earlier societies of horse-using people (Lawrence, 1998).

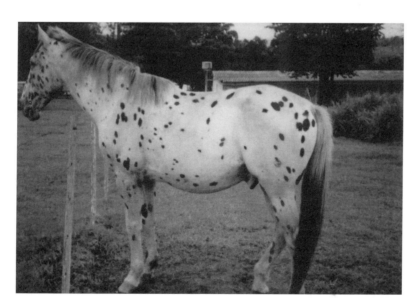

Fig. 8.10. Fenced in and alone. Photo: A.F. Fraser.

9 Rest, Work and Transportation

Introduction

The activities of the horse's body wax and wane throughout the animal's life. As the animal ages, its physical construction deteriorates and its dynamism diminishes. Most notably, in its very old age, a horse's main activity is eating. Responses become slow, and the fast gait may be used only when it is imperative to do so.

The fit horse has a kinetic drive that prevails throughout its life until old age. Under domesticated control the opportunity for gross action is often limited. A schedule of daily exercise must therefore be provided to enclosed or stabled horses. The given schedule may not always coincide with the horse's urge for movement, and brisk activity may need to be generated by compulsory methods in the exercise period. Conventional forms of work can give a horse its exercise. Rest, including sleep, naturally counterbalances the activity of imposed work or general self-maintenance behaviourally. For the deepest sleep, the horse must lie down. While most will lie down in a stable, they lie down best when they are outdoors. This is a key factor in coping with the stresses of work (Forkman et al., 2001).

Rest can be taken in its simplest form of inactivity when the horse is well fed. When free from ingestive work, the animal can lounge and drowse on its feet. A master clocking system evidently exists in the brain with clues from the environment. By this means, diurnal rhythms of rest and sleep are scheduled. True sleep exists in two main forms:

- **Brain sleep.** This is a quiet state with slow brainwaves. This state is called slow-wave sleep (SWS). In this sleep the horse is capable of remaining upright with some support from the 'stay apparatus' of the fore- and hindlimbs and from the firm structure of the 'reciprocal apparatus' in the hindlimbs.
- **Body sleep.** This is a very deep sleep, in which the brainwaves paradoxically resemble normal wakefulness. From time to time in this state, the animal may move its eyeballs rapidly, and this movement can be noticed under the closed eyelids. Such rapid eye movement is characteristic of this form of sleep. For this reason it is technically referred to as REM sleep. Additionally, it is also called paradoxical sleep. Because there is profound bodily relaxation in REM sleep, it can only develop when the horse is lying down. Through a 'group effect', several horses often lie asleep at the same time outdoors, while one remains standing awake nearby.

Foals sleep much more than their mothers and they have a good amount of sleep in REM form. Mares remain close to their foals at this time. Periods of sleep in adults are usually short. They are punctuated by arousal that is stimulated by the upper brainstem. The reticular formation of the upper brainstem is the pacemaker for the sleep–wake cycle. In effect, this is a biological clock.

Horses are awake and alert for about 80% of daylight time. Most of them will sleep or drowse on two or more occasions during daylight. During the night hours, horses typically drowse or sleep in several short periods, adding up to about one-third of the night. Periods of REM sleep at this time may only last for about 5 min per session. Lounging occurs during daylight or night and is a state of wakeful rest.

Horses may not sleep for 2 or 3 days in a row in new quarters. Sleep deprivation can be a problem for any horse subjected to changes in its accommodations or given inadequate stable space, or transported over long distances. Even if it is quite well cared for in all other respects, it is not humane to deprive a horse of a sleeping facility (Coumbe, 2001).

Rest and Sleep

Horses employ episodes of inactivity to punctuate energy-consuming activities and so cause resting behavioural phases and rhythms. Inactive behaviour is very functional as a tactic of temporal organization and self-conservation. In their simplest forms, self-conserving tactics include drowsing, ad hoc resting and short-term inactivity.

In the horse's inactive behaviour, various forms are observed. In this variation, some similarities occur with other species and some species-specific characteristics also occur. The horse exhibits both forms of deep sleep, namely SWS and paradoxical sleep, in which there is REM. Deep sleep is much more obvious in the horse in a natural state: outdoors. In familiar outdoor territory, horses are most well adapted to their environment. All forms of rest and inactivity, such as idling and sleep, flourish as one behavioural phenomenon. Melatonin seems to be the hormone of sleep. It is produced in the pineal gland and is present in higher quantities in plasma at night. Melatonin levels appear to be the link between the photoperiod and diurnal cycles of sleep and inactivity. Day length influences the relative amounts of body serotonin, a precursor to melatonin, and melatonin present in the pineal gland. These influence the organism's resting behaviour. The build-up of serotonin may induce drowsiness and sleep. Clinically, tryptophan, a precursor of serotonin, may be used to induce sleep.

Resting and sleeping are forms of physical conservation, which may occupy about a third of a horse's life. Since activity tends to have fixed diurnal patterns, it is found that episodes of inactivity, which permit rest and sleep, have equivalent patterns. The nature of sleep in horses has been clearly documented, showing that both SWS and paradoxical (or REM) sleep regularly occur. These two forms of deep sleep have been likened to sleep of the mind and sleep of the body, respectively. Drowsing is another notable resting method. All forms of rest represent a major need in equine self-maintenance and well-being (Hickman, 1987).

Patterns

Management practices can affect equine sleep patterns. When moved from stable to pasture, horses do not usually lie down during the first night, and total sleep time remains low for a month. If horses are tied too short in a stall so that they cannot lie down, they will not have REM sleep. Horses stabled only at night may or may not sleep during the day. Care must be taken not to deprive horses of sleep, as can occur when they are transported long distances and must be tied short in stalls for support. Diet also affects rest time in horses. For example, if oats are substituted for hay, total recumbency time increases.

Horses are polyphasic animals with regards to sleep and rest periods: 95% of horses have two or more such periods per day. The total length of time spent recumbent per day is approximately 2.5 h, with time variations associated with age and management. Twice as much time is spent in sternal recumbency as is spent in lateral recumbency, and normal adult horses rarely spend more than 30 min continuously in lateral recumbency; the mean time spent continuously in this position is 23 min. The adult horse normally rests slightly on one side of its chest, with one foreleg and one hind leg underneath the body.

During the day the horse is fully awake about 80% of the time. At night the horse is awake 60% of the time, but drowses for 20% of the night, in several separate periods. Stabled horses are recumbent for 2 h/day, in four or five periods, while ponies are recumbent for 5 h/day. SWS occupies 2 h/day and REM sleep occurs in about nine periods of 5 min duration. Many horses accumulate 6–7 h of rest during each 24-h period. Some of this sleep is accumulated during the hours of daylight and is largely achieved in the standing position. Typically, periods of sleep are short and irregularly spaced with rest.

Lying, Rising and Standing

Horses rise and lie down in specific ways. In descent the forelegs are flexed first, then all four limbs. The head and neck are used for balance as the animal lowers itself. All the legs are gathered together under the body, the knees and hocks are bent and the chest and forequarters make contact with the ground before the hindquarters.

Adult horses do not lie for very long periods. Mares with young foals tend to lie longer than usual when the foal is nearby and sleeping in full lateral recumbency. Mature horses are unable to lie in this flat-out posture for long periods of time before their respiratory functions become impaired. The full weight on the thorax of the horse, when laid flat, appears to be such that circulation to the lungs becomes inefficient after about 15 min. This is not the case among foals and young horses, however, and these subjects can be seen to spend many hours in the day sleeping socially on their sides at full stretch.

Young horses, and foals in particular, lie in sleep more than older ones (see Fig. 9.1). In particular, they spend a larger fraction of their time in REM sleep (for which recumbency is needed). The time spent in REM and total sleeping time vary among adults, but are relatively stable for any one individual. Lost REM time disturbs animals, and there is some reason to believe that REM sleep is important in some specific way. It seems that brain tissue in the REM state performs some essential function for which it has little or no opportunity in either the waking or the SWS state. Perhaps in the REM state the memory traces required for long-term storage of memory are being consolidated. Certainly learning can be hindered by depriving an animal of lying in REM sleep. In the REM state the forebrain is aroused, although disconnected from the lower CNS. Disconnection implies that sensory stimuli are less readily registered and that motor commands are not reaching lower motor circuits, as shown by decreased muscle tone. The brief movements frequently made in REM sleep are considered to originate from the brainstem. The disconnection does not permit sufficient motor control to hold the animal upright.

In lateral recumbency the upper limb is invariably anterior to the lower forelimb, which is usually flexed. The hindlimbs are usually extended, with the upper limb slightly posterior to the lower limb. In sternal recumbency, horses do not lie symmetrically. Their hindquarters are rotated, with the lateral surface of the bottom limb on the ground. A horse seldom remains lying when approached; a standing horse is better able to flee. To rise, the horse extends the upper foreleg. The forequarters are raised so that the lower foreleg can also be extended. At the same time both hindlimbs begin to extend. The main thrust of rising comes from the hindlimbs.

Standing and Resting

Horses may be able to drowse and even engage in SWS while standing, by means of the unique stay apparatus of the equine hindlimbs. Uniquely in the horse, the action of the hock is linked to the action of the stifle joint above it. Both joints work in harmony, as the result of a special arrangement in the equine hind leg, called 'the reciprocal apparatus'. When either the stifle or the hock flexes or extends, the other joint reciprocates with similar action. The reciprocal apparatus consists of two long muscular bands running down the front and the back of the hindlimb. One extends from a point above the stifle to a point below the hock at the front. The other extends from the back of the thigh bone to the point of the hock joint. Although these bands are muscles, they are composed mostly of tough fibrous tissue and serve largely as pulleys down the front and back of the leg, enclosing both stifle and hock joints in a fibrous parallelogram in which both joints are forced to move in unison because they are tied in to their reciprocal apparatus. When the stifle extends, the hock extends, and when the stifle flexes, the hock also flexes. In other words, both joints must extend and flex at the same time. Thus, if the stifle is fixed in unison, the leg distal to the stifle will bear the weight of the horse with little additional muscular effort.

A major benefit of the reciprocal apparatus to the horse is the ability of this mechanism to become fixed during upright rest. If the stifle joint is tightly held in extension, the hock is effortlessly fixed; the hind legs are then secured to support the posterior weight of the stationary horse with little effort. Further down the leg there is an associated assembly of flexible, fibrous, elastic ligaments that support the fetlock and the other foot joints. This supportive apparatus of the foot allows the fetlock to 'stay' or remain bent, without the foot becoming overextended or overstretched as it takes weight. The 'stay apparatus' goes down into the hoof and is present on both fore- and hind feet. It assists the horse in upright forms of resting, including light sleep.

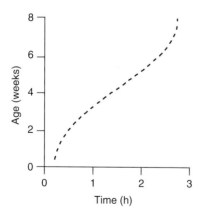

Fig. 9.1. Increasing durations of sleep periods commonly occurring in young foals.

The depth of sleep is estimated in terms of the intensity of stimulation, usually of a sound stimulus, required to awaken the sleeping animal. Light sleep is more common than deep sleep in horses. REM sleep occurs in all mammals, but not all the manifestations of REM sleep are exactly alike in all species. Animals are more difficult to arouse from REM than from other sleep states. Heartbeat and breathing tend to be more irregular and on average faster during REM than during non-REM sleep. Even though phasic movements are common, postural muscle tone diminishes, especially in the muscles of the trunk, neck and shoulder. As a result of this, the subject is unable to hold the head up in REM sleep. These multiple changes in cerebral and somatic functions show that REM sleep is in some fundamental way different from the other sleep stages. The chief effect in the horse is that an upright standing position cannot be employed in REM sleep, although it is possible in SWS.

Lounging and Drowsing

Although it is unusual to see all the members of a group of horses lying down at one time, they often rest simultaneously. The element of social facilitation, or group effect, is clearly a major factor operating in resting behaviour in most groups of horses. When they lie down together, they appear to surrender readily their individual, portable space during rest. Inactive behaviour, which excludes sleep, is very evident in the daily time budget of the horse. In the examination of inactive behaviour, various forms are seen in practice. In this variation, some similarities are seen with other species but some purely equine characteristics also occur.

Drowsing

A state of somnolence that is intermediate between wakefulness and SWS is drowsing. It is a definite state and one that the standing horse can frequently employ during periods of inactivity in the daytime and at night. Most horses accumulate about 2–3 h of drowsing per 24 h in phases of only a few minutes' duration (see Fig. 9.2). The horse switches quickly in and out of its short drowsing spells in a lounging phase (Ruckebusch, 1972). Table 9.1 illustrates various forms of resting behaviour.

Support apparatus

The equine hoof is extremely suitable for standing still on almost any surface. The horse's legs have special supporting structures well designed for stance. In the lower limb are arrangements of tendons and ligaments forming strong yet flexible supports. These help the horse to hold a stance for long periods without great effort. All four legs have the 'stay apparatus', which is mostly ligament. This apparatus supports the fetlocks. The forelegs also have a 'check' ligament for support.

The hind legs have a very unique supporting structure called the 'reciprocal apparatus'. It is both muscular and tendinous. Stretching on two sides from above the stifle to below the hock as a singular structure, this apparatus causes these two joints to flex or extend together in unison. For example, if the stifle is held extended, the lower leg will be fixed in position to support the horse without further muscular effort. Usually only one or the other limb has the reciprocal apparatus in operation for support at a given time. While one hindlimb is fixed for support, the other can be relaxed. By means of this apparatus, a horse is able to drowse or have SWS in a comfortable standing posture.

Lounging in the standing position is obviously less physiologically conservative than rest in a lying position. Sternal recumbency takes the weight off the horse's feet, limbs and their supportive musculature. Lateral sleep is comprehensively restful, additionally taking the weight off the head and neck. The neck functions in all other positions, and at all other times, as a large, mobile cantilever. Lounging serves behaviourally as the negative pole of the horse's characteristic dynamic bipolarity, vigorous pulling or running being the opposite pole in the equine character. Lounging is valuable in equine behaviour.

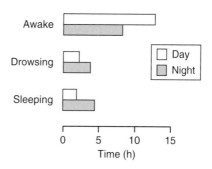

Fig. 9.2. Diurnal amounts of three states of consciousness in horses.

Table 9.1. Forms of resting behaviour in horses.

Term	Behavioural forms
Idling	Stationary standing for an extended time period with some limited limb-shifting and positional changing. The horse may be using available time free of active maintenance requirements. Idling may simply take the form of passively waiting for the next phase of an established husbandry routine, such as work.
Drowsing	A dormant state in which there are signs of light sleep with head movement and eye closure. The horse maintains this inactive state in one of certain variable postures. The horse usually has an upright stance. One hindlimb may be relaxed. Sitting on the sternum is another postural form of drowsing.
Resting	Rest is variously taken in a standing or recumbent posture with evident wakefulness. Rest in recumbency is seldom lateral. The forelegs are flexed with one beneath the thorax; the spinal column is held in a slight arc, in which the head may be held.
Sleeping	Sleep is seen as evident deep somnolence in extended recumbency. The usual sleep position is flat on the side with legs extended. True sleep occurs in the form of both 'brain sleep' and 'paradoxical sleep'. In the latter, rapid eye movement (REM) can be seen below the closed lids. Minor leg movements also occur, especially of the feet.

It is a tactic to manage the constant demand of bearing a heavy frame and trunk, and is periodically activated spontaneously or on demand.

In the typical lounging posture, the horse is stationary; the neck is extended; the head is slightly bowed; the eyes are open; the forelegs are vertical; and the front hooves are placed exactly beside each other. One hind leg is set back slightly and is weight-bearing, while the other is flexed; its foot is advanced and the toe of this hoof is in contact with the ground. The hindlimbs alternate in their arrangements, but the forelegs remain parallel to each other during the lounging period. In pairs or groups of horses, lounging is often performed simultaneously through social facilitation. Lounging sometimes leads into drowsing, which is a light sleep.

Drowsiness or somnolence may be defined as an intermediary state between wakefulness and SWS, characterized by a small decrease in muscular tone and respiratory rates. It is a stable, wakeful state, which ends in an abrupt transition to either wakefulness or

SWS. During their respective circadian cycles, different species exhibit different amounts of drowsing. The ratio of drowsing to total wakefulness is smallest in the horse, both during the 24-h period (9.06%) and during the night (26.63%). Horses exhibit a large number of drowsing periods and also record short drowsing durations, averaging approximately 3.71 min. They spend approximately 85% of the 24-h period in wakefulness, lounging or drowsing (Table 9.2). An equilibrium seems to exist between these two states. In the horse the shift is towards wakefulness; the proportion of drowsing can be increased in a single individual when in a protected environment.

Welfare Addendum

Disinclination to lie at rest is seen in horses with orthopaedic conditions and in old age. The normal sleep and resting characteristics of animals should be appreciated for purposes of assessing welfare and so that abnormalities can be detected. A horse

Table 9.2. Estimated average times (in hours) spent per day by 76 outdoor horses in states of drowsing, sleep and wakefulness.

Period of day	State			
	Lounging	Drowsing	Deep sleep	Wakefulness
Daylight	1.3	1.1	0.4	9.6
Night	0.8	0.9	3.7	6.2
Total	2.1	2.0	4.1	15.8

lying down at night in a normal posture is probably asleep. An adult horse that lies down a lot during the day (unless in the company of its foal or resting in sunshine) may be abnormal and should be carefully observed for other evidence of illness.

Some clinical conditions cause disturbed patterns of resting and sleep in horses. Significant clinical signs include sleeping fitfully and rising from resting postures frequently. Management practices should interfere as little as possible with normal circadian patterns of resting behaviour. Interruption of activity cycles and loss of sleep may play an important role in the aetiology of the stress-related diseases associated with newborn management, livestock transport, mixing of strange animals and introducing new horses into established groups.

Contemporary Horse Work

Large numbers of draught horses no longer work in fields and on roads as they once did historically up to 70 or so years ago, but some horses still work in haulage (see Figs 9.3 and 9.4). In particular the horse carriage trade has become an adjunct to tourism in many cities internationally and involves horses in a version of draught work. This work can be very demanding on many horses, and the carriage trade has become a source of concern for equine welfare's proponents. This concern can be fully justified on account of the scope that there is for erroneous horse

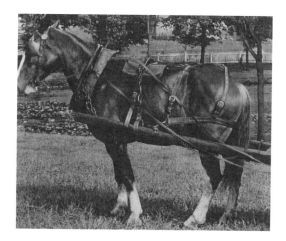

Fig. 9.4. Hard work in shafts. Photo: H. Hastie.

use in the course of the routine work involved. That most of this trade is carried out with few or no regulations relating to animal care is of further concern.

The sport of carriage driving and the various recreational activities that involve horses drawing wagons, carriages and carts are not comparable forms of horse work. In these activities the horses are not in continuing whole daily use and do not perform in city centres or among heavy traffic and exhaust fumes. Typically, the sport and recreational forms of horse vehicle haulage are done on natural surfaces in fields or parks under the supervision of stewards with high standards of horse use. These standards are largely respected. Such use does not represent a significant degree of work since the events are only occasional (see Fig. 9.5).

Horse riding, in recreation or sport, does not represent significant work, usually being within customary or imposed limits on times and distances. Common agreement determines that these are well within the ability of a fit riding horse. Nevertheless, any form of horse work, whether light or heavy, brief or chronic, monitored or private, requires welfare considerations to guard the animal's well-being. Some of these are contained within the welfare guidelines offered here for the carriage horse trade or for any horse in regular heavy work.

Carriage Horse Welfare

A most important component of a horse in carriage work is its characteristic behavioural nature, i.e. its basic temperament. As a part of its individuality every horse has a typical temperament, which is

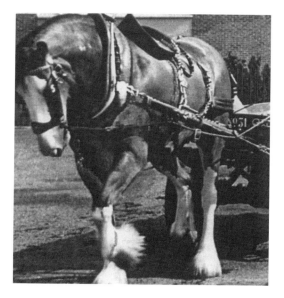

Fig. 9.3. Cold-blooded worker. Photo: H. Hastie.

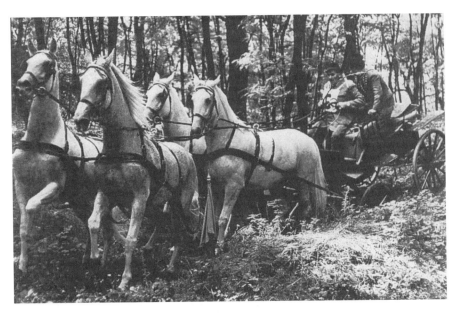

Fig. 9.5. Sport of cross-country carriage driving. Photo: S. Hlatky.

coexistent with the generic temperament of its breed or breed type. Allusion has been made to the contrasting forms of temperament usually featured in hot-blooded and cold-blood breeds, the racers and the haulers. The racers are quick to react and tend to react vigorously; they may react to slight stimuli and are somewhat defensive. The heavy-weight draught horse is essentially phlegmatic in its responsiveness. It normally has a stoic nature and reacts to its requirements with diffidence and easy compliance. Warm bloods, e.g. Standardbred, may lie between these extremes and could work in pairs (see Fig. 9.6a).

Knowledge of horse character makes it obvious that the basic features of racers and draught horses are different in terms of strength and temperament. In particular, they differ in suitability for draught work amid modern city conditions. It would be fair to add that there are no breeds of horse ideally suited to such work, but some are less suitable than others (see Fig. 9.6b).

In order to facilitate a horse's temperamental adjustment to busy street work, the animal should have a knowledgeable and sympathetic driver, whose voice and rein handling are familiar to the animal. Regular vocal reassurances should be given to the horse, particularly when it is in traffic. The horse's bond with its driver can be strengthened by being fed regularly by this person. When working with pairs, at least one should have a calm temperament and abundant experience.

The temperament and the physique of a horse are combined in the totality of its identity. No two horses are exactly alike in all respects. Apart from physical variations, horses have differences in patience and tolerance, which are facets of temperament. The comprehensive temperament of a horse becomes revealed in due course to anyone who has paid close attention to the animal for a while. While the temperament of a horse cannot be determined in a short assessment, its physical type can indicate its likely tolerance of city stressors.

Physique and feet

The carriage horse must be physically suited for this type of work. The horse needs the physical capacity to utilize leverage. Both forequarters and hindquarters perform this work; the forelegs perform much of the support work while the hind legs generate most of the propulsion. Leverage is essential in assisting the animal to alter its centre of gravity in moving a load, and height aids in leverage.

Of critical importance to a working horse are healthy feet and good shoeing. It is obvious that

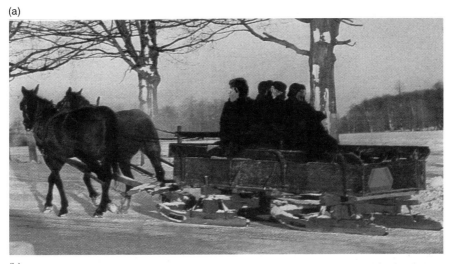

(a)

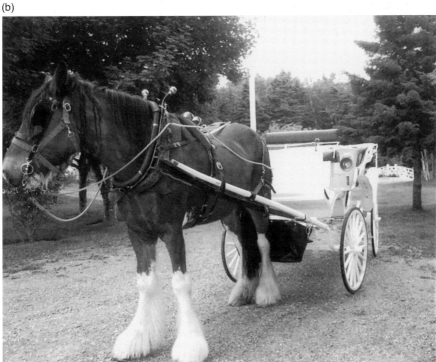

(b)

Fig. 9.6. (a) Sleigh-pulling by a pair of Standardbreds. Photo: C. Barker. (b) Carriage horse in suitable condition and of a suitable type (Clydesdale/Standardbred cross) in fitted harness. Photo: C. Halliday.

carriage horses need to be shod at all times of work and that their hooves need frequent and regular attention. The horny walls of the hoof grow continuously, but because of the slope of the hoof, it takes longer for the growing horn to reach the toe than the heel. It requires about 12 months for the horn to grow from its origin at the coronet down to ground level at the toe. This hoof growth rate indicates that trimming is regularly needed to have the hooves properly sloped.

Correct angulation between the ground, the foot and the leg depends on hoof trimming. In a forefoot the angle between the toe and the ground should be 45°. In the hind foot it should be 55°. A good stance and a sound manner of limb action require the normal hoof shapes to be maintained. Horses permanently involved in heavy traction are at great risk of developing navicular disease. The incorrect angulation of foot and pastern can be a predisposing factor. Circumstances leading to the pastern being overextended are a basic cause of the disease, which is essentially progressive degeneration of a sesamoid bone, called the navicular bone. This is a very small, boat-shaped bone at the back of the joint between the second and third phalanges. It lies just above the bulb of the heel and acts as a roller over which the deep flexor tendon passes (see Fig. 9.7). When the tendon flexes, it pressures the navicular. Excessive pressure cuts off the navicular's blood supply. Frequent recurrences of this cause degeneration of this bone, which then becomes a seat of

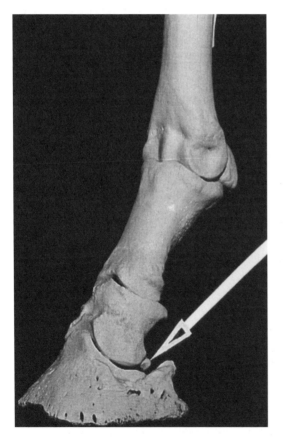

Fig. 9.7. Location of the navicular bone. Photo: A.F. Fraser.

pain. To relieve this pain, the horse at rest points the toe of the affected hoof on the ground, relaxing the ligament by flexing the pastern. Poor welfare, in the form of chronic ill use, is responsible.

Conditioning

A period of conditioning is essential to accustom the horse gradually to harness work before it is put to regular use. During winter it is common for idle horses to be fed only a maintenance diet. Any idle horse that is due to be given carriage use should be put on gradually increasing rations. Before the scheduled work the horse should receive extra exercise and the grain ration should be slowly built up to full work level. It is an important component of conditioning to have the horse harnessed on several occasions and fully exercised before real use.

A new horse would need to be given proper training and a full dress rehearsal: perhaps led by hand on the outward journey and driven on the homeward stage. During this test there would be opportunities to observe the animal's tolerance of civic stimuli and environmental stressors. Such tolerance is the key element in a horse's temperamental suitability for work in the tourist carriage trade in a city centre, which is such an unnatural location for any horse.

Short sessions of carriage-pulling in its own harness can be given to the horse while led by hand. This can build up until the horse is performing a half-day of light work, then a half-day of heavier work. For all of this conditioning to be complete, about 2 or 3 weeks would be required. An unfit horse, although otherwise healthy, should never be made to do a full day of work. As an aspect of fitness, the horse's skin must be progressively conditioned by harness contact.

Harness

When acquiring a new harness the horse in question should be properly measured for neck size, girth, weight, length and height. These and any other specific measurements that might be needed should be given to the manufacturer or supplier of the harness. A new harness may not be sufficiently supple for immediate use. It may need to be worked by hand for a while before it is suitable to be put on the horse. Even then, the application of the new harness should be done critically to ascertain any defects in the fitting. These would obviously need to be rectified before use (see Fig. 9.8). It should never be assumed that ill-fitting harnesses will duly adapt to the horse or that the horse will adapt to them in time.

All harnesses should fit the horse properly without any general friction or localized pressure points. The contact between horse and harness should be smooth or soft. Slight movement of a harness on the horse is inevitable and necessary but should be minimal. Security within the harness is essential for safety.

When using an old harness on a horse, there should be dress rehearsals and any ill-fitting feature should be rectified. Modifications to old harnesses should be completed before attempting to use them for work. Old leather should be de-greased and washed before applying it to the animal. The inner faces of collars and saddles that are not new must be in good condition; suitably sanitized and de-greased. When in use, all harnesses should be under continuous inspection. Straps can snap, fasteners can break and projections can develop – all in the course of wear and tear. The user cannot allow an impending weakness in the harness to create an accident. After removal, all harnesses should be made clean, especially the surfaces against the horse. Sweat and grease require immediate removal. All harnesses should then be hung up in their clean state.

Harness sores

When a horse has begun sweating freely in its harness, it should be stopped. The sweat should be wiped off as much as possible, from the neck, shoulder, back and sides, using a clean, dry towel. Sweat also accumulates beneath the collar and saddle, which should also be wiped. Movement of the saddle and harness over sweat can lead to sores. These can develop quickly and take a long time to heal. A few minutes of preventative care can save weeks of recovery from such saddle sores and collar chafing. A harness on top of sweat is a bad interface. Herein lies one of the great vulnerabilities of this animal during summertime work. Saddle galls are formed from uneven pressure of the saddle or back pad. In addition, girth galls can develop behind the elbow from badly fastened girths, when, for example, a fold of skin has been caught underneath the girth. When first formed, harness sores are reddened, moist, painful abrasions on the skin. They can later develop into ulcers.

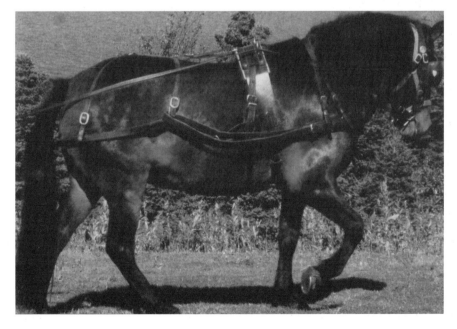

Fig. 9.8. Horse in new harness/horse strappings for carriage work. Photo: R. Butler.

Sweating

It is an important fact that no other animal can sweat as liberally as the horse. Working in heat, horses readily lose body salts (electrolytes) and become dehydrated from sweat loss. The fluid loss in sweating can be up to 15 l/day. Electrolytes, especially potassium and sodium chloride, are drained from the horse's body in the outpouring of sweat from work and heat. With the necessary increase in the daily intake of water goes the need for an intake of electrolytes to prevent excessive water loss, to maintain the appetite and to assist muscle function. If chloride loss is excessive, a state of 'alkalosis' can develop. This causes heavy and prolonged breathing following hard work. Supplementation with an electrolyte mixture of potassium chloride and sodium chloride can correct the problem. Three full tablespoons of common salt plus 'trace elements' daily in food would provide enough electrolytes for a normally active horse.

Rehydration fluid can be given over the tongue for prompt restoration of electrolytes in severe cases of sweat loss. It is essential to provide adequate drinking water to a horse receiving electrolyte therapy, in order to help the horse cope with the thirst that will develop. Carriage horses should be given shade and not worked in a temperature of 30 °C (86 °F) or higher. Humidity must also be taken into consideration. 'Misting' a horse with a fine spray of cool water can help a heated horse. In addition, they can be allowed to drink more if not recently fed. As aforementioned, all sweat should be removed promptly with a clean, dry towel.

Heat stroke

Heavy traction on paved city streets in the heat of summer puts a horse at great risk of heat stroke. In a temperature around 30 °C (86 °F) and above the horse can experience heat exhaustion in its work. It can also receive extra radiated and extreme heat from the street and surrounding buildings. In such conditions the horse will develop hyperthermia, with trembling and rapid breathing. Sweating ceases and unsteadiness develops if the hyperthermia progresses. The horse may soon collapse with heat stroke, and the subject's rectal temperature can rise from 38 to 42 °C (100 to 109 °F). The mucous membranes of the mouth are then bright red. Heat stroke is now severe and can soon be fatal. Heroic

first aid must be instituted immediately. Buckets of cold water should be thrown over the entire body surface as the harness is being removed and arrangements are being made to get the horse shaded. A hosepipe connected to a source of water must be brought to the scene, and water should be continuously hosed over the animal for about half an hour while its temperature is being monitored. The hosing should be continued until its temperature returns to normal and consciousness is restored. When the horse is able to rise, it should be taken home by horse trailer and given appropriate care. Monitoring of temperature should continue, as hyperthermia can return. Horses can deal much better with recreational sleigh work.

Drying

Rain is another weather factor that can be a problem. A wet horse should be taken home and quickly dried to prevent chilling. Drying off is emergency care to ensure that the horse's well-being is defended against a health challenge. Sudden, rapid and excessive loss of body heat can quickly predispose the horse to chilling and a flare-up of any infection that might be dormant.

No brushing should be done on a wet horse. As soon as it has been put into shelter and its tack removed, it should have all the surface moisture wiped off with a horse scraper. Hot-air drying must not be considered; it is contra-indicated. A sweat scraper should be taken over fleshy areas very firmly and repeatedly with slow, downward actions, yet it should be used more carefully over bony parts. After scraping, the horse should be rubbed down with thick wisps of hay to dry off the coat finally. The wisps are discarded and replaced as drying progresses. Wisping can be sustained for about 15 min. An armful of clean, dry straw can then be spread over the horse's body, with a rug placed over it, secured with a surcingle. Drying will continue with the help of some air circulating through the straw. The rug curtails the risk of chilling.

The legs of the wet horse can be dealt with once the body has received the attention described. Brisk rubbing of the legs with hay wisps is done against the lie of the hair. Dry, fine sawdust can now be applied to the legs. Leg bandages can be put on over the sawdust and left on for an hour or so. When the rug, straw and bandages are removed, the horse needs basic grooming and a fresh, dry rug. Any mud on the legs should not be washed off but dried and brushed off later. If the legs are left wet they are liable to develop a variety of skin disorders, such as dermatitis (mud fever), moist eczema and cracked skin over the heels. A horse standing continuously on a wet, unhygienic surface is very likely to develop thrush, which is a degeneration of the frog with secondary bacterial infection. The affected frog is moist with a black discharge and has a characteristic foul odour. Thrush calls for veterinary attention.

Chilling

Carriage horses are sometimes used in the winter season. In cold weather they need to be suitably rugged to prevent chilling, which is stressful. Quarter rugs cover the back and rump. Rugs differ in the amount of insulation they offer. Some have a firm fabric side and a woollen side, which goes against the horse. Sometimes it is sufficient to have a folded blanket over the horse's rump. To keep horses warm and dry, there are quilted, sheepskin and waterproof varieties of rugs. It would be humane to consider using a hood on some winter days, as hoods can protect horses in cold weather. They cover the horse's head and the upper part of the neck; there are some styles that go all the way down the neck, which may also cover the face and the ears. They are secured in position by tapes under the jaw and neck. A headstall fits over the hood but a halter or bridle is kept underneath it. Slits can be made for blinkers if necessary. Although horses can tolerate very cold dry weather if they do not have to contend with wind, the stop and go nature of carriage work presents thermoregulatory problems. Carriage horses should not, therefore, be at work if the temperature or the wind chill factor drops to −20 °C (−4 °F) or lower.

Shelter

It will be obvious that some form of shade or shelter should be located at the hack line in all seasons. There should also be a feeding and watering facility. It would be desirable to have the latter location at a spot where the air would be as clean as possible and free from gross pollution from traffic. The cooperation of civic authorities in providing or permitting this would be a very reasonable request in the interest of horse welfare.

Street Work

The health of horses in the carriage trade is at risk from injuries, lameness and lung damage. Injuries from accidents of various kinds are well documented. Walking and jogging on hard surfaces creates abnormal stresses on hooves and legs, with lameness often developing. The constant inhalation of exhaust fumes in carriage-drawing work in dense traffic duly causes permanent respiratory disorders. The life expectancy of such horses is much less than in the general horse population. Horse welfare therefore emerges as of great concern in the carriage horse business, and matters are not helped when such horses are in the hands of inexperienced, untrained drivers.

In addition to the horses used in the modern tourist carriage trade, there is now a growing population of police horses on city streets. Horses have been used for a century in such work in major cities, and their effectiveness in such problems as crowd control has resulted in large numbers of other municipalities adopting a mounted police capability. Such horses are carefully selected for this work and are graduates of very exacting training courses, in which many fail. As a rule, the type of horse chosen is a cross of cold-blooded breeds. They are also particularly large and heavy geldings, which are considered 'bomb-proof' in their reactive ridden behaviour.

Various other horses still work the streets, but do so under saddle in easier forms of work than in the collar. They radiate their well-being. The aforementioned police horses are examples of the highest level of horse care, receiving, as they do, a regimen of attention that can be colloquially described as labour intensive. The people who use them supply the care, which involves feeding, grooming, cleaning, bedding, hoof care and health monitoring. The grooms are properly trained for these duties, following selection. The author has been involved in the veterinary aspects of police horse husbandry in different locations over some years and can make these observations from experience. In a similar category, military horses continue to have use in ceremonial functions and parades, adding the elements of formality, dignity and authority to such events. In the public eye, the level of their welfare is obviously high, and deservedly so, for the role that countless numbers of horses formerly played in wartime. As a general rule it can be stated that the modern ceremonial horse, in police, official or military service, exhibits the level of care that sets the benchmark in high-quality horse husbandry (see Fig. 9.9).

Under normal circumstances, police work is of a casual nature, serving in a PR role as an attractive spectacle in urban locations, where they can be viewed. For convenience of use, they are usually stabled far from fields in city core locations. Invariably there is a high standard of care afforded to these horses, and the author's experience with many has confirmed this as a general rule. Their husbandry is along conventional lines, with good nutrition and body care. While they are at work, they are typically perambulating at a slow or steady walk, quite close to moving traffic. This often constitutes their chief provision of exercise, although in some cases there is periodic access to a paddock for free movement.

All horses working on civic streets experience the same job-related strain, once often referred to in the alliterative phrase 'hammer, hammer, hammer on the hard highway'. Although well shod with good iron shoes, horses stepping continuously on very hard surfaces experience the transmitted shocks to joints of the lower limb. The shoes on street horses have caulkins projecting from the heels to provide a better grip when the foot hits the smooth surface. This has the effect of keeping the frog, on the concave sole of the foot, clear of the ground. With such lack of usage it atrophies progressively. The frog normally gets periodic pressure when the horse is moving on a soft surface that yields to the hoof in the limb's support phase. The frog gets use when there is absorbent pressure on it while going on sand, turf or soft ground. On soft substrates, the frog absorbs some of the weight within each footfall of the horse, especially when the animal is unshod.

The frog is an elastic, horny body in the form of an insensitive mass of keratinous tissue in the shape of a thick arrowhead. It is located between the bars by the heels and points towards the toe of the hoof. It is normally prominent enough to make contact with the ground, although it can shrink progressively with age and ill-use. With such atrophy it loses its natural involvement with hoof physiology. When the frog is functional, however, it takes some of the force of the impact of footfall, and through

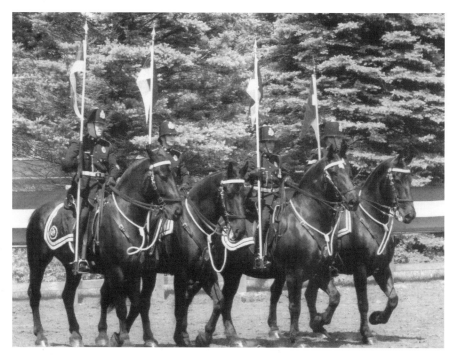

Fig. 9.9. Police horses (Percherons) on PR duty. Note top-grade condition. Photo: *The Telegram*, St John's, Newfoundland.

Chapter 9

its slightly spongy nature it transmits energy into the content of the hoof.

The horny inner wall of the hoof has numerous vertical, slender corrugations, which project into the profusion of the capillary-rich and sensitive laminae that constitute the 'quick' of the hoof. The hoof must be considered as an analogue of our middle digit, the nail and hoof being equivalent structures. During the swing phase, the capillary bed of the soft laminations of the quick is able to receive its maximal quantity of arterial blood pulsing through the foot. Extra pressure transmitted from the frog provides an additional boost to the perfusion of blood to the receiving surfaces on the internal face of the hoof. With the sudden pulsation of blood pressure within the hoof in the support phase, resulting from the frog's transmission of force, the venules arising from the capillaries in the very vascular quick are aided in their return of venous blood to the heart. In brief, the frog assists the circulation of the hoof, including that of its walls. The hoof walls receive nutritive fluid from the coronary band, down to their lower level at the inner 'white line', where the walls and sole are joined. This depends on blood flow to the region. When the frog is not functional, hoof circulation loses the assistance of this much-ignored organ. The hoof walls can become somewhat less nourished as a result. In due course, such a hoof wall can develop a crack.

The above circumstances add to the merit of regularly putting all street horses out to pasture. From a materialistic point of view, such breaks from work can extend the animal's length of service. To quote another old maxim among horse people, 'No hoof, no horse'. Pasture time ought to be in the animal's work contract, if only in an ethical attempt to provide behavioural corrective for their inevitable state of ethostasis, in which so much of their natural behaviour is prevented and made static by chronic behavioural restriction and physical restraint. Chosen for their placability, street horses are often middle aged. Some respiratory problems that may have been building up can suddenly embarrass the horse in this phase of life. Pulmonary emphysema or broken windedness can be concealed in an affected horse until the lung damage is extensive. Unfortunately, it may be in middle age that chronic obstructive pulmonary disease (COPD), from long-term inhalation of hay dust contaminated with mould and fungus, takes an irreversible hold of the horse, destroying its well-being permanently.

This is also a time when other problems might come to the surface, as, for example, when wear and tear on limbs and feet first arise.

Retirement from street work formerly meant prompt slaughter, but today there are a few places for such horses in the growing number of equine sanctuaries operated by charities, supported by public funds. The existence of such facilities points to progress in the public's appreciation for domestic animal welfare.

Transportation

The nature of the horse makes this animal particularly unsuitable for the standard methods of shipping livestock. Horses do not readily lend themselves to the packaging that is the essence of transportation. Their great talent is reactive running. Their forte is free flight. This is their method of operating in the wild in a wide variety of circumstances, from play to self-defence. Flight is the horse's modus operandi, and tight enclosure countermands this natural response to a frightening situation.

Present methods of horse transport usually involve visual and spatial limitation, with vibrations, motion and noise as cumulative stressors. Nothing could be invented that would be more unacceptable to the equine nature. The horse's predisposition to the stress and trauma of transportation makes this a key aspect of equine welfare.

Loading and unloading

Horses are most often transported by trailer or lorry. These vehicles vary in style from a single horsebox to very large trailers. Among the conventional trailers, some have end-loading or side-loading, or both. With both openings they can load via one and unload via the other. It helps a horse to enter if it can see a potential exit. The open-top type of trailer is best for short journeys in fair weather and it is a good trainer. Poorly managed or inexperienced horses can present difficulties on loading as a result of fear. They often shy back halfway into the trailer, when the fact of enclosure hits them. They are willing to hold that position, which gives them back some head space. Head shyness in horses has always been known but not fully appreciated as a major characteristic fear that occurs with loss, or threat of loss, of head room in transportation. It is inhumane to use excessive force on loading; this only increases fear. The animal should be restrained in position until its fear has subsided to the point where it can respond to customary commands. A wide-headed broom with a long handle may be pushed against the hindquarters to encourage the horse to load gradually.

Many horses become accustomed to road travelling and are then able to be loaded and unloaded without real difficulty. Other horses have great problems with transportation. It can be said of horse transport that anything that can go wrong will do so sooner or later if all preparations and precautions are not taken and taken seriously. To try to offset loading and unloading problems, the horse should be conditioned properly, given a suitable and familiar vehicle and, if possible, a good travelling companion. A placid and well-experienced horse or pony would be a first choice, but dogs and certain other animals familiar to the horse can provide this service. The companion should board the vehicle first. No person should travel inside the horse's compartment.

The loading ramp of the transporter should not be steep. Ideally it should be on a level with the floor of the vehicle, the horse ascending to it via a raised area with closed sides. Partitions should be placed at each side of the vehicle's ramp to prevent an attempt at escape. Other suitable arrangements should be in place to deal safely with any escape away from the handlers. The horse should be led on to the vehicle with a bridle and unloaded similarly. At unloading, many horses attempt to bolt out of the transporter. Full precautions must be made to control this, since serious injuries often result from precipitous unloading (FVE, 2001).

Certain protective items should be worn by the horse during its transport. These would depend on the particular conditions in each case, but leg and tail bandages plus a poll guard are advisable. In each case, ample consideration should be given to the various problems that the horse must face during a given journey. Sufficient time must be allowed for the procedures of loading and unloading, which are very critical points in horse transportation (EUSC AHAW, 2002; Broom, 2005).

Transit trauma

Horse transportation is plagued with inhumane practices and traumatic mishaps (Grandin, 2007). These begin with first loading, for which there is usually no prior training or conditioning. Typically, on loading, the horse is required to step up an inclined ramp, generally unstable, and into a vehicle with a dark interior. The horse will often jib or baulk partway into the vehicle or it may plunge inside before baulking and trying to retreat. It may attempt to 'rear', with limited head space. The handlers have the difficulty of controlling these reactions. Shouted commands and striking the horse are common but inhumane ways of forcing the horse into its assigned place. Once inside, it is then secured by the head collar. This scene can also occur in some horses with experience of transportation by trailer or truck.

Some horses panic immediately after they are secured, while some go berserk in transit, with a great risk of self-injury in either case. Injuries can also occur during unloading, when the horse may scramble rapidly to escape from the vehicle. Minor injuries are frequent. Serious transport injuries include the following:

- Head trauma, including fractures, cuts and abrasions of the head or face.
- Various limb injuries, including fractures.
- Raw tails from excessive rubbing.
- Muscle wastage from recumbency after a fall or an attempt at rest inside the vehicle. Death may follow.
- Broken necks occurring at unloading, resulting in death.

Transit stress

A range of illnesses can develop in horses during or after transportation, particularly if the journey has been long: more than a few hours, for example. Recovery can take place quickly with good care, but at other times the horse may not recover easily.

- Fatigue is common after a long period of shipping. This can last long enough to spoil a racing horse's prospects.
- Weight loss can be significant if the journey has been long.
- Diarrhoea can develop in some excited horses within the first hour of travel.
- Bowel stasis may develop in some cases where the journey has been long. Administration of mineral oil before the start of a long trip can prevent this.
- Transit tetany was not uncommon in former times, when there was heavy trading in large draught horses. This condition involves low calcium blood levels. Prompt intravenous treatment

with calcium and magnesium could effect a cure, but delay often meant death. Although this disorder is now rarely encountered, it could still occur.

- Trailer choke is an accident of ingestion that has become more common in recent years with a greater number of light horses being trailered. It has been observed that these cases develop as a result of the stressed horse eating rapidly in an abnormal, greedy fashion. Hay can become impacted in the throat. This is the result of giving a supply of hay to a horse being trailered to occupy it during the journey. This hay must be securely contained in a good hay net to prevent gorging.
- Equine colitis is a serious condition of the large bowel. Some cases occur after transportation. Emergency veterinary treatment is necessary.
- Respiratory infections may develop following transportation. The stress of this can predispose a horse to viral infection.

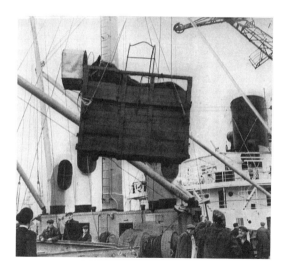

Fig. 9.10. Stallion being put on board in a custom-built crate. Photo: N. Fraser.

Air and sea travel

In horse transportation by sea or air, the risks as described above apply. A horse that is out of control on a plane can create a real crisis. Shooting with a 'free bullet' gun would be dangerous and it would be difficult to get close to the horse with a 'captive bolt' gun. Humane control could be carried out with an immobilizing drug, and the use of such should be made possible on any aircraft carrying a horse. The International Air Transport Association (IATA) sets out several conditions for the transport of horses by air. Long, enduring sea journeys with horses can involve deaths from trauma and stress, but every effort should be made for a comfortable stall for every horse in a vessel. Custom-built loading crates are required to get horses on board a ship or aeroplane (see Fig. 9.10).

It appears that many horses cannot escape the complex stress of travel in containment (Oikawa *et al.*, 2005). Those that do travel well show remarkable adaptation, and perhaps a high degree of intelligence. A fortunate few are preconditioned for travel. Long-distance travelling is particularly stressful (Appleby *et al.*, 2008).

Travel preparation

The protection of horses from the trauma and stress of transportation requires much consideration for each horse, adequate planning and proper preparation of the vehicle in which the animal will travel. Protective clothing can include helmets, hoods, leg wraps, boots, blankets and tail bandages. The horse might be given well-considered tranquillizers. The horse should be well hydrated and oral electrolytes can be given. A dose of mineral oil may also be beneficial and shoes should be removed.

The travel vehicle should be high enough to provide head room. It should also be in perfect condition, with no protruding objects in any part of the horse's space. Ventilation should be adequate. Suitable bedding must be provided, such as straw or rubber matting. Appropriate rest stops must be planned, with water provided at each stop. Periodic inspection of every horse should be carried out, and the first of these should be done within the first 15 min of the journey. The trailer connection should also be checked periodically. Sudden braking or swerving of the vehicle can be very dangerous, and speed should therefore be appropriate for the live cargo as well as for road and traffic conditions.

Transport conditioning

Pre-training or preconditioning of the horse would be in the animal's best interest. Step-wise introduction to a ramp and a trailer's interior could be given to a young horse, since it is very likely that it will be subjected to significant transportation at some point. Over a period of 2 weeks, a horse can be trained to enter and remain in a stationary trailer for a long length of time. An open-top trailer would be ideal for this training. It could be taken on a very short trip, then slightly longer trips could follow. Each stage of progress would need to be promptly associated with a food reward. Transport conditioning is strongly advisable for any form of horse transportation. Proper horse care is a major feature of welfare in horse transport (Broom, 2000).

Welfare Addendum

Welfare requires that the availability of space appropriate for the comfort-directed actions of a horse, such as stretching, rising, lying and postural changes, should be incorporated into the design of any form of containment for travel purposes (EFSA AHAW, 2004). There is always a stress potential in circumstances of excessive restraint of horses. For air and sea travel in particular, the close restraint of individual horses deprives their inherent behaviour of many outlets. Some actions need to be accommodated, for example balancing such needs as good bedding and plenty of foot space.

Certain changes in posture occur frequently in horses while they are at rest. These changes have been termed 'comfort shifts', and these shifts are necessary to maintain resting periods during travel. These shifts can occur in either standing or lying positions. Typically, they involve some articular modification of the extremities or some degree of trunk relocation. Space is required for such shifting. The contained animal also needs space for reaction movements and basic acts of body care, such as scratching.

10 Breeding Function

In circumstances of free range, horses usually breed competently. In hand-breeding and close husbandry, however, many difficulties can arise for horse and handlers alike. An adequate knowledge of the natural features of equine reproductive behaviour should be known to all those who are actively involved in horse breeding (Langley, 1990; Davidson and Stabenfeldt, 2007).

General Overview of Breeding Activities

With some experience of breeding, a stallion always shows interest in any mare coming within its vicinity (see Fig. 10.1). When he can approach a mare freely, he tests her for oestrus by nosing her hindquarters and nipping at her sides. If the mare is not in her breeding state, she will invariably react negatively to a stallion's intrusion into her presence by rearing and kicking back, vocalizing loudly with squeals, switching her tail and holding her ears back tightly. If the mare is clearly non-receptive, the experienced stallion will soon withdraw from her (Kiley-Worthington, 1999).

When the mare and the stallion have been haltered to each other in 'hand-breeding', those in charge of the animals must be able to recognize and understand these negative reactions and lead the horses away from each other quickly. Persisting in attempts to have the animals breed will probably result in the stallion being injured. Mares for breeding must be unshod, as a serious injury can be inflicted on a stallion if held behind a mare, should she kick back suddenly (Knottenbelt et al., 2001).

Some inexperienced females, even in heat, might kick back in alarm, probably due to the strangeness of the breeding situation and the sudden intrusion of the stallion into her individual space. For this reason, some horse breeders fit breeding hobbles on the mare's hind feet before the stallion is brought to her. This can provide safety to the male, but the female can be subjected to the stallion's vigorous biting. By far the better arrangement is to have a firm barrier – a 'teasing board' – between the two horses. When the stallion can reach over the barrier with his head and carry out his teasing or testing performance, the mare is able to react negatively or positively to the stimulation without risk of injury to either horse. A fence is not suitable as a teasing barrier. In fact, it would be extremely unsafe for the stallion in particular, since it might put a leg between horizontal spars and become entrapped, with very traumatic results.

The signs of oestrus in the mare are normally fairly obvious (see Table 10.1). The principal signs are most apparent when she is stimulated by the stallion's activities. In summary, these signs are: (i) standing still at the stallion's approach; (ii) raising the tail; and (iii) everting the lower portion of the vulva in a winking fashion. Additional signs include: (iv) passing small quantities of urine and mucus; and (v) raising the heels of one or the other hind hoof. Some of these oestrous signs can be shown occasionally by mares that are not in true oestrus when they are 'teased'. Teasing for a period of a few minutes should bring out the full oestrous display if the mare is properly in heat (Davies-Morel, 2000). Further aspects of oestrus will be discussed in a following section.

Stud protocol

In some Thoroughbred breeding studs in particular, there is a regular routine that the staff follow. During breeding there is fast action and many moving parts. The situation can offer immediate danger to any of the handlers. They should therefore wear protective clothing, such as industrial gloves and helmets (e.g. construction hats), plus suitable clothing that will not flap about. After it is confirmed that the mare is in heat, she is led to a spacious, well-bedded enclosure and held there by a groom. Another attendant lifts one of the mare's forelegs and straps the cannon to the forearm of the leg, so that the knee is flexed. The attendant holds the end

---

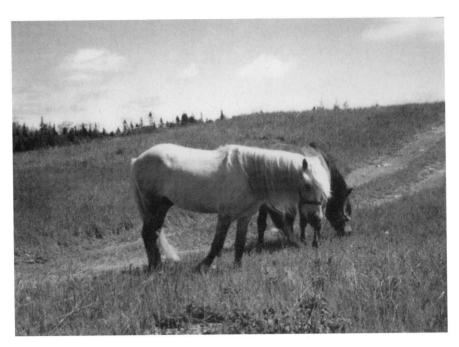

Fig. 10.1. Grey stallion in bond with oestrous mare. Photo: C. George.

Table 10.1. Inverse incidences of displays in oestrus versus non-oestrus in mares in stallion presence.

Display components	Incidence in oestrus	Incidence in non-oestrus
Remained calm and stationary	xxxxx	x
Raised tail away from perineum	xxxxx	x
Winked clitoral area	xxxxx	x
Postured with a hind foot out	xxxx	x
Urinated promptly	xxx	x
Moved position reactively	xx	xxxxx
Held ears back stiffly	x	xxxxx
Switched tail vigorously	x	xxxxx

xxxxx, over 80%; xxxx, 61–80%; xxx, 41–60%; xx, 21–40%; x, 1–20%.

of this strap. This prevents the mare from kicking back. The stallion's groom then leads the stallion to the rear of the mare, in line with her. It often takes a second attempt by the stallion to mount the mare before he covers her. Sometimes the stallion's groom will guide the animal's penis for intromission to be accomplished (see Fig. 10.2). When the stallion has finished serving the mare, he dismounts slowly. At this time the stallion's penis is still extruded but progressively flaccid. A further attendant may then splash it with lukewarm water and wash it with a sponge. At the same time, the mare's flexed foreleg is quickly released and she is smartly led away from the stallion, the breeding being completed.

Variations of the breeding routine include such procedures as applying a leather neck cover to the mare or a muzzle on the stallion to prevent him from biting the mare; holding up the mare's fore foot only briefly at the start of covering and bandaging the mare's tail with a thoroughly clean bandage. Sometimes after service, as the mare is led away, she is slapped on the belly to discourage her from sinking her hindquarters and straining to expel the ejaculate. Seminal volume aids fertilization because

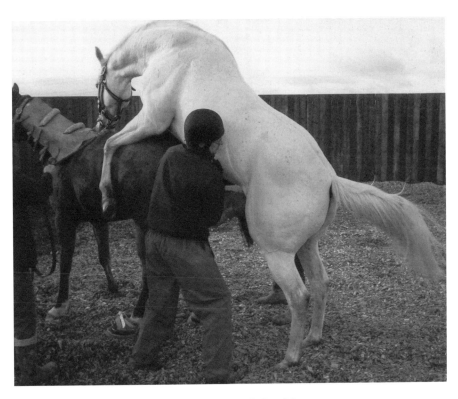

Fig. 10.2. Assisted breeding with some safety features. Photo: D. Dugdale.

the site of the insemination is chiefly intravaginal and intracervical. A small quantity goes directly into the uterus. A pool of semen must be located in the fornix and is drawn into the cervix from there, before passing into the uterus. Massive numbers of spermatozoa are lost in this process, but enough survive to be capable of fertilizing the mare if she ovulates within a day or so. Stallion spermatozoa can retain a fertilizing capacity for about 24 h in the mare's fallopian tubes.

In hand-breeding, repeated covering is usual. If the mare appears to continue in oestrus for a further 2 days, it is usual to have her bred again by the same stallion. Repeated hand-breeding is usually continued at 2-day intervals for as long as the mare remains in heat. The duration of oestrus normally varies anywhere from 3 to 10 days. In summertime, the duration of the oestrous display is more consistent, usually about 4 or 5 days. The oestrous display at this time is less ambiguous than at a much later time, such as winter. In natural breeding, with the mare and stallion running together, uncertainty regarding ovulation presents no problem. The stallion will breed the mare repeatedly for as long as she remains receptive. Furthermore, heats are often short under natural conditions with a stallion constantly present. Evidently the stallion's activities have a positive influence on the mare's breeding physiology. This phenomenon is termed 'biostimulation'.

Practical use of biostimulation is made in some extensive Thoroughbred breeding operations by including a small pony stallion in a herd of brood mares. The pony circulates among the mares, investigating them and detecting any in heat. While it will attempt to mount any mares in oestrus, the pony is not of sufficient stature to breed them. He will consort with an oestrous mare, allowing her to be identified and removed for mating.

Male sexual behaviour

Nipping and biting occur in the pre-coital actions of the stallion. This activity is prominent in its intense courtship activities. Ordinarily it prompts the female to move forward, but in oestrus, the female responds with a stationary stance. This facilitates mating and provides reciprocal stimulation for the stallion. He then maintains close body contact and association with the mare. Both sexes, therefore, contribute to the temporary alliance in a courting bond.

When breeding in free range, the stallion separates the mare from the harem several days before oestrus, keeping her under surveillance until standing oestrus occurs. The herd stallion keeps other males away from the mare during this time and will fight to protect her. In order to assess the mare's receptivity, the stallion will typically sniff or nuzzle the mare's perineum. The oestrous mare urinates in response; the stallion then shows the flehmen reaction and various vocalizations occur in both partners. Before the stallion mounts, he may move his head across the mare's rump, nip her flanks, hindquarters and hind legs, and toss his mane vigorously, seemingly in a display of intent.

Variations occur in the level of libido among stallions. Some characteristics of breeding virility are related to the stallion's breed type. Usually a lower level of libido is found in cold-blooded horses than in hot- and warm-blooded breeds. A high level of libido is more common at the start of the breeding season. Stallions that are not allowed to breed lose their libido dramatically. Libido also diminishes with ageing. Some stallions practise masturbation by bringing the erect penis into contact with the abdomen and thrusting until ejaculation occurs. This habit reduces libido (McDonnell, 1989).

In their pre-coital behaviour stallions focus on the oestrous mare, nosing her perineum, showing flehmen, sometimes repeatedly nipping and biting her hindquarters down to the level of her shanks and nipping along the sides of her trunk. He may even push her. Finally he extrudes the penis fully. Thereafter, several 'false' mounting attempts usually occur before the stallion makes a determined effort to 'cover' the mare. The penis becomes fully erect after the pre-coital phase. All components of male serving behaviour are very characteristic of every stallion (see Fig. 10.3).

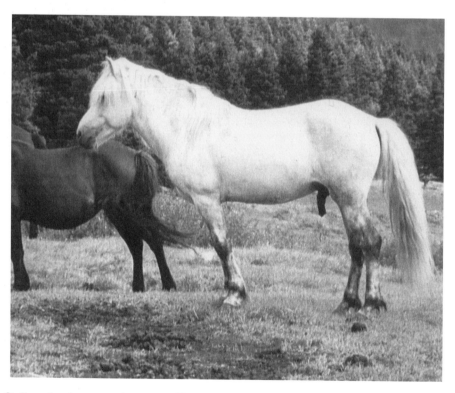

Fig. 10.3. Stallion attending pro-oestrous mare. Photo: M.Roberts.

Chapter 10

One of the chief components of the male display is the aforementioned olfactory reflex known as flehmen (flaring). During this display the animal fully extends the head and neck, contracts the nostrils, raises the upper lip and takes shallow respirations (see Figs 10.4 and 10.5). It occurs most usually subsequent to smelling urine and nosing the female perineum, and is a form of odour testing. Schneider first reported the reflex in 1930 and descriptively termed it flehmen. He observed it in horses and in a variety of ungulates in a zoological collection.

Coital regimen

In covering, the stallion quickly lines up behind the mare. After some pre-copulatory activity, the stallion achieves penile erection and mounting occurs. 'False mounting' attempts by the stallion are usual actions. In these, the stallion only covers the mare partially and dismounts without any forelimb clasping or pelvic thrusting movements. False

mounts show that the mechanics of mounting and of intromission are separately controlled. False mountings are very notable in the mating pattern of the stallion. Stallions will mount female donkeys, and jackasses will readily mount mares. Such interspecies coitus allows mules to be bred. The mule is a cross between a jackass and a mare. Blindfolding one or both animals is often done before covering.

After mounting and as covering progresses, there is tight gripping of the receptive mare by the forelegs of the stud. His legs become strongly adducted into the female's flanks. Repeated thrusting pelvic movements are required to enable the penis to locate and enter the vulva and to achieve intromission. The stallion's clasping increases in intensity at intromission of the penis. The covering position is complete when he quickly moves his hind feet forward, close to the hind feet of the mare, and his back becomes arched. When the stallion is securely mounted with intromission, the neck is lowered, allowing his mouth to rest against the mare's crest

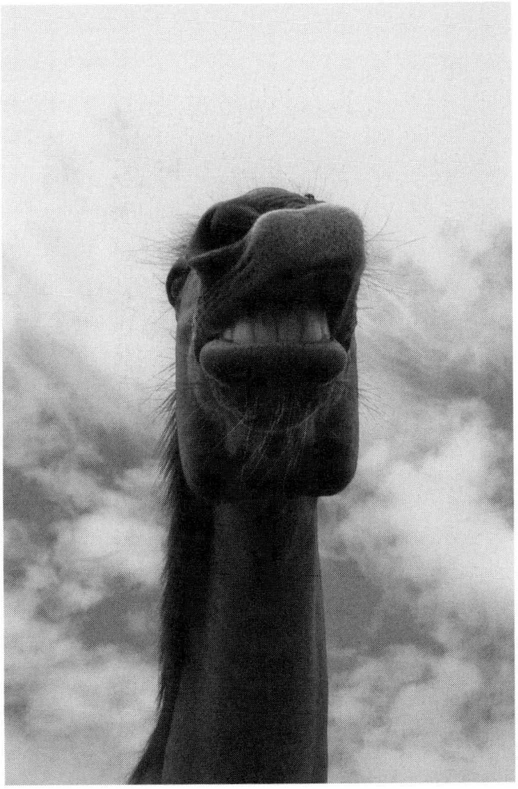

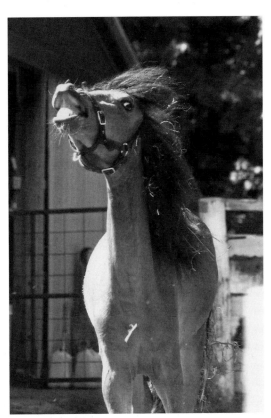

Fig. 10.4. Lip curl at start of flehmen. Photo: Melanie MacDonald.

Fig. 10.5. Total posture in flehmen. Photo: Melanie MacDonald.

or alongside her neck. Biting of these areas may occur, and in some cases this can be severe (see Fig. 10.6). The erection of the stud's penis becomes maximal once intromission is achieved. Several pelvic thrusts occur before ejaculation. Following this natural insemination, the stallion remains stationary on the mare for a brief period, before dismounting by sliding backwards, then slipping aside on to one forefoot. Table 10.2 illustrates some characteristics of stallion coverage.

Horse copulations occur promptly at the start of the mare's oestrus, but repeated matings are spread over subsequent days while the mare is in heat (Collery, 1969). Repeat mating thus varies between pairs; some may mate only a few times, while others may mate numerous times. Occurrences of mating are fewest during any warm period of the day. Night-time breeding has a high occurrence in freely breeding horses. Morning appears to be the diurnal period in which most copulations occur naturally,

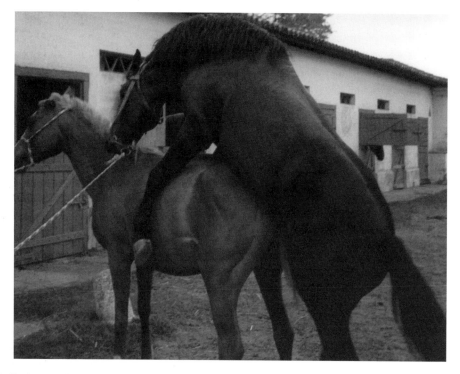

Fig. 10.6. Equine copulation. Note stallion's oral grip on mare's crest, plus clasp of the thorax. Photo: A.F. Fraser.

Table 10.2. Characteristics of stallion coverage.

Feature	Reaction time	Pre-coital behaviour	Manner of intromission	Duration of intromission and site of insemination	Repeat matings
Norm	Averages about 3–4 min	Nuzzles perineum	One to four mounts Several pelvic oscillations	30 s Intra-cervical	About three times daily
Additional	Varies with age and season	Bites croup region Penis fully erect	Inactive phase during insemination	Intra-uterine in some cases	Five to ten times per oestrus in pasture breeding

Chapter 10

in wild horses for example. Both mare and stallion make contributions to coitus. Coital behaviour progresses from pre-coital activity to the components of copulation, which include mounting, intromission and insemination. An experienced stallion soon mounts a presented mare as a result of positive conditioning. The time between presentation and mounting is the behavioural 'reaction time' (Fraser and Broom, 1990). Figure 10.7 illustrates common seasonal reaction times.

It is estimated that at least seven thrusts are needed to bring about ejaculation. Pelvic oscillations cease just prior to ejaculation; the cessation of thrusting is an external sign of its onset. The tail then commonly begins a series of up–down, flexing motions (tail flagging). About 30 s after copulation first begins, most stallions have achieved ejaculation and begin to dismount. Copulation times of 12–26 s commonly occur in ponies. Thoroughbred stallions average 30 s. After dismounting there is usually a refractory period of about 20 min. The penis is withdrawn into the sheath in 1 min. During the main part of the breeding season, most stallions can copulate three times or more per day without difficulty (see Fig. 10.8). At free-breeding, stallions have a common range of five to ten matings on each mare during her oestrus (Samper, 2000).

Although sexual reaction times in stallions can be influenced by various somatic and psychological factors, estimation of the reaction time provides a simple and ordinarily reliable measurement of libido. The first reaction times of most stallions remain almost constant, averaging 2–3 min. After the first ejaculation, reaction time increases with successive copulations as repeated breeding progresses. It has been found that the mean reaction time of four random observations spaced well apart gives an extremely reliable indication of the long-term sexual performance of the subject and its libido.

Stallions experienced in breeding may retain interest in mares and exhibit sexual behaviour subsequent to castration through a persistence in libido. The cryptorchid, or rig horse, which typically has only one testicle descended into the scrotum, shows normal stallion behaviour. Even after the removal of the descended testicle, the sexual behaviour persists. If such an animal acquires breeding experience, he is likely to become very difficult to manage. After surgical removal of the retained testicle, the animal's libido is quickly reduced, but it may not disappear entirely for a long time.

After they have acquired sexual experience, stallions exhibit strong attraction to any available mare, testing the mare's receptivity to mating. When a breeding stallion and a group of mares are at pasture or free-ranging, the stallion's sexual curiosity is constantly in evidence. Sexually experienced stallions will approach any mare, searching for receptive individuals, testing all mares that they encounter for olfactory, tactile, visual and auditory cues of sexual responsiveness. On being tested by the stallion, responses of mares not in oestrus indicate negative reaction. Only while in standing oestrus will an unrestrained mare facilitate mounting and permit intromission. The mare in non-oestrus will kick or show other signs of aggression as well as withdrawal. Most experienced stallions will determine the mare's receptivity with caution and only show fuller arousal if the behavioural feedback from the mare is positive. The stallion has immediate motivation (Hogan, 2005).

Various anomalies

Inhibition factors can develop and influence a stallion's behaviour adversely as a result of negative conditioning. Stallions experiencing arthritic discomfort or any pain during sexual mounting will, in time, have their breeding behaviour impaired. It is also strongly suspected that temperamental factors can cause sexual inhibition in stallions in the

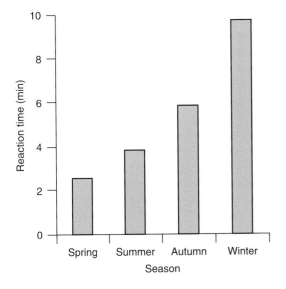

Fig. 10.7. Common seasonal reaction times of stallions in perennial-breeding studs.

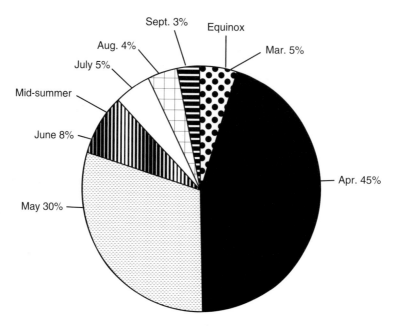

Fig. 10.8. Percentage matings in breeding season in Nordic pony mares.

course of breeding experience that has been unsatisfactory. Some pathological causes and congenital malfunctions occur, but in more cases psychogenic factors are responsible for or contribute to aberrant sexual performance. A stallion can acquire a severe inhibition towards sexual activity. An injury or psychological trauma during breeding is a common cause. Where management procedures, pain or unpleasant experiences have contributed to a problem in mating behaviour, resolution of the problem is often possible. Stallions respond well to retraining, and recoveries may not require treatment with drugs, as they can resolve spontaneously with breeding rest and careful management. Alteration of certain environmental conditions, such as a change in handlers, breeding site or methodology, may achieve success. Dysfunctional stallions sometimes regain breeding ability through improved welfare. Retraining that involves very considerate management and patient handling can restore sexual capability in some cases.

Colts

Colt foals will frequently mount others in play when just a few weeks old, but fillies engage in this behaviour less frequently. Although colts can produce an erection of the penis at 2–3 months of age,

they can only achieve successful mating by about 15 months old. Under natural conditions young colts do not have much opportunity to breed. If an equine group contains a stallion and breeding mares, the stallion will drive the younger male animals to the perimeter of the group. He will not show any aggressive attitudes towards them if they remain there. The stallion attempts to herd a group of brood mares together to form a 'harem' (McDonnell, 2002). Often the size of the harems among horses is about seven to eight mares. When a mare is in heat among other horses, the stallion may lower his neck and extend his head aggressively to drive and separate the individuals, swinging his neck from side to side and threatening to bite. The young colts in the herd form a bachelor group after splitting off from the herd at about 1–2 years of age. Fillies may occasionally join a bachelor group.

Female sexual behaviour

Oestrus is the behavioural state when the female seeks and accepts the male. The behavioural features are synchronized with various physiological changes of the entire genital system essential for mating and fertilization. The signs of female equine oestrus are characteristic and include frequent urination, straddling posture and repeated extrusion of the clitoris. Behaviour in general is altered when the mare is 'in heat'. Her usual routines of behaviour are disturbed during overt oestrus and typically there is a reduction in ingestive and resting behaviour, while locomotor, investigative and vocal behaviour is increased (Asa, 1986).

Variations occur in the degree of receptivity in oestrous mares. Most mares permit numerous matings per heat period, while other mares in physiological oestrus will not accept a stallion. Older mares are usually more receptive than maiden ones. The duration of receptive oestrus is variable, commonly ranging from 4 days to 2 weeks (Davidson and Stabenfeldt, 2007).

Olfactory, visual, auditory and tactile stimuli are supplied to the mares by association with an active stallion. This phenomenon of biostimulation is especially effective during the transition from the non-breeding season to the breeding season, namely springtime. Biostimulation provided by the presence of a stallion in a group of mares, in addition to inducing oestrus, has the added effect of stimulating most of the female population simultaneously. Thus, oestrus that has been prompted by biostimulation shows some general synchronization in this breeding method. Biostimulation not only affects the overall behavioural display of oestrus, there may also be an improvement in group fertility following such stimulation. 'Shy breeders' are also facilitated in their breeding by the effect of biostimulation, which results from the normal manner of a stallion.

With free and continuing access to a brood mare, a stallion can detect the state of oncoming heat with the aid of her pheromones (Wyatt, 2003). He will then focus his full attention on that animal until she is fully receptive. This attention appears to bring out clear signs of oestrus in a mare, which can be readily detected by staff on their daily inspections. The major clue is, of course, the close alliance of a mare with a pony. The little stallion simply functions as a 'teaser'. Mares that are clearly seen to be in heat are taken out of the band for service.

When bands of mares are assembled for breeding, a usual number is 16–20. If the members of the band are put together around the same time, the group settles down quickly – following a few introductory scuffles. If any further addition to an established herd is to be made, it must not be done by simply putting the newcomer rudely into the band without

any preparation. A newcomer would be assaulted by several in the socially fixed group. A technique exists to deal with this problem. It has sometimes been called partnering. It is essentially the formation of a pair outside the band, which will act in mutual defence when placed later in the established group. This is often done as follows. Out of the socially fixed group, one animal is selected to partner the newcomer. Ideally, the chosen mare should be one that has been observed to have some dominance within the group. The newcomer is placed in a separate pasture with the selected mare, where various exchanges, such as nose to nose checking, take place between the two horses before they accept each other's company. Horses are always keen to acquire the continuous company of a companion. The two mares soon form a bond of close association. Within a couple of weeks this bond will have become quite firmly established and the pair can then be put into the main group. When the other mares come to investigate and challenge the intruding bonded pair, particularly the newcomer, the pair will react together and repel individuals emerging from the group aggressively. The entire group is then soon united socially.

The experiences of horse breeders and the findings of many field studies have shown that when mares are 'teased' with restrained males, the display of oestrus is increased. This substantiates the modern view that oestrus is not under endogenous control alone and that its manifestation is subject, in part, to environmental factors, including biostimulation. The term oestrus applies principally to behaviour but it must be acknowledged that it also describes some internal physiological processes. The two facets of oestrus can occur separately in mares, but it is normal for them to exist simultaneously. When oestrus is displayed, behaviour in general changes, and many of the animal's usual behavioural routines become disturbed, e.g. there are often alterations and reductions in feeding and resting patterns. These are secondary to the essential characteristic of oestrous behaviour, which is the acceptance of coitus.

The duration and intensity of oestrus have been observed to alter with seasons (see Fig. 10.9). Oestrous periodicity occurs more regularly during the breeding season and with shorter cycles than at other times. No other ungulate species has a normal oestrous cycle so notoriously irregular in duration as the horse. This irregularity is found in the horse at all latitudes. It can be taken as very characteristic

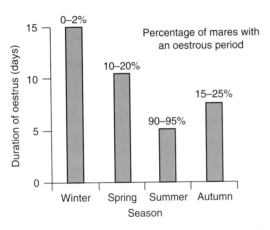

0–2%

Percentage of mares with
an oestrous period

10–20%

15–25%

90–95%

Fig. 10.9. Histogram of modal seasonal incidence and duration of oestrus in ponies and cold-blooded horses in northern latitudes.

of the domesticated horse. Although the mare usually remains in heat for a full week, it can last much longer. Shorter heats more often occur as the breeding season progresses.

The mare is the best-known example of a species showing early oestrus after parturition. This early heat is called the 'foal heat' and occurs, on average, about 9 days after the birth of the foal. The foal heat is often short but is commonly displayed intensively. Some considerable variation occurs in the occurrence of foal heats. The earliest heat noted was on the 4th day and the latest on the 132nd day after foaling.

The average duration of oestrus in the mare is commonly given as 6 days, but wide variations in duration are common. Some workers in equine infertility have suggested that oestrus exceeding 10 days in duration is abnormally protracted. Certainly, infertility is common in protracted oestruses of this nature, owing to the inevitable delay in ovulation. It is thought that many cases of this type are more common at the onset of the breeding season and are also more common in fillies.

Excessive oestrus

Excessive displays of oestrus or 'nymphomania' are not frequently encountered in mares. This condition is not associated with true cystic ovarian disease (in contrast to cattle). Nymphomania seems to be a condition of 'transient persistence' of one or more follicles, which eventually regress or ovulate spontaneously. The term nymphomania is sometimes used by horse breeders to distinguish between excessive oestrous manifestations and normal oestrus. Normal oestrus can recur in infertile mares so regularly and frequently that a history of polyoestrous may be given. This encourages an incorrect, speculative diagnosis of nymphomania.

Sexual maturity may be more variable in mares than has been generally recognized. There is no doubt that there is great variation in the age at which young mares attain normal ovarian activity, as evidenced by polyoestrous. It is a paradox that many mares that show very marked irregularity in oestrous cycles are found to have functionally normal ovaries. These findings show that variations in the oestrous cycle are completely unreliable as a means of diagnosing ovarian dysfunction – a fact of some clinical importance. In a large number of observed cases of mares showing aberrations in oestrous cycles, it has been found that not one case was considered analogous to the typical cystic ovarian condition common in cattle. The regular repetition of long oestruses in mares that do not become pregnant (e.g. from infertility) can give the appearance of oestrous excess, or nymphomania. Suspicion of the latter as a pathological condition is often unfounded, being merely a physiological consequence of non-pregnancy in most cases (Davidson and Stabenfeldt, 2007).

Absence of oestrus

Anoestrus is the condition in which a female animal fails to show cyclic recurrence of oestrus. Anoestrus normally occurs when the animal is pregnant or when it is in its non-breeding season. Seasonal anoestrus is common in the winter in northern countries. European countries often report an incidence of about 50% of winter anoestrus in mares. The incidence in North America is at least as high as this, and in Canada it is considered normal for most mares to be in seasonal anoestrus during the winter.

Prolonged activity of corpora lutea in non-pregnant mares has become recognized clinically as a common cause of anoestrus. The incidence of this condition within the breeding season is evidently quite high in most regions and breeds. Some studies indicate that the condition of spontaneous extension of luteal activity affects the majority of barren mares at some time each year.

The protracted luteal phase typically occurs after a normal oestrus in which there has been ovulation. The subsequent dioestrous phase, in which there is an active corpus luteum, extends far beyond the normal 12–18-day limit and the mare goes into anoestrus. Protracted luteal phases typically range from 1 to 3 months in duration, and average 2 months. The phase ends with resolution of the condition taking place spontaneously and normal oestrous cycles recommencing. The condition is of highest incidence in mid-summer, but cases occur in all months of the year. Treatment with prostaglandin is usually successful. The condition should be suspected if a mare exhibits oestrus, is not mated, and then fails to return to oestrus in the normal time (Asa *et al.*, 1979). The condition can also occur in mares that have been mated but have not conceived. The syndrome is quite different from normal seasonal anoestrus, in which there is no corpus luteum found on rectal palpation.

Quiescent oestrus

The recognition and detection of ovarian changes in oestrus has made possible the discovery that, in many cases, the ovaries can undergo oestrous changes without the subject showing signs of oestrous behaviour. This demands separate recognition of the two aspects of the female mating state, i.e. the discrete physiological and the overt behavioural. Anomalous oestrus is evident in the condition known as 'silent heat', in which behavioural oestrus can be so subdued as to be virtually undetectable. This state is also referred to as 'sub-oestrus'. It constitutes a problem in commercial horse breeding. Its incidence has been estimated in mares at 7%.

Non-fertile oestrus

In contrast to silent heat, some mares can have behavioural oestrus without ovulation. In some cases, oestrus is associated with follicle formation, but the follicles fail to mature completely and ovulate. As many as 40% of infertile mares in one study were found to have this form of ovarian dysfunction. It must therefore be recognized as one of the more common causes of infertility in the horse. This oestrous dysfunction may occur in otherwise normal brood mares at any time, but particularly when environmental conditions in general are unsatisfactory. For example, there may be unsatisfactory nutrition or management.

Oestrus in the mare can, in some cases, be shown without associated follicular development in either ovary. In some of these cases, the behavioural signs

of oestrus can be quite intense. At the present time, no satisfactory explanation for this condition can be given, but exogenous oestrogens in the animal's diet might be responsible in some cases. Again, in some cases, there may be small follicles present in the substance of the ovary, which may not be palpable but might have endocrine function. Heat may occur occasionally during gestation in some animals. There have been several reports of mares showing heat while in advanced pregnancy.

It is clear that manifestation of oestrus in the mare is not only due to internal, endogenous factors but also to external, exogenous stimulation. The latter stimulation is complex, involving odour, sound, sight and touch. Earlier it was supposed that oestrus was entirely under endogenous control, but it is very evident that exogenous factors are of considerable importance and that this is a responsibility of management. The failure of oestrus during the breeding season can often be attributed to the absence of facilitating exogenous factors and the presence of environmental stressors (McGreevy, 2004).

The phenomenon of seasonal breeding is not constant. For example, Thoroughbred mares do not have an absolute anoestrous season in winter in England, where only about 50% of mares go into true anoestrus at this period.

Climate and Daylight

Temperature can also affect seasonal reproductive behaviour. Some stallions do not breed well in heat. At some point, an increasing ambient temperature will make it difficult for an animal to dissipate heat, and hyperthermia will tend to develop. Discomfort due to climatic heat can be aggravated by heat increments within the animal as a result of physical activities. Clearly, it is physiologically appropriate that there be limitations on activity during hyperthermia at any level. The decline in male sexual activity with increasing environmental temperatures therefore has homeostatic significance. It is most likely that the control of this homeostatic mechanism is placed in the hypothalamus (Robinson, 2007).

With the exception of the latter thermal factor, the tropics, as regions of maximum climatic stability, do not restrict reproductive activity to the same extent as do many other climates and regions of the globe. Brief or chance changes in weather such as cold, rain or heat can be responsible for temporary arrest in breeding behaviour in horses in temperate climates.

Both adverse and favourable weather conditions can affect breeding activities in animals, free-living horses included. When a season offers improved weather conditions, the nutrition available to local animals will probably be improved in consequence. This more favourable environment can facilitate breeding responses in some cases, as the animal is provided with increased valuable energy through its improved diet.

Photoperiod

In spite of weather, photoperiodism is the outstanding environmental cue for reproductive responses of a seasonal nature. The study of photoperiodic responses has revealed that some developmental processes are controlled by the length of day. Day length can control the annual cycle of oestrous periods. Certainly in the horse, photoperiodic responses are due to the length of daylight per day more than to light quality. Breeding responses induced by photoperiodism can be produced when the length of natural day is extended by artificial lighting of very low intensity. Experiments of this nature have shown that the duration of the photoperiod is more important than the intensity of light.

It has been observed that mares of the Shetland breed, a breed with a very restricted breeding season, can be made to undergo oestrous rhythm by irradiation with strong artificial light. Similarly, it has been shown that Korean mares have been successfully bred outside their normal breeding season following treatment with increased artificial illumination.

The stimulus in the environment for seasonal breeding is long or lengthening daytime. The animal's own physiological characteristics produce the rhythm, and the exogenous factors in the environment initiate the endogenous rhythm. The horse breeding season is in different months in northern and southern hemispheres for these reasons. The breeding season of the horse appears to be controlled not by a single factor, such as periodicity, but by a combination of external stimuli, including behavioural, which act in different ways. Compound stimulation influences the sense organs and the internal rhythms of the individual. Relevant stimulation operates through the exteroceptors, the limbic system, the hypothalamus and the pituitary.

In order to observe the effects of natural photoperiods and their related climates on equine reproduction, the author has collected bulk data on horse breeding in the contrasting geographical locations of the islands of Iceland and Jamaica, over a number of years of visitation and residence there, respectively. The breeding was done in Iceland with herds of mares; each herd having the continuing company of its own proven stallion. In Jamaica, the pasture breeding methods varied. The breeding showed emphatic differences of reproductive seasonality in Iceland, which touches the Arctic Circle, and perenniality in Jamaica, in the tropics. Such differences are largely in accord with general expectation and are illustrated in Figs 10.10–10.13. Verification of this biological feature with recorded data on this scale has not previously been confirmed in contrasting ecologies.

Some interesting factors emerge that relate to sharp seasonality. One is the evident spread of fertile puberty in maiden fillies in Iceland. This may be due, in part, to the short breeding season of 2 months, which may cause slow-maturing females to miss a season or two. Again, a special restraint on breeding is evident in the fact that some brood mares in Iceland miss a year, in spite of spending that season with the herd stallion. Remarkably, these barren mares are the first to become pregnant in the following year, compared with the rest of the herd. The foaling of these previously barren,

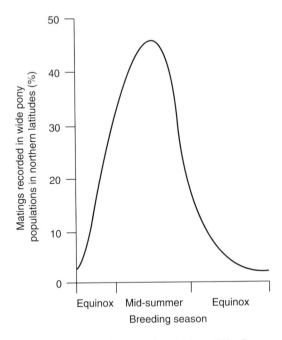

Fig. 10.10. Matings in general population of Nordic ponies (Icelandic, Fiord, Shetland, Highland), showing post-equinoctial breeding season.

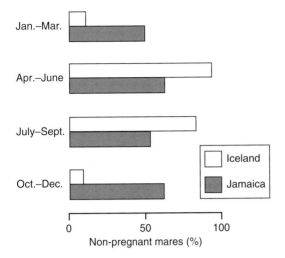

Fig. 10.11. Perennial proportions of non-pregnant mares with an oestrous cycle in the northern and tropical islands of Iceland and Jamaica.

infertile mares usually occurs 1 full month ahead of the others. In addition, the mare that missed a year of breeding is more fertile; as a group, they have a pregnancy rate of 97%, versus 82% in the other group. The data on the latter phenomenon of increased fertility in mares that were barren in the previous breeding season are derived from the Department of Agriculture in Iceland.

In their various breeds, the Nordic ponies, as an equine race, exhibit seasonality in their reproductive functions. Even Thoroughbred stallions show an element of breeding seasonality in their libido. The latter is indicated in their reaction times when taken to an oestrous mare, as shown in Fig. 10.7. Even in the Jamaican mares there appears to be a marginally higher (non-significant) incidence of oestrus in the period from April to June. At the Jamaican latitude of 17°N, there is a slightly increasing amount of daily light and sunshine in that period. This suspicion of minimal equine seasonality in this ecological situation adds some weight to the idea that all horses have an inherent capacity to have their breeding functions sensitized by climatic factors, including photoperiodic change (see Fig. 10.13).

Complexity of equine stimulation

The nature of the light stimulus for the horse in natural seasonal breeding is complex, involving both a daily quantity of light and the relative quantities of light each day, which change daily as the season progresses. In addition, there is light intensity, which increases day by day. It has been known for some time that the relative length of the daily light period is a factor in determining breeding behaviour in some animals. Seasonal breeding, for instance, is largely determined by changes in the daily photoperiod. Light quality and intensity inform the horse of its breeding time; horses begin their sexual activities during that portion of the

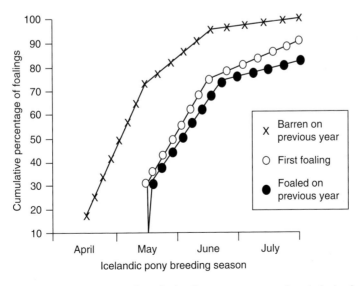

Fig. 10.12. Rates of foaling in three categories of 150 Icelandic pony mares on a farm in Iceland.

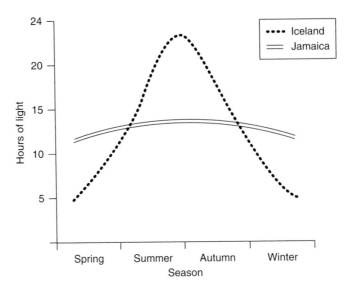

Fig. 10.13. Diagram of contrasting photoperiods on the islands of Iceland and Jamaica.

year when light is becoming stronger and the amount of light time greater each successive day.

Although it is generally believed that daily fluctuations in the photoperiod emphasize the change taking place in daily light supply, it is also clear that a fixed, minimal photoperiod is important. Seasonal breeding can be maintained as long as there is an adequate quantity of light (contrasting with dark) being delivered daily. When the photoperiod fails to provide adequate stimulation for horses, a refractory period develops, during which their breeding behaviour is arrested or diminished in most breeds.

The environment acts as a time-giver for the inherent rhythm. Within each breed or type of horse, the better developed the endogenous factor (or inherent rhythm) the more the time-giver will function merely as a synchronizer. Endogenous rhythm is apparently inherited rather than learned,

such as the dependence of cyclical activity on the internal 'physiological clock'. Some examples of the initiating stimuli include changes in light/dark and light intensity; even the lunar cycles may impart accuracy to the timing of the internal rhythm.

It is very clear that breeding periodicity results from internal and external factors, as discussed. The breeding season depends on the interaction of environment and internal rhythm. In the horse, the facilitation of sexual behaviour is dependent on a wide range of factors, including neural mechanisms, hormones, pheromones and the sensory reception of a variety of stimuli. These bring the animal into a state of breeding capability, which then often overshadows other classes of behaviour by its high degree of motivation. In the case of the Jamaican mares, some were bred to jackasses (to produce mules); however, this did not appear to affect their oestrous motivation, i.e. their receptivity.

11 Mare/Foal Dynamics

The most critical occasion in equine life is the time of parturition and neonatal vitalization. This is spread over 1 full day, in which there is a timetable of numerous behavioural challenges for the mare and foal. In this period there are also various risks to the well-being and life of both. In natural breeding, first births are commonly at 3 years of age. This situation warrants matters of welfare to be focused on it. Included in this requirement are continuous monitoring and knowledgeable attendance to ensure good horse midwifery. An investment of such animal care greatly improves the prospects of a successful equine reproduction (Davies-Morel, 2000).

Vital circumstances precede the actual birth; they are important for a natural delivery of the fetal foal. While these do not allow significant manipulation, they need to be understood in the event that formal obstetrical intervention becomes necessary. Normal fetal activity in the broad pre-partum period needs to be appreciated to create a concept of fetal work preceding its birth. Such work is a demand on the resources of the fetus, even before it is subjected to the intense pressure of expulsion by a singularly powerful maternal subject (Davidson and Stabenfeldt, 2007).

Fetal Behaviour

Fetal activity is a very specialized area of behavioural study. Some 'action patterns' of fetal behaviour appear in the neonate. This shows how some behaviour is the result of truly innate programming. An appreciation of the late prenatal activity of a fetus is enlightening and useful in its optimum management at birth. As an example, the mature fetus engages in a considerable amount of oral activity, including sucking and swallowing. This fact should dispel the notion that the 'suck reflex' of the foal is a phenomenon that comes into existence for the first time postnatally. In the limited space of the uterus, the fetus is able to produce remarkable and various actions. Some of this activity appears in action patterns such as pandiculation. Fetal inertia has been recognized as a condition associated with malposture at birth (Fraser, 1977).

Fetal movements are important, as they probably relate to fetal well-being and perinatal competence. Fetal kinesis indicates forms of movement in confined space essential to normal physical function. Studies on equine fetal kinesis have been based on Doppler ultrasound, scanning ultrasound, physical palpation and radiography. It has been seen in radiography that the principal features of fetal kinesis include simple and complex movements and that the function of terminal fetal kinesis is a radical change of posture (A.F. Fraser et al., 1975).

Some of the terms used in describing fetal actions need to be made clear. The principal terms are posture, position, prone, supine, presentation and righting. The definitions of these and other terms are given below. Posture is the relation of extremities to the trunk (i.e. flexion or extension). Position is a bodily attitude of the fetus in relation to the maternal spine and is chiefly either prone or supine. Prone means situated with dorsum towards the maternal spine. Supine means lying on the back with dorsum towards the maternal belly floor. Presentation is taken to indicate that the fetus is in the birth position, lying in the uterus with respect to the birth canal. When it is in this location and position, with the fetal poll fully into the pelvis, the fetus does not retreat from the pelvis. This is termed engagement. Righting is the complex movement of the fetus during the day before birth, directing the fetus towards the maternal pelvis and resulting in adjustment of the fetal birth posture. Fetal kinesis refers to detectable movement of the fetus. Simple fetal movement means one to three individual actions within the movement. Gross fetal activity refers to mass action in lengthy phases. Complex fetal movement means approximately four to six (or more) individual components in the movement of the fetus. Engagement means that the fetal skull is entirely within the pelvis.

Equine birth posture is achieved through the efforts of terminal fetal kinesis. The latter is characterized by the complex fetal movements in the processes of righting. In its pre-partum activity the fetus is changed in position from the supine to prone. Presentation is occasionally, and probably accidentally, changed from the posterior to the anterior. Postural change is notable in the pre-partum extension of the head and neck and in carpal extension.

The effects of complex fetal movements in subjects at full term involve 'righting behaviour'. In the equine fetus this involves a change from a supine position to a prone position, with the fetal spinal column resting on the maternal abdominal floor. The principal acts in righting behaviour cause a change from general flexion to strategic extension of certain parts. In the equine subject, this occurs before or during first-stage labour.

Further specific postural features of note during the second stage include extension of the head and forelimbs, with compression of the elbows against the thorax. The hindlimbs remain flexed at the stifles and hocks while pushed by uterine and abdominal contractions towards the maternal pelvis. Upon contact with the pelvic brim, the stifles move instantly from full flexion to full extension in association with the hocks, which also convert to extension with the aid of the reciprocal apparatus, described in Chapter 9. The delivery of the hindquarters is much faster in comparison to the forequarters.

Parturient Timing

Over 80% of mares foal at night and they are capable of delaying parturition if unsettled. The mare at parturition delivers a vulnerable neonate into an environment that, under its original conditions, contained predators. Thus the time of parturition appears, in many instances, to be so arranged as to limit the vulnerability of the neonate. Most births take place at night, and the young animals are active and mobilized by morning. It seems that parturient times are arranged in nature so that the neonate will not remain weak and vulnerable for too long but will grow quickly in a period of optimum nutrition and favourable weather. These time factors dictate terms in the equine species and, as a result, some degree of synchronized parturition can be observed. This synchronization may be diurnal or seasonal. The records on the foalings of Icelandic

mares have been studied, with interesting data, illustrated in Fig. 11.1.

Icelandic records of foaling mares that had early access to stallions in free-breeding systems indicate that 3 years of age appears to be the natural age of first foaling (see Fig. 11.2).

Data on the foaling seasons in Icelandic mares show that some brood mares miss a year of breeding,

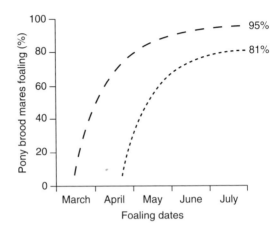

Fig. 11.1. Annual foaling of Icelandic mares classified by prior breeding status. Barren (*n* = 21); gravid (*n* = 120). All mares in same herd (*n* = 141). – – –, Barren in preceding year; - - -, gravid in preceding year.

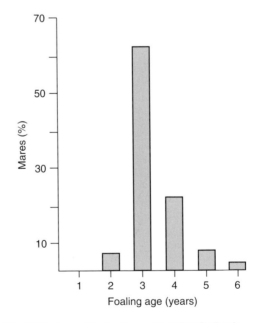

Fig. 11.2. Ages of Icelandic mares at first foaling in records of 218 births.

in spite of being in a herd of mares with a breeding stallion. Such mares have their fertility restored in the following year. In the next breeding season they are evidently the first to conceive and have a higher conception rate than mares that foaled in the previous season. They even had a higher fertility rate than maidens breeding for the first time.

In a study by the author, records were taken on the birth times of Thoroughbred and pony foals. Of these, 30 were fillies and 24 were colts (see Fig. 11.3). Most of the births occurred at night between 6 in the evening and midnight. A smaller number of births occurred just before dawn. A significant number of fillies were born in the evening hours, but the colts tended to be born throughout the later hours of the night. In fact, only 50% of the colts were born before midnight. This pattern of gender foaling times has been confirmed in other observations (see Fig. 11.4). This tendency for female foals to have evening births allows fillies maximum time to find their feet and become capable of running by dawn. Since fillies are more important in reproducing the species than the

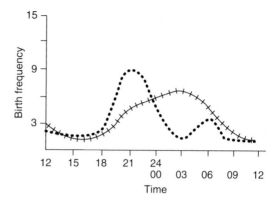

Fig. 11.4. Course of birth times in 106 mares, according to sex of foal. +++, Colts; •••, fillies.

colts, this birth timing arrangement might be a primitive characteristic to ensure the herd's perpetuation; such perpetuation requires that most of the breeding females reproduce. Only about 10% of males ever become involved in natural equine breeding during their lives.

In the interests of equine welfare, it is important to anticipate the time of a foal's birth so that supervision can be planned, as well as assistance provided to the mare or foal should it be necessary. Just prior to birth, the unborn foal is very still. This is after its birth position has been achieved. The full engagement of the equine fetus in the birth canal occurs several hours before birth. This engagement of the fetus creates a lull before the birth storm. The entire fetal head becomes located within the pelvis of the mare when engagement is fully established. Both forelegs are extended (Knottenbelt *et al.*, 2001). Figure 11.5 illustrates recorded foaling times.

There is very clear evidence that the time of parturition is not determined entirely by a fixed gestation period, but is arranged so as to be centred around a period in the early summer in which the nutritional potential of the environment is usually greatest. So it is found that mares mated early in the breeding season will often have a longer gestation period than those bred late in the season. The average gestation period is 8 days longer for mares foaling in the spring than for mares foaling in the autumn. This phenomenon is observed in a considerable variety of breeds. Clearly some temporal factor is utilized by these mares in their time of foaling. It could be that the lunar cycle imparts clues to the timing of an internal rhythm that has an annual register (Schulkin,

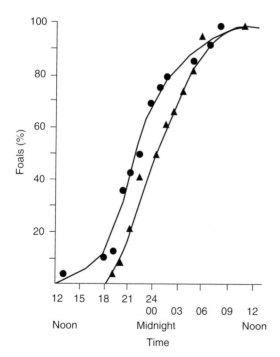

Fig. 11.3. Cumulative frequencies of colt and filly births in diurnal time frame. ▲, Colts (*n* = 24); ●, fillies (*n* = 30).

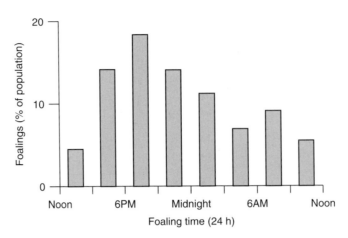

Fig. 11.5. Histogram of foaling times in 180 Thoroughbred mares recorded over a 3-year period in one Canadian stud farm.

1999; Smolensky, 2001). Perhaps the mare needs to sense or experience 12 lunar cycles for optimal control of gestation.

It is general knowledge that gestation in horses is approximately 11 months. Thoroughbred mares in England have an average gestation (based on last service by the stallion) of 340.7 days, with a range of 327–357 days for 95% of the mares. Australian records on the duration of pregnancy in Thoroughbred mares (based on ovulation to parturition) are from 315 to 387 days. Some foals are carried for more than a year. The average gestation period in a wider population gives slightly shorter durations in smaller breeds of horses than in larger breeds. The average gestation for ponies in general is approximately 12 lunar months, i.e. 336 days. Exogenous factors, such as season and nutrition, interacting with endogenous factors, such as the sex of the foal and individual variation of the mare, can affect gestation. For example, well-fed mares have slightly shorter gestations than mares that are on poorer nutrition.

Behavioural Phases of Parturition

Parturient behaviour is characterized by a series of connected episodes. Equine labour is divided into three classical stages. The first stage refers to the dilation of the cervix; the second to the expulsion of the fetus; and the third to foal grooming and the passage of the afterbirth. The behavioural phases of parturition include these three stages of labour, plus other periods pre- and postpartum (Table 11.1).

Oxytocin is the key hormone in the onset of labour, but the obstruction of its effects in equine parturition is phenomenal. It is known that epinephrine (adrenaline) can block the actions of oxytocin, and it is recognized also that epinephrine is freely produced in the roused subject via the sympathetic system. As a result, imminent parturition can be postponed from a time of considerable environmental disturbances to another of minimal disturbance. Many horses in their pre-partum phase are affected by this phenomenon, with 'false starts'. Behavioural signs of approaching birth in stabled mares usually follow a well-established pattern. Increasing restlessness and other evidence of a build-up of pain constitute the predominant indications of the impending birth.

It is of some real value in horse breeding to recognize the span of the pre-partum phase and its end. The time of birth can be correctly anticipated in many cases. Such forewarning facilitates the husbandry of parturient mares and their foals. Physical evidence is of great value in the recognition of impending parturition in mares, but careful evaluation of any behavioural evidence can also be significant in determining the probable end of the mare's pre-partum phase and the imminent birth phase. This initial phase, however, may last for minutes or hours (Gore *et al.*, 2008).

Aside from some reduction in general social activity, there is very little significance in the animal's behaviour in the pre-partum phase until parturition is very close. When parturition is near, free-living mares will separate themselves from the main group and select a site where the birth will

Table 11.1. Principal parturient events in mares.

Immediate pre-partum period	Parturition	Postpartum period
Anatomical changes		
Tumefaction of teats	Cervix enlarges and becomes effaced during first stage	Rapid resolution of any oedema; tumefaction fades from teats and vulva
Cervix reduced to thin, soft ring	Allantochorion ruptures as second stage begins	
Udder distended	Amnion usually remains intact in this stage	Uterine involution is very rapid, and is virtually completed in 8 days
Vulva becomes flaccid		
'Waxing' of teats indicates imminent foaling	Rapid placental dehiscence and expulsion in an inside-out form	
Behaviour		
Becomes shy of interruption	First stage: restlessness, aimless walking, tail swishing, kicking, pawing at bedding, crouching, straddling, kneeling	Lies out flat on side for about 10–20 min
Ceases to eat immediately before foaling		Does not eat fetal membranes, but grooms foal overall
Whisking of tail is shown as first-stage parturition commences	Second stage: lies down to strain powerfully and regularly to expel fetus	Attention directed at foal
Usually withholds birth until night	Birth may have short arrest with vaginal band across forehead of fetus	Reacts to invasion of foal space
	Expulsion lasts 10–30 min	
Miscellaneous		
Pulse rate increases (e.g. to 60)	Parturition often occurs at night (80% of foalings)	Third stage: transfusion of blood from placenta to foal during postpartum pause
Patchy sweating on flanks begins as an early development during first-stage labour	Patchy sweating continues throughout first stage (1–4 h)	Expels membranes within 4 h
	Expulsive (second) stage lasts only 10–30 min	Grooms foal
	'Water bag' (amnion) relatively late in rupturing	Abnormal delay likely to induce metritis/laminitis
		Oestrus shown by 9th day ('foal heat')

occur. Mares at pasture may withdraw from the grazing group when birth is only an hour or two away, but in some cases the mare may simply fail to keep up with the grazing movement. When they are at free-range, mares usually leave their social group or let the group move on, showing varying degrees of isolation at foaling.

Parturition

About 4 h before the birth, sweating is evident at the mare's elbows and on the flanks. Sometimes there is unusually high elevation of the head preceding the initiation of the birth process, namely the first stage of labour. As this commences, the behaviour of the mare includes intermittent restlessness, circling movements, looking around at the flanks, raising the tail and getting up then lying down repeatedly. Feeding ceases abruptly with the onset of this stage.

Increasingly, the mare rises and lies down, rolls on the ground and slaps the tail against the perineum. Periodically in this stage the mare assumes a typical straddling and crouching posture and passes urine at the same time. The mare often shows flehmen soon after the first fluid has been passed. It is clear to an observer that the animal is exhibiting discomfort stemming from within. While physical evidence is of great value in the recognition of impending parturition in mares, behavioural evidence can be more significant in determining the probable end of the mare's first stage and the imminent second stage. The initial stage may last for minutes or several hours, however.

Second stage of labour

During birth, the posture of the dam varies a great deal. In some cases the mother is recumbent throughout birth; in others, there is alternate lying and standing; while in others, lying, standing and crouching may be observed. The duration of the second stage of labour is usually much shorter than the first stage. The transition from first to second is dependent on the opening of the cervix and the escape of uterine content into the vaginal passage. As a result of this development, the outer fetal membrane, the chorion, still adherent to the uterine wall, extrudes into the canal and becomes torn with pressure. When this occurs, the chorionic fluid is released through the birth canal and helps to lubricate it. Some mares investigate the allantoic fluid discharge and may then exhibit flehmen. A tendency to lick the fluid, their skin and nearby objects is common about this time.

In the second stage, straining occurs for the first time. With severe straining now started, the mare soon goes down flat on her side. The straining efforts increase in number and recur more regularly as the second stage of labour advances. The inner sac and the fetus now slip further into the vaginal passage. This allows the amniotic sac, containing the fetus, to bulge through the vagina and enforce more dilation. Now the fetus enters the birth canal. These latter events advance the second stage, accelerating the expulsive efforts of the mare. Repeated straining occurs, with voluntary and involuntary muscular contractions of the abdomen wall and uterus. The manner and degree of straining vary from one mare to another, but in all cases the expulsive efforts become intensified and soon the water bag, or amniotic sac, becomes extruded unburst. The bouts of straining become progressively more vigorous until the foal's feet and nose have appeared outside the vulva.

The fetus is now wedge-like, and this form is quite clearly appropriate for expulsion. There is a postural feature of protective significance. It has not always been recognized that in the natural birth posture, the elbows of the foal remain flexed and retracted, covering a substantial area of the chest. With the elbows bent in this way, the chest is given reinforcement. The chest of the fetus can benefit from this supportive 'scaffolding'. The pressures exerted by the mare during birth are sufficiently great to slow the heart rate of the fetus and even fracture its ribs in rare cases. During the birth the fetal heart rate drops very suddenly when the dam is exerting her full expulsive forces. As the foal passes through the pelvis, the reinforcement of the flexed elbow may be of value to protect heart action in the foal. In addition, the upper leg bones provide support that can protect the foal's chest against the external pressure from the surrounding birth passage when it is being pushed out.

In cases of birth difficulty (dystocia) requiring simple traction, it may be undesirable to apply great force to the forelimbs alone. This will extend the elbow joints and expose the chest wall. Intrapartum pressure on an 'unprotected' thorax could impede heart function in the foal. This could cause cardiac damage or arrest in some cases, if such pressure is continued. With traction, the head should be included with the forelimbs. Any significant amount of traction should be applied equally to the head and the limbs to permit normal posture during the critical stage of expulsion. The value of simple forelimb traction in not questioned in an emergency if the procedure can result in prompt birth. The posture of the fetus with the elbow and shoulder joint extensions as the result of such traction is evidently not the natural one.

Sternal recumbency is maintained with the early expulsive efforts. Many mares stand and change positions as the fetal forelegs and muzzle protrude from the vulva. Severe straining increases now and the mare soon lays down, flat on her side. The straining efforts increase in number and regularity as the process of birth advances further into fetal expulsion. At this time, mares often elevate their extended upper hindlimb during expulsion efforts. Incomplete rolling movements may also occur and this is quite normal; however, birth difficulty or dystocia is shown in very protracted lateral recumbency. Mares, while lying out flat, may periodically lift the head off the ground, turning it towards the flank. This can be evidence of dystocia. Such a sign is a common indicator of a very serious state, one calling for expert intervention (Bertone, 1994). Under natural conditions, prolonged dystocia often proves to be fatal to an unaided dam.

In the course of a normal birth, the difficult passage of the foal's forehead through the taut rim of the mare's vulva opening (the fetal 'head band') causes a delay. Once the head is out, the rate of passage of the foal is accelerated. The shoulders of the foal follow the head in a few minutes. Further straining produces the trunk, and the mare's vigorous straining usually ceases when the foal's trunk is through. Soon after, the remainder of the foal, except its hind feet, slips out. With the fetal hindquarters expelled, there occurs a resting period. Both the mare and foal lie still. The foal's hind feet remain within the recumbent mother's pelvis. The actions of the foal's head now rupture the amniotic sac and the foal breathes. The second stage is then complete, after about a quarter of an hour from its start.

The foal's expulsion is nearly always completed while the mare is in lateral recumbency with legs extended, rarely while standing. The mare usually lies at rest for a further quarter of an hour, with the second stage of foaling terminated. However, an important passive phase is now due, as the terminal phase of the natural second stage of equine parturition.

Postnatal pause

In a postpartum pause, the foal's long umbilical cord is still intact while the mare remains recumbent. This delay before the umbilical cord breaks allows time for the important transfer of about a litre of placental blood to the foal. Severance of the cord prematurely will deprive the foal of considerable blood volume, depriving it of cerebral oxygen as a result of a diminished quantity of blood to the brain.

In time, after its birth, the foal pulls its hind feet free of the birth canal and the membranes. Its movements accomplish severance of the umbilical cord in a natural and normal fashion. The cord breaks about 3 cm from the foal's abdomen. In the postnatal pause, virtually all of the blood from the placenta passes into the foal's circulation. This transfusion is very important for the foal's well-being. Only a small amount of blood remains in the placenta when the cord ruptures after the pause, but 1000–1500 ml of blood can be recovered from the placenta when the cord is prematurely ruptured. This loss to the foal represents about a third of its potential blood volume. Sufficient blood pressure is necessary to fill the capillaries in the lungs and to create the hydraulic pressure needed to expand the lungs to produce proper aeration. Circulatory dysfunction and anoxia can occur if blood pressure is low. Such circumstances are likely to cause one of the various syndromes of neonatal incompetence that go under the term 'neonatal maladjustment syndrome', to be described in Chapter 12.

Some mares may rise from the recumbency of foaling within 5 min, but such mares have usually been disturbed. Most mares do not rise until about 15 min after the birth. Some even remain lying up to 40 min. After the mare eventually rises, she begins a prolonged period of licking her foal. Steady licking may last 30 min. The licking proceeds over the foal's body: first its head and upper surfaces, then its lower surface and limbs. The mare commences her strong social attachment to her foal during this grooming. The association between a mare and her newborn foal allows the blending of their own 'critical periods', when they bond quickly and durably (see Fig. 11.6).

The premature removal of the foal from its own dam to be raised by a human leads to unusual social attachment to humans. The optimum time for an appropriate relationship with humans to be formed in foals is after normal weaning. Since horses are behaviourally competent at birth, interaction of the foal and mare is essential from birth to weaning. If the attachment of humans has been very exclusive, such hand-raised foals may later relate sexually to humans. They resist human control and can become 'problem' animals.

During the critical period, sudden perceptive developments occur. Prompt bonding establishes the maternal–neonate unit, which operates largely in the interests of the foal as it becomes the focal subject of the mare. She now has a new behavioural role with the acceptance and maintenance of the foal. As in some other 'new role' situations, increased and special hormone levels have behaviourally primed the animal. Maternal care develops very quickly and is characterized by collaborative care-giving conduct, directed exclusively to her new foal. In some cases a mare will not accept her foal. Rarely a mare will show aggression to her newborn foal. Such problem cases seldom become resolved and the foal has to be reared as an orphan.

Third stage

Grooming by the mother is an activity that is part of the third stage. It is clearly well-motivated behaviour. Both dam and offspring make specific vocalizations during grooming, and this is important to the development of the maternal neonatal bond. When the newborn has been well attended, the grooming phase ceases. The mare's attention is not constant, however. When not attending the foal, a mare may nibble at hay or straw, smell and lick objects smeared with birth fluids and become occupied with discharging the placenta. She may show some restlessness and signs resembling colic prior to the passage of the fetal membranes. Expulsion of the afterbirth often coincides with grooming and occurs, on average, 60 min after delivery, concluding the third stage of labour. If the

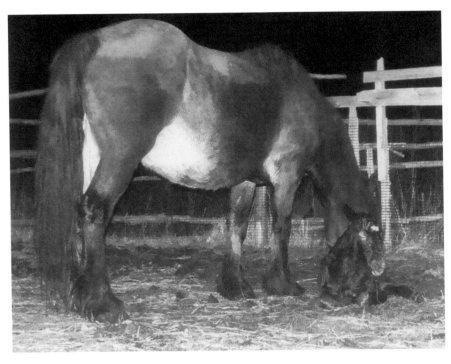

Fig. 11.6. Third stage of parturition: grooming wet foal; placenta emerging. Photo: R. Butler.

afterbirth has not been passed within 4 h, there is a health crisis and emergency veterinary attention is needed to remove the retained placenta and forestall sepsis and laminitis.

A natural and facilitating form of stimulation is manifest in the early care-giving behaviour by the mare, as shown from the time of birth. It seems triggered in part by the taste and smell of the allantoic fluid. Mares sniff the ground where these fluids have fallen and show flehmen. Sometimes they appear to be seeking a foal before labour is completed, once they have received such stimulation. Evidently the maternal behaviour of the mare can become facilitated by olfaction even before birth of her own foal has occurred. Following the birth, odour plays a large part in the establishment of a strong bond between a mare and her newborn foal. This bond is dependent firstly on recognition through odour. Although odour is the principal means by which early recognition occurs between mare and foal, visual recognition soon takes over as the secondary means of mutual identification to facilitate nursing behaviour.

Prior to nursing, the mare grooms the recumbent foal; such grooming can be considered as a component of the mare's third and final stage of the parturient process. The other component of this process is expulsion of the afterbirth. Frequently, this coincides with the grooming of the neonate. The afterbirth expulsion is usually a progressive event, requiring a period of about 5–15 min to be completed after it has started. During expulsion the afterbirth hangs from the mare, eventually reaching the ground. At this point, the mare may tread on it as she moves. This can cause the afterbirth to become stretched and torn. As a result, it is possible for some portion of the afterbirth to be left in the womb when the main part has become separated and discharged. This event may not be known until a raging sepsis develops in the affected mare. To avoid such an accident it is advised practice to tie up the hanging afterbirth so that it does not reach ground level (see Figs 11.7 and 11.8).

Neonatal Foal Functions

After its separation from the mare and its period of being groomed, the further well-being of the foal depends on the successful completion of

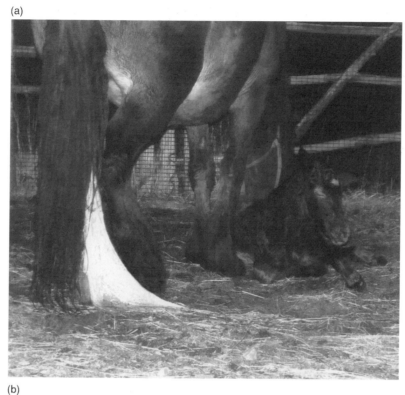

(b)

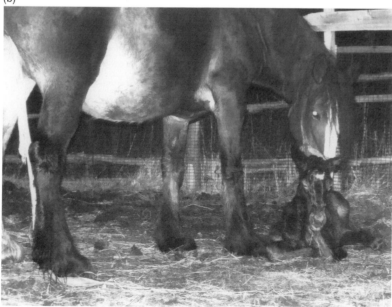

Fig. 11.7. (a) Mare shedding afterbirth. Night photo. (b) Mare standing on stretched afterbirth while grooming newborn foal. Night photo. Photos: R. Harnum.

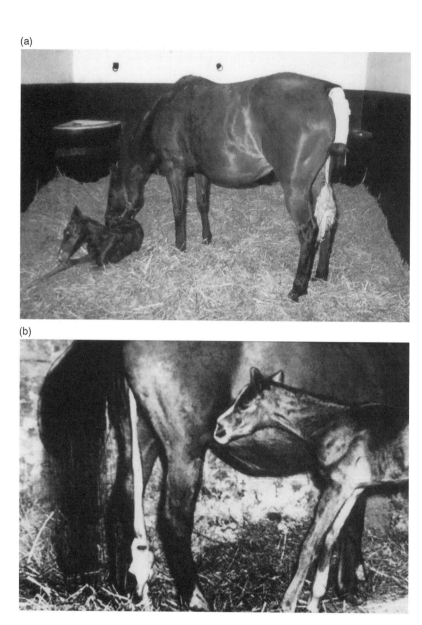

Fig. 11.8. (a) Thoroughbred mare grooming. Foal has one foreleg extended in preparation for first rising attempt. Photo: David Dugdale. (b) First teat-seeking approach. Note tied-up afterbirth. Photo: A.F. Fraser.

several steps in activity development. These follow a fairly specific order. The early steps in this development lead to kinetic competence and nutrition. The order of the six initial antigravity steps is as follows: head raising; sternal recumbency and ear movement; rising and quadrupedal stability; ambulation; maternal orientation; teat-seeking and suckling. The details of the antigravity actions are given in Table 11.2. These steps can be completed in 1 h. Some foals of large breeds may take 2 h to be able to suckle; however, delays beyond this time indicate a serious situation, which calls for assistance to the foal. The foal can be raised, helped to walk and suck the mare. The normal or commonly recognized time schedule for stance and suck is illustrated in Table 11.3.

Table 11.2. Postural characteristics of equine suckling. Equine suckling requires mutual physical fitment in a combination of mare–foal postures, as listed in A and B below.

A. Principal components of foal's nursing posture	B. Principal components of mare's suckling and let-down posture
I Full extension of head and neck with ears back	I Arrest of all other activity
II Some rotation of head towards mare's udder	II Alignment with foal's axis
III Stance in opposite alignment with mare	III Muzzle to foal's rump
IV Close intimate lateral contact with mare	IV Flexion of hind leg opposite to foal
V A slight rotation of hindquarters round mare's forequarter	V Stationary throughout full nursing period

Table 11.3. Times taken by 54 Thoroughbred foals (fillies and colts) to stand securely and to suck after birth (on one stud farm in one season).

Factor	Sex of foals	Number of foals	Mean (min)	Standard deviation	Statistical test
Stand after birth	Colts	24	71.0	30.0	0.02[a]
	Fillies	30	54.4	17.8	0.02
Suck after standing	Colts	24	52.2	32.5	0.31
	Fillies	30	43.5	29.2	0.31
Suck after birth	Colts	30	123.2	49.6	0.03[a]
	Fillies	24	98.0	27.1	0.03

[a]Fillies took less time than the colts ($P < 0.05$). The analyses of times to standing and to sucking suggest that the time from birth to sucking is a continuous process. This observation is based on the smaller coefficient of variation (i.e. SD/mean) for the time from birth to suck than on the time from birth to stand, plus from stand to suck.

After success at feeding, basic functions are programmed into the neonate's activities, consolidating its viability. These functions and their daily incidences are given in Fig. 11.9.

Mare–foal relationship

Following the grooming, the mother has learned much of the identity of her young. Olfactory, gustatory, visual and auditory recognition have become established and will be reinforced thereafter. While the newborn is exploring its immediate environment in the course of teat-seeking, the mare receives its approaches passively. She also shows positive behaviour in accommodating the foal. This accommodation is not always obvious, as superficially the mare's behaviour is one of inactivity. Typically, the mare takes a stationary position immediately adjacent to the newborn and will hold this position, permitting the progressive exploratory approaches of the young animal (see Fig. 11.10). Occasionally the dam may make an alteration in position or stance to correct the young animal's orientation, relative to herself. From this time on, the maternal subject will give care to the young animal and defend it with much intensity, if she has parental drive (Clutton-Brock, 1991). Mares do not immediately know their own foals after birth; however, bonding becomes firmly established in 2 h, and alien foals can be fostered on to mares for up to 3–4 days after birth. Early foal recognition is largely based on smell (Wolski *et al.*, 1980).

The maternal attitude towards the foal resembles recognition of the latter as an extension of herself. The foal facilitates this by maintaining an intimate association with its mother, by vocalizing for assistance or support and by numerous nursing attempts. As a result, the mare is motivated in all her maternal behaviour by a strong maternal

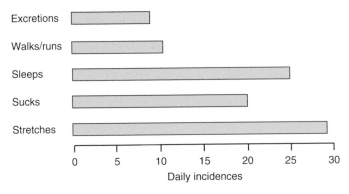

Fig. 11.9. Incidences of basic functions in foals during first 3 days after birth.

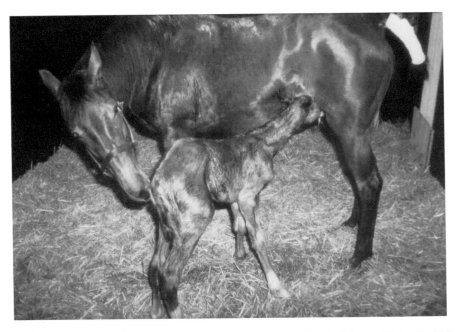

Fig. 11.10. Parturition completed: afterbirth shed; mare in suckling posture; foal in first suck. Photo: David Dugdale.

drive of care-giving behaviour. Socially subordinate mares have less suckling motivation, i.e. poorer epimiletic function. Foals with subordinate mares have interrupted sucklings and do more nuzzling and perisuckling activities, e.g. pushing the udder. Some of these foals have abnormal oral behaviour before weaning, and others, following weaning. Some foals spend twice as much time nuzzling as they do suckling (Nicol and Badnell-Waters, 2005).

Suckling behaviour

The nursing and suckling behaviours relate to the transference of milk from the mammary gland of the mare to the stomach of the foal; this transfer of essential material is not done by simple mechanics. Milk release is dependent on an ejection process in the mare. The milk-ejection reflex is commonly termed the milk 'let-down'. This is associated with a sudden rise in milk pressure in the mammary gland. The full reflex path is a neuroendocrine arc that commences with udder stimulation and passes via peripheral and central nervous systems to the hypothalamus and the posterior pituitary (Nelson, 2000). Here the arc is continued with the output of oxytocin into the general bloodstream and to the udder, where a sudden rise in milk pressure then occurs. With the establishment of this pressure, there is milk 'let-down' and the foal can readily suck out milk.

The mechanism clearly requires initial activation, e.g. by stimulation of the udder by the foal and its presence. It also requires time for oxytocin to circulate in the bloodstream. Although the principal stimulus to milk 'let-down' is undoubtedly local physical stimulation of the mammary gland, there appear also to be visual factors and various other factors, such as odour and, most importantly, conditioning. The let-down of milk can be prevented by stress factors due mainly to epinephrine release. The complex mechanism involved in 'let-down' makes it vulnerable to loud noises or other disturbing stimuli. The resulting release of epinephrine acts directly on the mammary gland (Mason, 1975; Malyshenko, 1982).

Suckling refers to the behaviour of the dam and her foal while feeding. The mare has a unique suckling posture, which relates to the fact that the mammary gland located in the inguinal region is closely suspended. Since the mare's mammary gland is not very accessible, the foal is required to extend and rotate its head and neck to reach it while retaining its 'parallel and opposite' position with the mare (see Fig. 11.11). The mare soon develops a nursing posture in which she flexes the hindlimb on the side opposite to the foal. The effect of this is to tilt her pelvis slightly in such a way that her udder is directed at her foal as it sucks. It appears that this udder-tilting coincides with the milk let-down. Figure 11.9 illustrates incidences of suckling amongst other basic functions.

During suckling, the foal's orientation is not always parallel to the mare's body and not fully in physical contact with her. In these instances of neonatal disorientation, some mares have not cooperated in suckling and the milk 'let-down' may fail.

In the first day of nursing activities, the maternal subject may feed the neonate hourly throughout the day and night, but as the young animal becomes a few weeks old, the mother's nursings may become less frequent. At this time, although most mothers will have accommodated their young on the demand of care-seeking, the maternal–offspring association may undergo some equalization, in which the mother may not permit suckling on every instance.

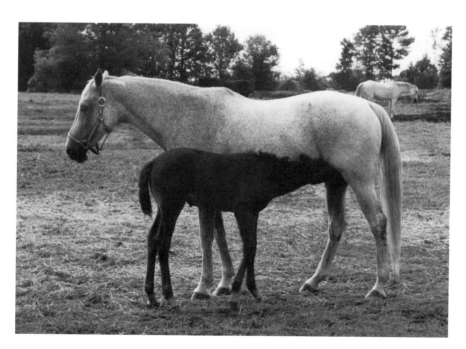

Fig. 11.11. Exact suckling position. Photo: Stefanie Smith.

Weaning takes place naturally at about 9 months of age, but is more usually imposed on the foal at about 6 months of age, or even earlier.

Foals from restricted environments display fear responses to novelty more than foals from groups. Naturally mothered foals in novel situations are much more active and vocal than orphan foals. Unlike foals from naturally reared groups, animals reared in isolation are slow to investigate a stimulus and often turn away to avoid one. Foals reared in isolation usually react negatively to a novel environment, withdrawing and avoiding interaction with it. Different rearing methods influence the response of foals to a novel environment in such a way that experience-deprived foals are deficient in curiosity. A deficit of this nature would not provide the horse as an adult with good survival prospects in a natural environment or make it a good recreational animal.

The exploratory behaviour of experience-deprived individuals, regardless of how it may be initiated, is characteristically brief. Incomplete exploration is a poor basis for adaptation, and an individual with such a deficit must be at a biological disadvantage in many situations. A major law of exploration can be drawn from all of this, along the following lines: experiential deprivation can result in deficiencies in understanding and curiosity; in addition, it may create a greater tendency to fearfulness. The needs of horses are various: some are merely elemental, such as a need for food or water; some are complex, such as a need for territory. Other needs are compound in nature, such as the need for body care and, not least, the need for association. The perceptive need is a collective one, where the requirement calls for multi-sensory stimulation. One of these is a tactile requirement, which has relevance in suckling.

Tactility

The report by de Mazieres (1993) provides evidence that horses can find pleasure in the tactility of grooming, particularly in the lower neck region. In the horse's general associative behaviour, a predilection for physical contact is very evident. Very close contact is a prominent feature in bonded pairs, with both partners contributing touch to the other. In the head overlay, which has already been described as a friendship display, the main feature is firm physical contact involving the ventral surfaces of the head and neck. Mutual grooming is another example of specific tactility in the horse. The bond between mare and foal involves keen bodily contacts (Pycock, 2001). The suckling postures jointly create maximal tactility for the pair. Among horses of inferior social status in a group, actual physical contact with others is avoided and resisted. The avoiders do not participate in the equine custom of readily making contact, in some manner, with others. Between dominant and subordinates, physical contact is not tolerated or attempted. When food is deposited for a group in winter conditions, communal feeding occurs at the site and this involves some physical contacting. Subordinates do not participate until the dominants have left the site (Ingolfsdottir and Sigurjonsdottir, 2008). Mares that are poor with contact do not readily form the intimate 'parallel and opposite' suckling position, and foals at feeding can be left in a slightly misaligned position. Under these conditions, the mare does not usually show the udder tilting and opposite hindlimb flexion of the classical milk-letdown posture. These foals have the nursing difficulties described by Nicol and Badnell-Waters (2005). Tactility is important for foals in their development of confidence (Figs 11.12 and 11.13).

The mare may not always have a good influence on the foal; she may not be properly trained herself. Under such circumstances the mare can exhibit fractiousness and the foal will learn her negative reactions. If the mare has a poor temperament, her foal may have a predisposition to the same. This should not be allowed to become consolidated by bad experience. Very early weaning would be in order in such a case. The foal could then be given an older, placid partner to serve as a more exemplary associate and a model. This might be helpful, to some extent, in modifying the inherent temperament of an aggressive and non-compliant foal. The view is taken, however, that temperament is principally a heritable trait in the horse, stemming from its parentage (McGrogan et al., 2008). At the same time, it is not necessary to have any negative reactivity in the foal reinforced by association with any established disordered behaviour.

The young foal does not graze very efficiently until it is several weeks old. By about the end of the first week of life, however, the foal has begun to nibble food in association with its dam. The essential feeding habits of their mares are learned by the

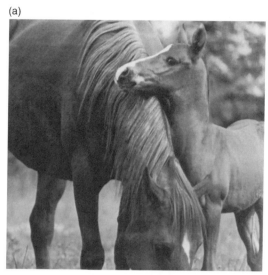

(a)

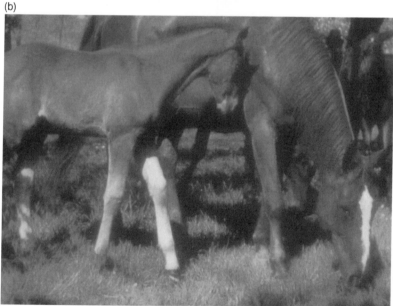

(b)

Fig. 11.12. Tactility in care-seeking aids bonding (epimiletic behaviour). (a) Head overlay. (b) Close contact with mare's trunk. Photos: A.F. Fraser.

young foals. Group size and leadership may also influence grazing by dictating the timing of group feeding.

In the course of their development, young mammals proceed from ingestion by milk sucking to ingestion by chewing. Young foals grazing with their mares will begin to eat grass tops as their capacity for grazing develops. Nursing foals are quick to develop the ability to ingest dry feed presented as a supplement to natural milk. This infant feed is usually a compound, and when it is made available it is usually behind a barrier, below which they can creep but which prevents the mother's access. Rapidly growing foals benefit greatly from the opportunity to supplement their diets by 'creep' feeding and forage-on-offer.

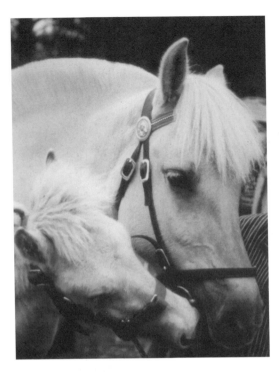

Fig. 11.13. Foal in care-seeking (nose-to-nose contact). Photo: B. Flatlandsmo.

Abnormal Maternal Behaviour

Occasionally maternal behaviour fails to develop with parturition. The mare may fail to show the normal epimeletic or care-giving responses, such as proper grooming and suckling of the newborn foal. Again, a number of abnormalities in maternal behaviour occur as very real forms of aggression towards the newborn. In these aggressive activities the dam will drive the newborn away when it approaches and she may also strike out at it with actions that are injurious to the vulnerable foal. Such maternal rejection of the neonate is a curious syndrome, which has been given no satisfactory explanation regarding its cause, although it has been noted in many different animals. It can be postulated, however, that it might be associated with a neuropeptide deficiency at this critical time (Gibbs, 1986a,b; Insel, 1992). A failure of oxytocin release is a possibility since this hormone has a role in affiliation and is sometimes necessary as a therapeutic supplement in some clinical parturient situations (Pavord and Pavord, 2002). Much of the abnormal rejection of the newborn happens while it is still in its critical period, when imprinting should occur. Such events also deprive the newborn animal of intake of colostrum, which, for optimum passive immunity, should be ingested promptly after birth under stress-free conditions (Gerros, 2002). It is believed that the causes of several neonatal diseases are complicated by such behavioural malfunction. Foal rejection is not a rare event. Houpt and Olm (1984) reported on 23 cases of mares rejecting their foals.

Abnormal Parturition

The term dystocia means difficulty or failure of the parturient dam to effect the delivery of the foal. It is a mishap that can occur occasionally (Mair *et al.*, 1998). Various factors, such as malposture, malposition, an oversized fetus or restrictive pelvic outlet, can cause dystocia. In all such cases the parturient behaviour of the mare remains unproductive. Persistence of the behaviour of pain ends with the establishment of uterine inertia. This condition may rarely be primary but usually it is secondary, developing as the consequence of uterine fatigue and at a rate that varies greatly between individuals. Before the onset of uterine inertia, cases of dystocia are likely to reveal behavioural evidence of the disorder. For example, dystocia is shown in protracted lateral recumbency. Mares, while lying out flat, may periodically lift the head off the ground, turning it towards the flank. This is strong evidence of dystocia. Such a sign is an indicator of a very serious state, one calling for expert intervention. As stated, dystocia often proves fatal to the unaided dam under natural conditions.

Occasionally, in a posterior presentation, two hind feet extend out of the birth canal (Fig. 11.14). The soles of the fetal hooves are directed inwards, covered with the gelatinous, protective pads, the eponychium. Again, on occasion, the fetal tail can appear in a case of breech presentation. All abnormal presentations require expert attention.

On rare occasions, mares may have twins (see Fig. 11.15). They usually suffer from some degree of dysmaturity; one being more affected than the other. The latter may survive, but the less mature foal commonly dies in spite of receiving good care. For this reason, mares of value are sometimes examined a while after breeding to detect for twin embryos; if discovered, one is ruptured.

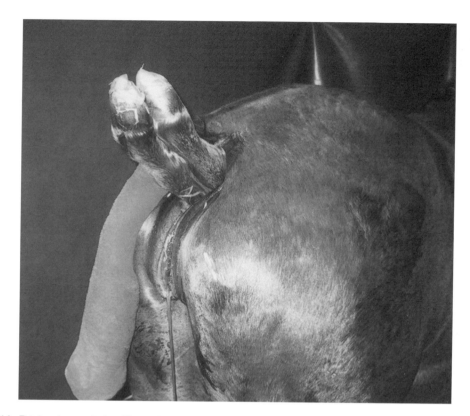

Fig. 11.14. Fetal malpresentation. Photo: David Dugdale.

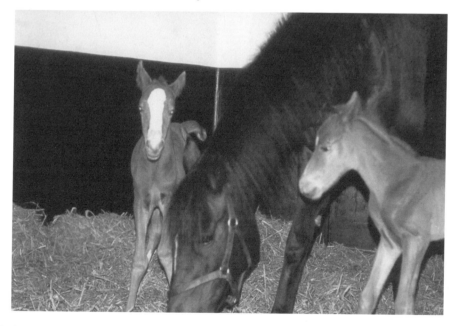

Fig. 11.15. A rare event: twin foals showing a promising degree of viability. Note one foreleg not yet straightened. Photo: David Dugdale.

Welfare Addendum

1. In the course of supervising an equine birth, an attendant should not interfere with the normal process of fetal expulsion or foal behaviour unless the norms of these developments are not occurring.

2. If the foal's head is not passing through the rim of the vulva after numerous expulsive attempts by the mare, she can be assisted by manual expansion of the vulva, stretching its upper rim and forcing it over the forehead of the foal.

3. Assisting the foal to stand is justified after a third fall by the foal in its rising attempt. The foal's tail can be gripped to lift its hindquarters. The thorax can then be raised by hand.

4. Premature separation of the umbilical cord from the placental membranes is ill-advised. The traumatically severed cord can leak 100–200 ml of blood from the foal.

5. The 'postnatal pause' precedes antigravity tonicity and should not be interrupted (see text).

6. Any sign of illness in a newborn foal should be regarded as an emergency and such a foal requires intense professional care (Freeman and Slusher, 2002).

12 Foal Function and Welfare

Many endeavours in the care of a foal are the work of the mare, but that is not the end of this essential service. Human participation is also needed (Palmer, 2007). For example, immediate attention should be paid to the clearance of the foal's nostrils at birth. Its respiratory tract might be blocked with thick fluid, and assisted respiration may be needed. The foal can be lifted up by the hind parts; gravity may clear the air passages. If there is no heartbeat, brisk rubbing of the foal's chest can stimulate heart action by expressing blood out of the heart repeatedly. Insertion of a tube into the trachea and strong suction can help some desperate cases of breathing difficulty. A simpler method in an attempt to stimulate breathing is to run a straw up the foal's nostril. Oxygen can be given if breathing is delayed.

Sometimes attention to the foal is required before it is born. Antenatal care for the mare has benefit for the foal. During her pregnancy the mare should receive good nutrition and health support. Regular worming is required. A special worming treatment should be provided before foaling in the interest of the foal in its first weeks of exploring around the mare and her droppings. For similar reasons, the mare should be made clean before foaling (Davidson and Stabenfeldt, 2007).

Immunity

Some critical need for vaccination of the mare may occur at a time or in a place of an infectious outbreak. In addition, it is desirable to have the mare's immunity against tetanus, influenza and strangles boosted about a month before the estimated foaling date (an intranasal vaccine against influenza can be administered easily with an applicator and is very effective in generating immunity). The mare's immunity from vaccination will be passed on, to some degree, to the foal via the colostrum (Yang and Glasser, 2000). Such vaccination can be of great value to the foal indirectly and it also provides health support to the mare. Close to her foaling date, the mare's level of general immunity (which will go into her colostrum prior to the birth) can be determined by a laboratory test of her blood serum. This test could reveal any anti-red blood cell (RBC) factors if present. Such anti-RBC immunity will seriously affect the foal if it drinks the mother's colostrum (Gore et al., 2008).

The activities of the mare, including any forced exercise, should be of a controlled nature during the late stage of pregnancy. The mare has a form of placentation that is unique to the equine species (epitheliochorial). Her placenta has a diffuse and intimate contact between the lining of her uterus and the outer fetal membrane. When the fetus is large and surrounded with its supportive fluids, the uterus has a heavy load. If the mare is very active in the late stages of pregnancy, this load can put a strain on the placentation. Fast galloping in an advanced stage of pregnancy may cause a placental injury. Such injury can cause a slight separation of the outer fetal membrane from the uterine lining. In the event of such placental injury, there can be a fairly large leakage of blood from this membrane, which in reality is part of the fetal foal's circulatory system. Fetal blood cells, including RBCs, will then come into contact with the mare's womb. They will be absorbed from there by the mare's circulatory system and will pass to her immune system. If the mare and the foal have the same type of RBC, this simple, but unnecessary, accident will cause no problem. Should the foal have a blood type differing from the mare's, the RBCs will be detected as foreign matter by the mare's immune system. Antibodies against the foal's RBCs will be produced in response by the mare and ultimately secreted into her colostrum. Since there is no mixing of whole blood between the mare and the fetus across the microcotyledons (the units of nutrient exchange in the placenta), the fetal foal will continue to develop normally. It will be unharmed by the antibody that has been produced by its mother to destroy its different RBCs.

When the foal's blood group is not the same as its mother's, it is because the stallion and mare have different groups and the fetus has acquired the stallion's group. Horses have nine blood groups. When the mare's blood type is A/Q negative and the stallion's is A/Q positive, the foal can be A/Q positive. On exposure to these alien factors carried on RBCs, the mare produces antibodies to A/Q positive RBCs. At the time of imminent birth, the mare's antibodies accumulate in her udder's secretions to form colostrum. By this means the newborn normally acquires immediate and valuable immunity to the infections or vaccinations that the mare has endured. With its mother's colostrum absorbed, the foal can face its mother's infected world. With antibodies to its RBCs in its mother's colostrum, however, the foal's fate is in doubt. It will suffer destruction of its RBCs (haemolysis) if it drinks its mother's colostrum. Only expert intervention can possibly save it if the problem is recognized. If such a foal is left with its mother for company, it must be muzzled for 36 h, by which time the danger of haemolytic disease will have passed.

Haemolytic disease

The first signs of haemolytic disease may be seen as early as 8 h or as late as 5 days after birth. The foal, once active, becomes lethargic. It shows laboured breathing, disinclination to stand or to feed from its mother. It has a pounding heart; its urine becomes blood tainted; and the interior of its mouth shows jaundice. Badly affected foals can die within 1 to 2 days of this disease – neonatal iso-erythrolysis (Ahmed and Schurig, 2007).

The condition is extremely uncommon in young mares. Repeated placental injuries are needed to boost the mare's immunity to danger level in successive pregnancies. In large measure, it is a Thoroughbred problem, although it can occur in other breeds. It can be anticipated by a test of the mare's blood serum or if she has shown this problem previously. The foal can be taken from its mother at birth and fostered for 36 h or it can be bottle-fed with stored and safe colostrum during this time. Frozen colostrum must be thawed carefully. It must never be thawed by microwave, as this would destroy the immunoglobulin content. About 3 l (6 pints) of pure colostrum should be given in four doses in the first 10 h of the foal's life.

The mare should be repeatedly milk-stripped by hand. In 36 h she will be safe and her foal can be returned to her.

Foals that are not too seriously affected by this condition of haemolysis should be quickly treated with antibiotics and kept comfortably rested until their RBC levels have been returned to normal. Severe cases will require a blood transfusion to survive. Whole blood from the mare or sire cannot be used, as the foal has absorbed immunity against its father's blood, while the mother's blood can only do more and final damage. One technique that has been found to be effective (if all the technology is available) is to transfuse the foal with saline-washed RBCs from its mother.

Neonatal protection

The question of the foal's immunities being derived from its mother is an important matter. If the foal does not suckle the mare quickly and thoroughly in its first few hours of life, it may not receive the full benefit of the immunity factors in the milk. Some mares leak too much colostrum before the foal is born or able to suck, and this depletes the antibody content of her milk. Again, some mares may not provide all that is needed to give the foal protection in its environment. Added protection against infection may be desirable for the newborn foal. A special method of giving the foal its mother's immunity is to transfer an amount of the mother's blood plasma into the foal's bloodstream by veterinary attention. Alternatively, plasma can be obtained from another horse living in the same stable since it would probably have a general immunity similar to the mother. Any donor must be in good health. Plasma can also be purchased commercially. When the foal is 1 day old, its blood can be tested to determine if it has good immunity. Cover against infection can be given by way of an antibiotic injection to the foal immediately after its birth (Koterba et al., 1990a,b).

Another prophylactic procedure, which should be routine, is quick antiseptic treatment of the foal's umbilical stump. Any good antiseptic can be used. The traditional method is to soak the stump with tincture of iodine. This can be done by putting a small glass of tincture of iodine over the cord remnant, holding it firmly against the abdominal connection – the navel – and shaking the iodine around this site. The iodine is antiseptic and it also dries the remnant of cord. This can be followed later with an antibiotic spray over the area. If the spray is coloured, the area treated can be better seen. This can be repeated daily. Hygiene in the foal's environment is an extremely important practice to prevent foal sickness (Gregory, 2004).

An untreated umbilicus is an open route for infection. This infection will later cause such joints as the hock and knee to become inflamed. It can create sepsis elsewhere and cause septicaemia. A particular form of septicaemia in foals can develop in the first week of life from mixed bacterial infection from the immediate environment. Affected foals show increasing weakness, loss of the suck reflex, an inability to stand, diarrhoea, then coma and death. Preventative measures against this septicaemic disease include good hygiene at foaling, disinfection of the umbilicus and navel (as described) and the administration of a prophylactic antibiotic (as mentioned above). The navel can be repeatedly treated over the first few days for antisepsis.

Diarrhoea in young foals is a serious matter (O'Connor, 1987). It can indicate enteritis from a specific bacterial infection (Grinberg et al., 2003). Again, an unhygienic environment can be the source, although at times the overconsumption of milk can be the cause. Prompt treatment with electrolytes is needed to deal with the fluid loss, and appropriate antibiotics will be needed also.

A catalogue of potential diseases in foals as they grow older cannot be given here. This is a vast sphere of veterinary medicine. It can be emphasized that good care takes into account the maintenance of hygiene, and close monitoring of the foal and mare for evidence of normal behaviour. Illnesses begin with a departure from normal activities or normal appearances. It is therefore of vital importance to know what is normal in both respects and for veterinary attention to be quickly obtained when abnormality is observed (Russell and Wilkins, 2006).

Activity Norms

Of particular importance is the normal series of events indicating vitality in the foal. Irregularities here can indicate the need for the speedy provision of procedures for foal care. Human intervention can be imperative in such ways as assistance to the newborn foal during its standing attempts (after it has repeatedly failed to the point of exhaustion) or to suck (when it has failed in teat-seeking). The root of the foal's tail can serve as a handle. With

the tail grasped, the foal's hindquarters can be raised and supported until the foal is up on all its legs and standing steady. By holding the tail with one hand and steering with the other hand on one side of its chest, the foal can be guided to the mare's udder and then pressed against her side for full contact to be established.

At times, an indifferent mother may need to be held for the foal. A hostile mare may need to be restrained with a foreleg up to help the foal teat-seek and suckle. In any crisis of this type, the full knowledge of normality will make clear what should be happening. Any delay or difficulty in defecation in the foal has to be treated as a critical matter. An enema of a commercial type can be used or veterinary treatment may be necessary. Some horse breeders give enemas to all newborn foals as a matter of routine. The early clearance of meconium is vital (Koterba et al., 1990a,b).

The newborn foal behaves in a set pattern of development. Initially it rotates on to its sternum, makes struggling leg movements, tilts its face upwards and displays erect ears. Rising attempts soon follow in an antigravity drive after birth, as indicated in Chapter 11. The foal attempts to become upright, with antigravity tonicity obtained. In these standing attempts, it will fall several times, but its efforts continue. The newborn pony foal is usually stable on its feet within half an hour of birth, while larger breeds usually take longer. Once securely on its feet and able to move around, the foal begins to pay keen attention to its immediate environment (Fig. 12.1) and to its mother in particular. The mother responds positively, and from then on there is a balanced reciprocity between mare and foal in the attention they pay to each other. Almost all of the foal's activities are initially concerned with teat-seeking. In its teat-seeking activity, the foal's actions are initially random in their direction; a certain amount of exploratory activity is required before the mammary region of the dam is found (see Fig. 11.10).

Many breeders of horses are in favour of mares foaling in the open. With most mares at pasture foaling at night, their foals are able to trot and move well by daybreak. In all events, a mare keeps her newborn at her side and greatly limits the direct contact her foal has with other horses. This facilitates the maternal protection of the foal. The full suckling link-up between mare and foal is a vital development that contains several features providing evidence of mutual well-being. This suckling

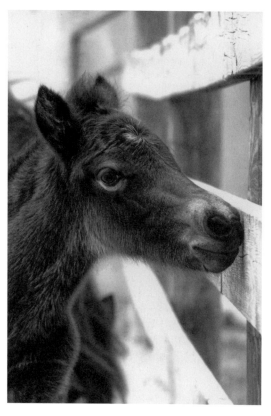

Fig. 12.1. Neonatal foal investigating its immediate environment. Photo: Melanie MacDonald.

its mother, moving under her neck, tail and body. Tactile contact is a feature of the foal's relationship with its dam. Early environmental experiences affect later well-being (Gluckman *et al.*, 2005).

Survival of the foal depends on the successful completion of several steps in activity development according to a fairly specific time schedule. The initial steps in this development lead to kinetic competence and nutrition. The goal is primary mobility. As previously indicated, the steps, collectively, are: (i) head raising; (ii) recumbent coordination; (iii) rising and quadrupedal stability and defecation; (iv) ambulation; (v) maternal orientation; and (vi) teat-seeking and suckling. These behavioural steps can be done in 1 h and normally should be completed well within 3 h (see Table 12.1).

When ingestion of colostrum has been achieved, the development of the foal enters a further series of steps relating to consolidation. In these consolidating steps the foal lies, sleeps, rises, stretches its legs and urinates. Except for urination, some of these latter activities can occur by the second hour of postnatal life. Increasing coordination of physical activities is featured during this time, such as sudden short runs and little jumps. Such activity is termed saltation, which has been described in Chapter 7. Deficits in all of these norms would indicate a need for intensive care, such as assistance to rise, to ingest milk or an enema to pass fetal

link-up includes the behavioural features described in Chapter 11.

It is in the first few hours postpartum that mare and foal learn to recognize one another. This recognition is based on their full senses, using visual, auditory, olfactory, gustatory and tactile clues. The mutual recognition becomes the basis of the intense, close attachment that typifies the relationship between the mare and her foal from the outset of the latter's life (Houpt, 2002). For the neonatal foal's life, the initial behaviour of its mother is vitally important. The dam's care helps adjustment to the particular environment into which the foal is born. The dam becomes very protective of her newborn foal if any intruders approach. Sheltering and herding of the foal is exhibited keenly. An increase in aggression heralds the intensely protective attitude that the dam will later show regarding her foal. For its part in the reinforcement of the bond, the foal makes a great deal of physical contact with

Table 12.1. Epigenesis of antigravity tonicity (AGT) in the newborn foal.

Sequence of AGT items	Specific behavioural items of antigravity tonicity
1	Rotation on to sternum from lateral recumbency
2	Raising head and slight elevation of neck
3	Erection of ears from floppy state
4	Foreleg extension forward
5	Partial elevation of hindquarters
6	Head and neck upwards extension
7	Elevating thrust of hindlimbs
8	Full hindlimb extension and forward stretch of forelimbs
9	Initial attempt to stand on all limbs in half-up position
10	One, two or three falls and re-risings
11	Stability of stance on all limbs
12	Some tentative steps forward, then competent walk

faeces (meconium). Behavioural evidence of retained meconium is persistent tenesmus, the straining to defecate (Fig. 12.2). Congenital anomalies can be present in rare cases and confound development. Veterinary examination would be needed to identify these and advise on humane action in each given case (Beech, 1985).

Well-being in the foal is established when each of the neonatal norms has been achieved. The chief indicators of foal well-being include standing, suckling, defecation and holistic stretching. Full stretching follows the first episode of sleep, about 2–4 h after birth, and is shown either lying or standing as follows: extension of limbs, throwing back the head and neck, and stiffening the trunk and spine. Some of these actions are key events and deserve some detailed emphasis, as illustrated in Tables 12.2–12.4 and Figs 12.3–12.6.

Once the ability to rise and stand is complete, oral activity emerges (Nicol and Badnell-Waters, 2005). By trial-and-error activities the foal locates and investigates the mare's limbs and ventral regions, the mare's inguinal region and ultimately her mammary gland. The trial-and-error activities in the foal's teat-seeking behaviour are often extended over a substantial period of time. With highly successful foals it may be complete within 30 min. In others it may take several hours. Yet in other, rare instances, there may be total failure. In the phases after sucklings, most foals engage in sudden jumps or short runs; this type of spontaneous, sudden activity is evidence of competent activation.

A number of foals suffer retention of meconium. If this problem is not relieved promptly, the foal will soon develop a painful colic that can have a fatal result. Monitoring the norms of newborn foals is of particular value in the management of valued horses, when intensive care, if it is to be given to the young foal, must be provided promptly (Morresey, 2005) and good nursing given (Coumbe, 2001).

When maternal adoption has occurred and the foal has been suckled, it consolidates itself with more food, rest and exercise. The foal will have had its first sleep by 3 h. Sleep usually occurs after feeding, as well as some investigative acts or sudden bursts of activity. The latter often take the form of bucking, short runs or jumps. Sleep episodes are often of 20–25 min duration, lying in flat-out recumbency. During the first week, foals spend most of the day resting and sleeping. In the second week they rest and sleep half of the time. Paradoxical sleep is most noticeable, as a result of rapid eye movement

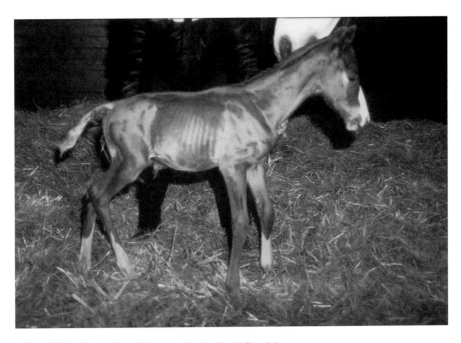

Fig. 12.2. Foal straining with swollen abdomen. Photo: David Dugdale.

Table 12.2. Timing of primary neonatal functions in foals of various breeds.

Primary functions	Time (min)
Head lifting and shaking	1–5
Sternal recumbency after chest rotation	5–10
Ear erection and mobility (ears pendulous at first)	5–10
Rising attempts (several)	10–20
Stance attained firmly	25–55
Walking	30–60
Defecation (passage of meconium)	30–60
Oral actions of a sucking nature	30–60
First successful suck and intake of milk	40–120

Table 12.3. Normal order and timing of the secondary neonatal functions in ponies.

Order	Functional activity	Features	Modal time postpartum (h)
1	Walk	Brief trot	0.5–1
2	Sleep	Session 20 min	1–2
3	Pandiculation	After sleep	2–3
4	Saltation	Spontaneous jumps	2–4
5	Urination	After three or four suckings	4–6

Table 12.4. Norms for quantitive functions in newborn foals.

Function	Normal frequencies (per day)
Number of urinations	4–10
Number of defecations	3–5
Number of walks	8–14
Duration of sleeps	20–25 min
Number of sucks	18–24
Duration of sucks	25–58 s
Number of pandiculations	40–60

and jerking of limbs. In this deep sleep they can be difficult to rouse and they clearly experience much more sound sleep than adult horses do.

Pandiculation

Attention should be paid to the phenomenon of systematic stretching in the equine neonate since this appears to relate to physical competence and well-being. Vigorous stretching actions involving the head and neck, the trunk, forelegs and hindquarters are performed by young foals numerous times daily from the first day of life onwards, using both extensor and tensor muscles. These inherent actions ensure that all major body parts of the foal are systematically extended, tightened and exercised, even without much locomotion of the foal.

Newborn foals sometimes have stiff or bent joints after their restrictive period in the womb. The systematic stretching assists the young foal in its orthopaedic development. This stretching occurs as brief exercises, performed quite casually when the foal is relaxed and undisturbed. These actions need a quiet and peaceful environment and are usually performed on rising after rest. Most stretching occurs as a series of actions as follows: flexion at the throat, arching of the neck, straightening of the back, elevation and movement of the tail, plus full extension of the

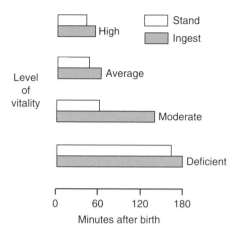

Fig. 12.3. Times taken for newborn foals to stand securely and suck successfully as indices of vitality.

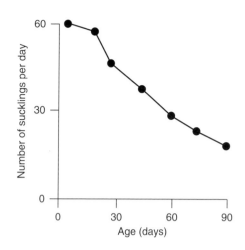

Fig. 12.5. Common suckling frequencies in foals up to 3 months of age.

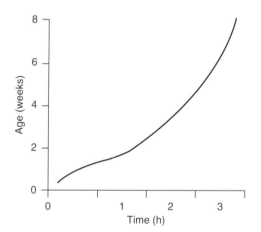

Fig. 12.4. Increasing durations of sleep periods commonly occurring in young foals.

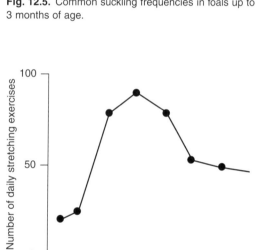

Fig. 12.6. Exercise by stretching in foals up to 7 days old.

forelimbs and then the hindlimbs. Extension of each hindlimb singly or in sequence is a related exercise.

This stretching phenomenon is termed pandiculation in human medicine. This stationary activity is vital to a foal's growth and joint correctness. It has as much effect on tendons, bones and joints as on muscles in the course of performance. An orthopaedic role for this is obvious. It is needed for self-development in the young animal, even more than in the adult. In fast-developing foals it is essential.

Foals that are most healthy perform pandiculation most often, about 50 times per day. Stressed or sick foals do not pandiculate vigorously or frequently, if at all. It is therefore a clear sign of good health and its absence a sign of illness. It is a positive signal of equine neonatal well-being.

Stretching usually occurs after the first deep or true sleep. A common time for this is about 4 h of age. Before the end of day one, foals sleep and stretch regularly. They frequently stretch during

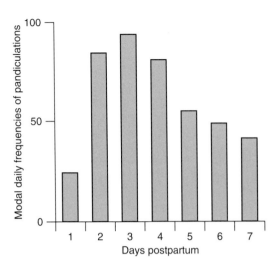

Fig. 12.7. Histogram of daily norms in Thoroughbred foal pandiculation in first week of life. Note general tonicity.

- Both hind legs extended straight out with both forelegs bent at the knees.
- Both forelegs extended straight out with hind legs resting flexed.
- Both hind legs and upper foreleg extended straight out with lower foreleg lying flexed at knee.
- Limbs outstretched, head and neck outstretched.
- Limbs outstretched, head drawn in to breast area.

Defecation

A vital part of the newborn foal's early functions is defecation. The foal normally passes the fetal faeces (meconium) about an hour after birth. With its first ingestion of milk, the foal's alimentary tract is fully operational, with peristalsis. Such propulsive action induces the expulsion of the material that has accumulated in the fetal intestines from prior physiological secretion and the swallowing of amniotic fluid. The meconial material may not be particularly soft at times, on account of its period of storage, and its expulsion can require some effort by the neonatal foal, whose abdominal musculature has not yet been strengthened by any significant exercise of the trunk. Occasionally the peristalsis only causes the meconium to become impacted in the terminal gut and the foal is unable to pass the material on schedule. It may succeed with a delayed defecation in a further hour or two, but failure is also possible. This can result in the potentially fatal pathology of total blockage of the large intestine. Behavioural evidence of this is the aforementioned tenesmus (Spiers, 1997), in which the animal persists in attempts to empty its terminal bowel. The straining is severe and the affected foal becomes distressed and increasingly weakened. A crisis has now developed (Madigan, 1991). Employment of enemas often resolves the problem if administered as soon as a delay is evident or when tenesmus has begun. In extreme cases surgery would be necessary, and veterinary evaluation of the foal's condition would determine this. Meconium can be recognized by its colour. It is not the usual colour of foal faeces, being blackish or greenish (Pavord and Pavord, 2002).

sleep and during recumbency, as well as in the upright position. Stretching becomes significantly more frequent over days two, three and four (see Fig. 12.7). This is precisely the time when the foal's legs straighten, if they have been born with contracted tendons. Episodes of stretching may occur while the foal is standing or lying and they may be full or partial in their display. The variety of performances is evident in the following list.

Stretching acts in foal behaviour (eyes closed in most cases)

Standing upright with:

- Neck upraised and head pulled down close to breast area. Back straight.
- One hind leg and then the other extended to the rear. Neck arched. Back straight.
- Both hind legs extended to the rear. Neck arched. Back straight.
- All four legs straight and stiff, with neck arched and head pulled in to breast. Back straight.
- All four legs straight and stiff with back 'humped' and head pulled in to breast.
- Both forelegs and head outstretched.
- Standing with head outstretched and yawning.

Lying outstretched on one side with:

- All four limbs stiffly extended straight out at right angles to the body.

Sidedness

When they are lying out flat, most foals lie on one particular side. They usually maintain this one-sidedness throughout the first week of life. By the second week they adopt the opposite side for lying on for a day or two, after which they alternate their lying sides randomly. A minority of foals will persist in lying on one side exclusively throughout the first 2 weeks after birth. In these cases the lower limbs do not get stretched to the same extent as the upper limbs. These foals could benefit from being turned over, especially if a lower leg is not perfectly straightened, as in contracted tendons or minor states of valgus or varus, in which the limb is slightly bent outwards or inwards. Some horses remain one-sided in their preferred actions until this is trained out of them, e.g. unable to change a lead. McGreevy and Thomson (2006) found persistent motor laterality in numerous performance horses. Among many Thoroughbreds, they found a strong preference for left laterality.

Birth Trauma

Failure to meet the temporal norms in neonatal development is common in a non-infectious condition of foals, which is termed the neonatal maladjustment syndrome (NMS). This condition includes abnormal foals commonly termed barkers, dummies, wanderers and convulsives. Foals with NMS are characterized by failure to develop or by very late development in activity or consolidation. Their appearance at birth is normal, but the signs of maladjustment soon appear. The first sign is loss of attachment to the mare and loss of sucking ability. The syndrome progresses into hyperexcitability, apparent blindness, grinding of teeth, aimless wandering and severe muscular contractions. Some of these foals also make barking sounds. Extended rigidity develops, before recumbency and coma. NMS occurs chiefly in Thoroughbreds, but it may appear in similar breeds.

The immediate cause of NMS is known to be brain damage, including haemorrhage. It is believed that this is due to increased blood pressure within the skull during birth. Now it is known that chest damage can be involved. Half of NMS cases die. Less severely affected cases can survive with intense care. The latter would include supplemented ventilation, artificial feeding, warmth, fluid supply, rotation of the foal's body regularly and physical assistance in movement. As to the mental competence of survivors, nothing is known. The condition draws attention to the intrapartum care of foals, and of Thoroughbred foals in particular. A danger point occurs when the vulvar rim

is tight around the neck of the fetus. Severe lasting pressure on the neck can result in haemorrhages in the eye (Munroe, 1999, 2000a). Additionally, damage to the hyaloid apparatus can occur (Munroe, 2000b). Hypoxia in the newborn foal can cause severe brain damage (Kaur and Ling, 2009).

No other breed of horse obtains the foaling assistance given to the Thoroughbred. In some studs, foaling teams of staff are on hand around the clock during the foaling season (winter–spring). Thoroughbred foals can have great commercial value – hence the close attention.

The mare's birth canal needs some time to expand fully for delivery. The fetal head can do some of the work to effect this expansion bit by bit, while the shoulders will cause further expansion. A time factor is involved in this process. A reasonable period of labour must be permitted to prepare and dilate the cervix, vagina and vulva for the natural passage of the fetus. Traction on the fetal foal's limbs is a common form of assistance at foaling. If this is applied too hastily or too vigorously, there will be an above-normal pressure on the foal's head, neck and chest as it is drawn through the birth passage. It is already known that there can be severe damage to the foal's rib cage during birth by forced leg traction (Jean et al., 1999; Rossdale, 1999).

Premature traction on the fetal foal must now be seen as a dangerous routine. The normal birth process described in the chapter on foaling can be taken as the norm. Outside of that norm, assistance may be necessary, but if the birth is progressing normally it could be wise to let nature take its course. Assisted deliveries are a minefield of disputation, but caesarean section in the mare, if this is the alternative in equine dystocia, is a major undertaking and difficult to organize on short notice at present. It is an option, however, in equine dystocia cases that are intractable and constitute an emergency (Orsini and Divers, 1998).

Orphan Foal Care

Some unfortunate foals may be orphaned or unable to keep to the development timetable through a deficiency in the mare's milk supply. In either case there is a feeding crisis for the foal, requiring an immediate course of action. It is important for the foal to receive colostrum within the first 10 h after birth. It could be administered by a feeding bottle. The foal should also be kept warm and comfortable.

Ideally a foster mare in milk could be found for the motherless foal. A mare with a placid disposition would be best, but a milking mare suitably controlled could feed the foal in a crisis. The foal and the foster mare should be supervised at all times until a bond is formed.

In the absence of a nurse mare, a milking goat can be used, as horses and goats can accept each other. The goat can be held on a raised surface to allow the foal access to the goat's udder. The foal would need to be taught to feed in this situation. Artificial mare's milk can be obtained commercially if fostering fails. The foal should be fed by bottle at regular intervals of about 2 h for the first 2 weeks of life. As it gets older, it could be fed at longer intervals, with greater amounts of milk each time. The feed should be warm for the young foal. A suitable starting quantity is 250–500 ml (0.5–1 pint) per feed. Eventually the foal should be given 10% of its body weight per day.

By 1 month of age, an attempt should be made to get an orphan foal to drink its ration of milk from a clean bucket. This simplifies the feeding work. The foal should be given an animal companion, ideally a small pony. When it is weaned it should be put in suitable equine company to prevent any unhorse-like behaviour from developing, such as non-compliance with humans in training or use (Sondergaard and Ladewig, 2004).

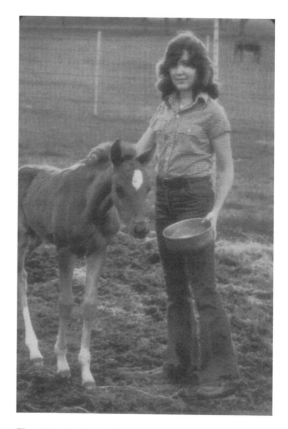

Fig. 12.8. Early gentling. Photo: Anonymous.

Protective Foal Care

All foals should receive human contact on a regular basis as soon as possible (Spier *et al.*, 2004). They will follow their mothers while the mares are being led for exercise. This is a useful first step. They can then be haltered in a few weeks and progressively handled. Early gentling takes the stress out of training at a later age (see Fig. 12.8).

Vaccination of the foal can be started at about 10 weeks of age (Cymbaluk, 2002). Worming young foals is very important; it is vital to worm them against bloodworms and roundworms (Valla, 1994).

By 3 months of age the growing foal requires extra rations of food (Fig. 12.9). Special 'creep' rations are produced and can be started at an early age. Food must be clean and fresh at all times. If the foal is on creep food when weaning is due at 5 or 6 months, there will be minimal weaning stress (Heleski *et al.*, 2002). Foals weaned early must be given a milk replacement. Quantities

needed range from 2 l (0.5 gal)/day, when the foal is only a few days old, to 15 l (4 gal)/day at 1 month old. Foals can learn quickly to drink reconstituted milk replacer from a bucket, but a nipple bucket may be needed for some individuals. All feeding items must be rigorously cleaned between each use.

Progressive weaning can be done in a variety of ways and should be spread out over a period of a week or so. The objective is to take as much stress as possible out of the double stress of the loss of the mother and the switch to dry food. The stress to the mare is lessened also by a gradual weaning process (Waran *et al.*, 2008). At the beginning of this process, the mare and foal can be separated from each other for a limited period of a few hours. If they are within sight or sound of each other at this time, the initial separation is much better tolerated. The amount and degree of separation are progressively increased daily. Since the loss of companionship is stressful at this time, the foal and

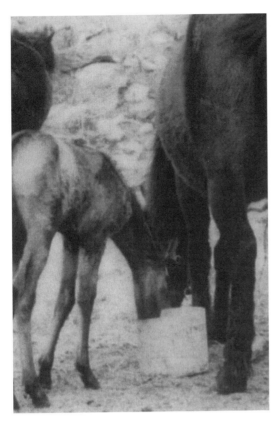

Fig. 12.9. Foal learning to eat solid food with its mother. Photo: A.F. Fraser.

Foal Training

While the foal is very young, long before its weaning, it should be handled as much as possible, until it is accustomed to human manipulation (Miller 1991; Simpson, 2002). It can be haltered within its first days and taught to be halter-led in the company of its mother. Regardless of haltering, foals learn about directed movement by following their mares when led out for walking exercise. The foal's feet should be picked up soon after its birth to check its legs and hooves for soundness. Thereafter the feet can be picked up frequently and checked; they can be lifted in order and tapped with something. This leg and foot handling should be done often enough to make the foal accept the procedure without reaction (Ligout *et al.*, 2008). This is the start of hoof care, which will be a major part of the animal's handling throughout its entire life. Continuous daily foot care allows the soles to be cleaned. Muddy pastures can cause frog and heel diseases if the feet are not cleaned and dried regularly. Grooming should also be performed on foals in training, as it can have a calming effect (de Mazieres, 1993).

Foals do not always learn handling routines quickly. Every handling lesson should be in the presence of the foal's mother, in which she is unable to intrude. Foals often require a span of time, such as a few days, between lessons, in order to absorb the experience. This facilitates training without difficulty (Williams *et al.*, 2002). No training session should continue if the foal is firmly showing negative reaction. Nevertheless, the foal must be eventually taught to accept human authority, and will do so through its developmental plasticity (Bateson *et al.*, 2004).

The essence of foal training should be steady progression. The handling of the foal's body should advance to the more sensitive areas, such as the poll, ears, belly and male genitals. Only when these areas can be handled at any time without reaction can that aspect of training be considered complete. Another handling procedure is the periodic opening of the foal's mouth to inspect teeth. Of further importance are lessons in straight backing-up for several steps. Gentle pushing while the head is controlled is the means of starting the foal on this important manoeuvre.

Some degree of grooming is desirable in training. At some advanced stage in its handling education, the foal can be given a girth from time to time. Convenient girth material would be stable

mare should be provided their own company at the weaning intervals. Abrupt weaning, without any conditioning, is not humane (Nicol *et al.*, 2005). The stress can diminish immunity (Yang and Glasser, 2000) and result in illnesses (Broom and Kirkden, 2004).

When the weaning process is completed, the mare's udder should not be stripped out. The pressure within the udder, as it stocks up, inhibits milk production. Maintaining the foal in a weaning paddock in suitable company allows it to be supervised, handled, wormed, vaccinated, fed and watered properly. Its hooves can also be trimmed before it goes into its next step in life, where it is its own individual young horse. As foals learn to socialize, they often make repeated snapping actions close to the mouths of strange horses. They seek social acceptance by this gesture, which is usually successful. They may react negatively to the presence of a strange person (Minero *et al.*, 2009).

bandages. The long-range objective in all of this is to take away as much stress as possible from the realities of the animal's later life. Even as a 2-year-old youth, it could find itself being treated as an experienced adult. Conditioning is essentially what foal training is. The concept of conditioning the foal for adult life is the basic guide in humane foal education (Visser *et al.*, 2008).

The foal's bond with its mother can aid in its training. For example, if the mare is accustomed to harness work, the foal can be her partner in such work. In the mare–foal partnership there is scope to teach the foal many things to which the mare is already fully accustomed. Human contact in general is one such thing (Gore *et al.*, 2008).

As the foal matures but is still feeding off its mother, it wanders from her at pasture for increasing distances (Fig. 12.10). If a young foal, e.g. less than 2 months old, is observed to be separated from its mother by a significant distance, it may be hungry and in need of attention.

Foal Protection

With the mare safely delivered of her foal, attention shifts to the transitory progression of the neonate from a nascent fetus to an ambulant individual. The progress is shown in a concatenation of discrete behavioural events with temporal values. They indicate vitality and they form the norms of neonatal development. These need to be monitored for verification of foal well-being (Fraser, 1989). The

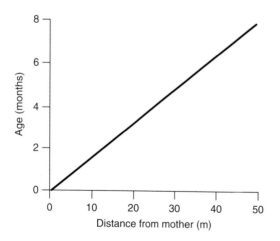

Fig. 12.10. Correlation of age with limits of distance between foals and mothers.

monitoring of well-being in the horse is, of course, an ongoing feature in its general care, but for the foal, it is a major, continuing requirement, at least until weaning has been completed. Without attempting to review the vast areas of veterinary medicine that relate to foal diseases and disorders, some of the chief examples can be dealt with here in three groups, namely parturient sequelae, neonatal infections and foal pathological states.

Parturient sequelae

1. Several salient disorders relate to the birth process (Morresey, 2005). During its expulsion the equine fetus is subjected to powerful forces of voluntary and involuntary contractions by the mare (Rossdale, 1999). The horse has the strongest abdominal wall among all domestic livestock, and the foaling mare's voluntary straining stems from her abdominal musculature. This pressure is known to have caused fractured ribs in Thoroughbred fetuses, often with fatal results (Jean *et al.*, 1999). Forced extraction of the fetus before the full expansion of the birth canal adds to the intrapelvic pressure, which can contribute to fetal trauma.

2. Compression during delivery is believed to be the cause of bladder rupture, another congenital, non-genetic dysfunction, which becomes apparent on the foal's second day. The signs include arrest of feeding, depression, vain attempts to urinate, swollen abdomen and respiratory difficulties. Eventually, these symptoms lead to coma, and death in about a week. Surgery can repair the bladder and save the foal if performed by the third day of the evident dysfunction (Russell and Wilkins, 2006).

Neonatal infections

A great variety of neonatal dysfunctions and infections can affect foals even after normal birth (Palmer, 2007). These usually destroy the foal's well-being and threaten its life.

1. An infected umbilicus is a common cause of early foal illness. Pyosepticaemia neonatorum results from umbilical infection and will quickly cause death if not treated promptly and appropriately with a suitable antibiotic, supportive therapy and good nursing (Freeman and Slusher, 2002). Alternatively, the infection may settle in the umbilicus or limb joints, creating localized inflammation there. Dipping the umbilical stump in 7% tincture

of iodine is the conventional and effective method of prevention and a welfare insurance.

2. Tetanus, with its characteristic and fatal stiffening, is a major risk for newborn foals. This warrants the administration of tetanus toxoid (not antiserum, since it can cause serum hepatitis). Pregnant mares can be vaccinated against tetanus about mid-term and given a booster a month before foaling. This will ensure passive immunity in the foal after it ingests the dam's colostrum.

3. Viral enteritis is a serious foal infection (Pilliner and Davies, 2004). It is most severe in foals under 1 week old and requires urgent treatment. As the condition is readily spread, an infected foal should be isolated and its faeces safely removed.

4. Pneumonia is a serious and often fatal disease of neonatal and older foals. The condition is highly contagious and may have a bacterial or viral cause. It requires immediate veterinary attention. High-quality management and good hygiene can do much to prevent foal pneumonia (Gore *et al.*, 2008).

5. A wide range of infectious bacterial conditions of a serious nature, but of less common occurrence, can cause severe illness in foals (Grinberg *et al.*, 2003). Any departure from normal healthy behaviour in a foal warrants prompt veterinary intervention. Hygiene in all forms can prevent much transmission of infection.

6. The 'shaker foal syndrome' is botulism. It is most common in Kentucky (Gore *et al.*, 2008) but, in theory, could occur anywhere. It is caused by the ingestion of spores of *Clostridium botulinum*, which may be present in hay or feed. The signs progress from weakness in movement to stilted gait, shaking, falling and paralysis. Death occurs in a few days from respiratory paralysis. Immunization of brood mares in a risky district can help in the control of this remarkable condition (Cymbaluk, 2002).

Foal pathological states

1. A great range of uncommon congenital anomalies of genetic origin are known to occur in certain horse breeds. These range from dysfunctional conditions of limbs, eyes, heart, brain, skull, anus, thyroid and neck, to colour (e.g. lavender foal syndrome in the Arabian breed, and the overolethal white syndrome in the Paint breed). Often these congenital anomalies are not amenable to treatment, and euthanasia is required to avoid unnecessary suffering.

2. About 50% of foals experience ulceration in the stomach or duodenum within their first 4 months (Gore *et al.*, 2008). Often there are no striking signs, but there may be slight signs of stomach pain, poor appetite, grinding teeth, frothy salivation, periods of diarrhoea and loss of condition (Herdt, 2007). Typically, such foals often lie on their backs. The cause is considered to be stress, and humane care is clearly the method of control (Gore *et al.*, 2008). Anti-ulcer medication is often an effective treatment.

The condition termed 'neonatal maladjustment syndrome' (NMS) is referred to under a variety of common terms, including barker foal, wandering foal, dummy foal and convulsive foal (Palmer and Rossdale, 1976). The cause is believed to be intrapartum hypoxia that affects some area of the brain. These common terms are descriptive of the principal behavioural signs. The condition has been found mainly in the Thoroughbred breed. The cause is unknown, but there is room to suspect premature separation of the neonate from its placenta. The latter is, of course, a major part of the circulatory system of the fetus. Because of the great value of many Thoroughbred foals, it is not unusual for birth attendants to rescue these foals promptly from the birthing mare in order to attend to it, by drying it and locating it in a safe and comfortable site until it can stand (Simpson, 2002).

Foals suffering NMS are unable to right or rotate themselves from a position of lateral recumbency to sternal lying. This is termed 'loss of the righting reflex'. Another sign is loss of the sucking reflex, following which there may be spasms of the neck, jerking movements, seizures, thrashing of the limbs and convulsions (Koterba *et al.*, 1990b). Respiratory distress and barking sounds then occur. Following this barker stage, the foal exhibits a dummy stage, in which it lies lifelessly and unresponsively before rising later and wandering aimlessly, showing no affinity with its mother and blindly bumping into objects. About 50% of NMS cases die, but the recovery of the others may be fairly complete in a number of weeks, especially if they receive high-quality veterinary care.

3. Neonatal isoerythrolysis is a serious illness in about 1 or 2% of foals, resulting in the destruction of its red blood cells by the mare's colostrum, as previously described. An affected foal shows abnormal sleepiness and lethargy on its second day (see Fig. 12.4 for norms of sleep). It may lie with its chin on the ground, gasping for air. The whites of

the eyes and the gums turn yellowish with the bilirubin from the haemolysis, which may be fatal. This condition calls for high-quality care and highly technical intervention, which may include transfusion. The responsible parentage of the foal should be noted for any further breedings to control this condition.

4. While some limb deformities in newborn foals are inherited defects (Wright *et al.*, 2002), others appear to be the result of a malposition of the limb of the fetus *in utero*. Some of these are corrected within 1 or 2 weeks by the foal's own stretching activities. Others involving hyperflexion or hypertension can require correction by veterinary attention and nursing (Stoneham, 2001).

Beyond the critical early days of foalhood and before the great stress of weaning, there lie other hazards for the young animal, including viral enteritis (Mair *et al.*, 1998). This disease has already been mentioned with reference to the neonate; however, this dysfunction more usually strikes at foals about 8 weeks of age, causing diarrhoea. The highly infectious faeces vary in the form of soft pats or green fluid. Electrolyte loss is severe. Prompt veterinary therapy is necessary (Pavord and Pavord, 2002). Brood mares can be vaccinated against the causal rotavirus, and the colostrum would then provide the foal passive immunity lasting about 3 months (O'Connor, 1987). Foals themselves need their appropriate vaccinations and this can be started at about 10 weeks of age. De-worming should also be carried out by this time.

Weaning Welfare

The separation of mare and young foal is emotionally disturbing for both, even for a short period. It is particularly stressful on the foal if the time away from its mare is extended and she is out of sight. The main features of the maternal absence that create stress in the foal are sudden severance of the bond, loss of physical contact and soon hunger and thirst. These stressors collectively have a very real effect on the foal's well-being if they are not promptly relieved by restoring the foal to its mare.

Foals weaned early must be given a milk replacement. Quantities needed range from 2 l (0.5 gal)/day, when the foal is only a few days old, to 15 l (4 gal)/day at 1 month old. Foals can learn quickly to drink reconstituted milk replacer from a bucket, but a nipple bucket may be needed for some individuals. All feeding items must be rigorously cleaned between each use.

The growing foal will soon need extra food in the form of special 'creep' rations, which are produced specifically for foals (Cunha, 1991). These can be started at an early age. Food must be clean and fresh at all times. If the foal is on creep food when weaning is due at 5 or 6 months, there will be minimal weaning stress. The foal suckles about every 2 h at this age (See Fig. 12.5). Before weaning can be considered, it should be verified that the foal is eating a sufficient quantity of solid feed for its age and size: about 2–4 kg of creep, plus grass or hay.

Sudden weaning is very stressful and impairs foal immunity (Ahmed and Shurig, 2007). Weaning stress can cause diarrhoea, marked loss of physical condition and a high susceptibility to infectious disease. If the foal is taken from the mother and isolated indoors, it shows extremely distressed behaviour until exhausted. If it is put outdoors in the company of familiar foals, its distress is less severe. It is somewhat better to remove the mother and leave the foal in its customary environment with other foals and horses with which it is familiar (Heleski *et al.*, 2002).

Abrupt weaning without good foal management and special preparation is not good welfare. From a welfare perspective, progressive weaning is the method of choice. Progressive weaning can be done in a variety of ways and should be spread out over a period of a week or so. The objective is to take as much strain as possible out of the stress of the loss of the mother.

At the beginning of this process, the mare and foal can be separated from each other for a limited period of a few hours. If they are within sight or sound of each other at this time, the initial separation is much better tolerated. The amount and degree of separation are then progressively increased daily. Since the loss of companionship is stressful at this time, the foal and mare should be kept together during the weaning intervals. Maintaining the foal in a weaning paddock in suitable company allows it to be supervised, handled, wormed, vaccinated, fed and watered properly, and have its hooves trimmed before it goes into its next step in life, where it is its own individual young horse and its foalhood has successfully concluded.

13 Development and Social Behaviour

At about half a day old, the newborn foal will have completed its normal biological timetable by achieving ambulatory and feeding competence, maternal attachment, performance of excretory functions and deep sleep. Its achievements also include the passive acquisition of the mare's immunities in her colostrum. The eponychial foot pads (which protected the intrauterine environment from sharp fetal limb actions) will have been removed from the hoof soles by the abrasions from walking. This removal of the large under-hoof pads helps with stability. The articulation of all its skeletal joints will have occurred and the foal now walks with distinct strides, going to its mother and inspecting its immediate surrounding.

When it is 1 day old, the foal can perform running gaits, particularly if it has outdoor freedom with its mother. Such runs can be fast and fairly lengthy. This latter achievement sets it up as a horse. Horse-like, it is bonded closely with a companion, its dam. The mare reciprocates, going where the foal goes, tilting her udder towards the suckling foal, and often places herself over it as it lies flat out in its numerous, short sleeping sessions (Fig. 13.1). In addition to its visits to its mother, the neonatal foal's essential musculoskeletal exercises in its first days stem mostly from the high frequency of pandiculations while it is lying down and from short episodes of saltatory activity, which appear as little kinetic sorties.

Saltation

The foal's first episode of saltation is often about 2 h after birth, in the form of jumping and dancing (Fraser, 1992). Additional forms of saltation in the day-old foal are featured as acts of kicking, hopping, trotting and running. When space permits, some of these actions are later included in bouts of play. Games develop between foals as such mutual activities lead to exchanges and contests. In itself,

the phenomenon of saltation obviously has a significant effect on the neonate's vascularization and strength. It increases heart rate, boosts blood flow and promotes haemodynamism and hypertrophy in musculature, relating to kinesis. The phenomenon counters the arrested activity in the foal's numerous sessions of sleep between sucklings. Since saltatory activities are functional for the foal's health, it is an adducible concept that its absence relates to poor health and therefore has monitoring value in the foal's well-being (Fig. 13.2).

General Play

Horse play is taken to be any substantial activity occurring spontaneously or reactively in horses that does not have relevance to basic maintenance or reproductive behaviour. It occurs in single subjects and in social groups of varying numbers. It is typically an activity of juvenile or young horses and is essentially kinetic in nature, usually taking the form of fast, short runs in which vigorous kicking and head waving may be expressed as saltation. When playing in pairs, there are also competitive activities, particularly in young subjects. These competitions include mock fights, with pushing, head to head rearing and biting. Competitive racing also occurs in pairs and sometimes in larger numbers (see Fig. 13.3). In young foals, mounting each other is shown by both sexes in bouts of social play. Play evidently has a role in social development (Hall, 1998).

The day-old foal will show sudden bursts of playful activity in the form of leaping in saltation. Saltatory play takes the form of jumping upwards, suddenly running about alone or in groups, chasing with much head tossing, sudden stops and starts, and kicking of the hind legs in the air. Foals play increasingly as they mature. Their play often begins with the foal nibbling at the legs of its mother. In addition to grooming with their dams, foals in

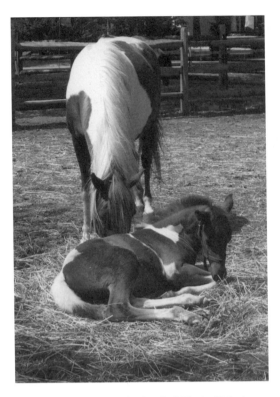

Fig. 13.1. Mare overseeing her foal. Photo: Melanie MacDonald.

one major method of harmonious integration between the foal and its ambience. It can therefore be presented as a system of particular importance to the equine species, which is so very reactive, kinetic and social. Play-fighting is a notable component of general play (Pellis and Pellis, 1998).

Foal play has certain rules that distinguish between these activities and the analogous ones that can occur in serious adult circumstances in later life. For example, the various play activities differ from the 'serious' counterpart activities in their accompanying emotions and in the duration of action. In the 'serious' situation, when an animal has fled beyond the reach of its opponent, flight ceases; again, when an animal has repelled its opponent, flight ceases. Such cessations are not observed in play, which may continue for extended periods. In the several manifestations of play, there is the single emotion of apparent pleasure, while in 'serious' situations there are the specific emotions of anger, fear, etc. Equine play is a good demonstration of play as a purely kinetic activity. For example, 75% of the kinetic activity of foals is in the form of play.

Play is central to behavioural epigenesis, both as a set of rules and as a mechanism for modifying these rules in response to individual play experiences (Fagen, 1976, 1981). The phenomenon of play could become a basic factor in the determination of conditions of welfare, particularly as it relates to the development of the athletic horse (Fig. 13.4). An absence of play in a young horse could indicate poor welfare. The kinetic ethos of the horse has been diverted in domestication into forms of work and recreational activities. The modern horse adopts these activities as analogues to natural play, which, incidentally, ensures the integration of the animal's use and its welfare under domestication. For example, running and chasing relate to racing; grouped movement may relate to team work in harness. Natural kinetic output may relate to racing and the various forms of riding.

Horse play facilitates social bonds. The pairing–bonding capacity of the horse is remarkable. Human bonding may be the secret of success in the way this animal has dealt competently with domestication while preserving its behavioural characteristics, such as reactiveness, more suitable to the wild state. It may be that such adult bonding is an outcome of play skill in the horse. This again would allude to the survival value of play: the behavioural phenomenon that is apparently both frivolous action and vital experience (Wong, 2000).

groups also groom one another. Grooming bouts often initiate play, and during initiation oral snapping actions can also be observed. Foals show that play is an important business and that it is a necessary part of life. As they grow it becomes most important as exercise. It functions as a means of practising and perfecting adult behavioural skills that may be necessary in later life for a wide range of actions. Play is clearly valuable for the development of normal behaviour and it occurs most often in healthy foals. In concise terms, it can be stated that play is the appearance in behaviour of a motivating force concerning action. It possesses evident conation (Bruner *et al.*, 1974).

Play Principles

Some learning is required by foals for their play. Although play movements are basically innate and patterned, they are not perfectly performed on the first occasion. Proficiency in play is attained remarkably quickly after foals learn the attributes of associates and environment. Play is evidently

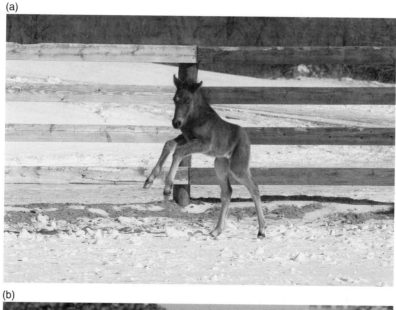

(a)

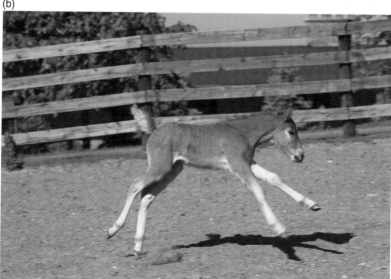

(b)

Fig. 13.2. (a and b) Neonatal saltation. Photos: Melanie MacDonald.

The principal functions of horse play appear to be the following:

- development of physical strength and endurance;
- promotion of development rates in physique;
- experience yielding awareness and behavioural adaptability;
- establishing and strengthening social bonds; and
- providing the exercise that is essential for health (Caanitz *et al.*, 1991).

Social play reflects biological adaptation in the service of fitness. Because of this, it is clear that play is neither essentially cooperative nor necessarily competitive, since partners are usually evenly matched and bonded. Typical activities are non-injurious and do not harm social relationships. It may help to establish lasting cooperation for individuals remaining in one group. Even when an older animal plays cooperatively with a young one,

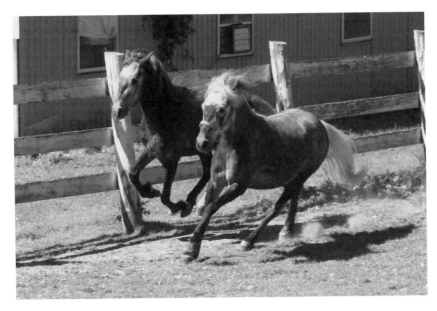

Fig. 13.3. Adult horses racing in play. Photo: Melanie MacDonald.

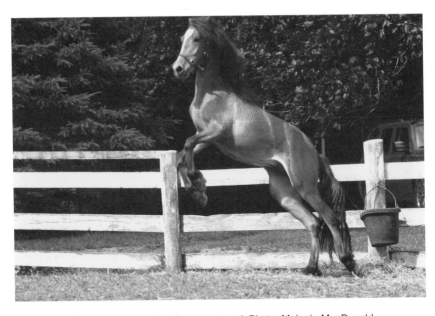

Fig. 13.4. Leaping upward in play. Note one hind foot on ground. Photo: Melanie MacDonald.

special communicative signals and stabilizing techniques ensure that play is fair to both participants, and the non-serious nature of play ensures that real injury is seldom inflicted. For example, no escape is truly achieved in a play-fight since real aggressive intent is absent.

Play has an emotional component. In particular, neuromuscular activity is evidently emotionally satisfying in foals when this factor is activated in playful sessions. The animals seem emotively reinforced in playing, as they play repeatedly and spontaneously. When play is denied, as in chronic confinement in the adult, an outburst of play activity is usually observed when these animals are released from work and put on pasture. Although the kinetic manifestations of play simulate those seen in the 'serious' activities of fight and avoidance, the evident emotions in these various activities differ between the 'serious' situation and play. In serious fight there is anger and in serious flight there is fear, whereas in play there is only the one very evident emotion of pleasure.

Review of Objectives in Horse Play

Certain parts of the neuromuscular system, such as those concerned with change of posture and walking, are adaptive in the newborn foal. An adaptive role for other parts of the neuromuscular system is not so evident. These latter parts are precisely those concerned in the phenomenal activities collectively called play. Play is composed of patterned behaviours. Similar patterns are traits that are typical of the species, not of a breed. Acts of play are simulations, and although non-serious in nature, they are strongly motivated. It can be seen that horse play is the projection into behaviour of a motivating force concerning action. Play facilitates the capability of the individual horse, as a mobile and social unit. It has a major role in the behavioural, social and physiological development of all horses.

The 'serious' adult activities of fight and flight are not functional in the foal, as the dam provides food and protection. The juvenile normally does not need to fight, nor does it need to initiate flight, yet although these serious activities are not needed, the neuromuscular requirements are already in existence and are thus included in playful practice. The development of dynamic skill begins in play and is kept through the whole life of the animal in many situations. Each component skill is characterized by its own rate of development and by its particular susceptibility to environmental influence. In addition, play can be seen as release of strain or stress and an outlet for positive expression.

General Laws of Horse Play

Twelve features that most exemplify the laws of horse play are listed below:

1. When ready to play, horses show a play appetite by looking for an opportunity to play and then initiating it.

2. Inhibitions control horse play and these avoid injuring the play partner.
3. Use of inanimate objects or individuals of other species as substitutes in play indicates a need for this activity.
4. A horse repeatedly returning to the stimulus source indicates that play has the character of habit.
5. Bouts of play are typically preceded by a signal of playful intent, such as nipping or pushing. These signals may recur during the bout to keep it continuing. This transmission of a playing mood to other individuals, particularly playmates, shows social facilitation as a play facilitator.
6. Short sequences and repetitious motor patterns are characteristic of brief bouts.
7. Sequences of play bouts may involve saltatory actions (see Fig. 13.5). Repeated actions in an exaggerated manner are very characteristic. These may be relatively unordered in sequence from one time to another.
8. Playful movements within the sequence may be repeated more often than they would usually be in 'serious' situations.
9. Movements within the sequence may not be completed and incomplete elements may be repeated, indicating that behavioural units in play are not essentially linked in a chain.
10. Play lacks a consummatory act as an end point. It usually winds down.
11. Horse play stops when a stronger stimulus or an important event becomes the focus of attention.
12. Play occurs in a relaxed motivational setting when it is not displaced by events or essential maintenance. The activity appears 'pleasurable' to the participants.

Vascularization

During repeated and extended play sessions there are accumulations of various benefits. Improved blood flow throughout the body and specifically to the voluntary musculature involved is the chief physical benefit. Vascularization is markedly influenced by the activities of vigorous play. In the foal, with the onset of postpartum life, a new situation arises regarding vascularity. Each system of the body is liable to make its own demands on an essentially limited blood supply. This supply is influenced by the work of the heart. Without the existence of play, the neuromuscular systems would be denied the heart's optimum activity, with consequent failure to obtain optimal blood supply for the foal. The physiological

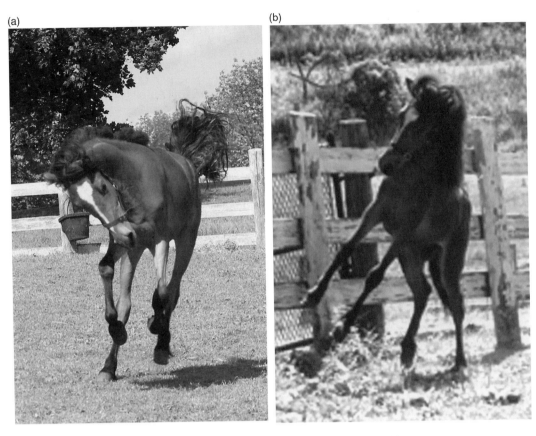

Fig. 13.5. (a and b) Adult horse showing playful saltation. Photos: Melanie MacDonald.

role of play is apparent because play does not occur in cold, wet weather, when haemodynamic factors are being fully used to maintain body temperature.

When voluntary muscles are deprived of optimal blood flow by the absence of play activity during prolonged confinement, there is usually an outburst of such activity on release of the affected foal. This can be presumed to indicate lasting tension in play motivation, which may relate physiologically to the needs of muscles for periodically increased vascularization. As a result of increased blood circulation during play, there is physiological benefit in general somatic development, creating, temporarily, a generalized hyperaemia. This contributes to the physiobehavioural development of the individual animal.

Social Foal Play

Play is beneficial in the early social integration of the foal in its group. Social play is common as pursuit and mock fighting. Pairs become formed as a result of a series of playful episodes and exchanges by two individuals. Neck overlapping is often shown by the pair, as well as joint scampering, and when the playful partnership has become established, a close bond is formed between the two. This binds them together in all circumstances. When the pair is part of a larger group, the twosome arrangement operates dynamically in their interests.

Playful activities in the foal occur at their best when a pair, a trio or group of foals can join in the activity together. Playful activities around the mother become reduced after the first week of life, by which time they prefer to play with others of their own age group.

Interactive play is displayed in the form of chasing and reverse chasing, and includes body contact in the form of pushing, biting, neck-wrestling, mutual rearing or riding (see Fig. 13.6). This form of play is

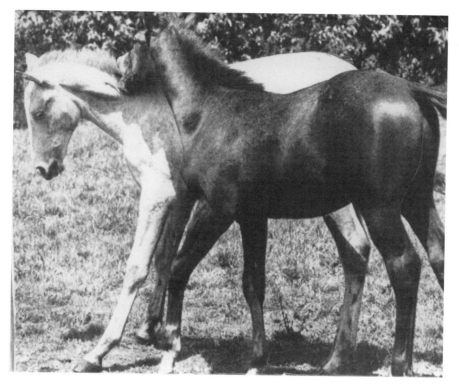

Fig. 13.6. Playful partnership. Photo: Anonymous.

especially frequent in group-living young horses and may merge into low-intensity agonistic fighting. Social interactions involving physical contact between young males can sometimes combine structural and functional characteristics of play with low-intensity agonistic fighting. This may determine position or rank in young horses just entering sub-adult society. The characteristics of fearfulness can emerge at this time (Lansade *et al.*, 2008).

Social play among foal groups usually increases with age. In social pairs or groups, foals groom one another. Grooming bouts often initiate play, and oral snapping actions are also seen in foals when they are initiating play. The commonest form of social play between foals involves nipping of the head and mane, gripping of the crest, rearing up towards one another, chasing, mounting and side-by-side fighting. Play tends to be more frequent in male than female foals; sex differences can be observed, with colts mounting more frequently and generally engaging in play more vigorously than fillies. A response of fillies to colt play is often withdrawal or aggression. Foals initiate play bouts

with each other more frequently as they mature and leave the mare. Foals 3–4 weeks of age often have play bouts lasting 10–15 min. Such bouts are usually initiated by one foal developing the bout from a mutual grooming episode by changes to acts of nipping. A bout may be ended mutually by the two foals separating or, more often, by the withdrawal of one foal.

As the foal develops into a more competent juvenile horse, play continues to be a prominent part of its behaviour. In juvenile play the same locomotor or manipulative behaviour is often repeated, with slight variation, at a given stage of mastery. Such behaviour contains saltatory items such as jumping vertically and running away from the mother, and then back to her suddenly. Saltation is reduced to a very low order of activity by 2 months of age. Various repetitive manipulations of objects occur in solitary play. Solitary play persists in lone foals and their social play may relate to other species of animals and humans.

It may be that juvenile experiences of play determine the best racehorses, providing they are organically sound in all respects. Play motivation is valuable since it can override physical fatigue, to a point. The level of this in an animal may be subject to mood and to the self-image of social status among the field of runners. Those further psychological features therefore add greater variability to racing success in horses. Even the best bred, best fed, and best trained could have their prospects influenced by early play-related and handling factors, which have lasting effects on physique and psyche (Ligout *et al.*, 2008).

Horse sports that entail much variety of pace and environment are capable of adding play motivation to the efforts of some animals. Events such as gymkhanas, cross-country running and point-to-point racing are examples. Even dressage, with its variety and formality, might evoke a play approach in some horses more than in others. Some forms of work for horses can contain elements of stimulation for this inherent inclination to take opportunities to play creatively. Thus, elements of play do extend into horse work, exercises in precision and power games, as well as the speed games of racing.

General Social Behaviour

One factor of major importance in horse behaviour is a social purpose. Social motivation is a strong force that maintains equine cohesion. The population strategies of horses are implemented by systems of collaborative behaviour, as in the 'group effect', also termed 'social facilitation', which influences communal activities. The various forms of association between individuals permit the organization of numbers of horses into social units and herds.

Social force brings discipline to all the individuals of a horse group, ensuring the mutual pursuit of tactics required for living, while social motives are manifestly related to common survival (Hamilton, 1964a). Among horses, the phenomena of social behaviour are found to be pursued with particular vigour. The evident need of the horse for company of its own kind makes it a very social animal and social features compose much of its ethos. Social capability with man was evidently a prototypic feature of horses. It is certainly essential to their efficient manipulation in husbandry. In the use of horses, their readiness to accept human association is a vital quality.

Horses readily form a social order. When they live in bands a clear social hierarchy becomes established, in which the older and larger animals are usually found to be high in the dominance order. Stallions can easily dominate geldings or mares, but do not always do so. A leader dictates the movement of the herd through the grazing area and maintains a vigilant role. As has been recognized down through the ages, socially dominant horses are sometimes found to have very aggressive temperaments. Individual mares are found to associate closely with certain individuals serving as close friends. Colts and fillies tend to separate from the mares and stallions. The stallion usually attacks members of the younger group if they approach too closely. As mentioned previously, a stallion will round up mares on the periphery of his herd or 'harem' but will ignore or repel fillies. Among free-living ponies, close groups of various sizes are formed. Most are family groups, with fillies remaining with their mothers for 2 or more years. Once they leave their mothers at the end of the mare–foal bond (Houpt, 2002), young mares tend to change groups, often joining older mares with foals. Young stallions in winter join bachelor groups in a loose social organization. Some members leave to form other groups for a period and then rejoin their original group. Some pairings change in time. Old stallions often live as solitary individuals.

Social Features

Various features of social behaviour are observed in domesticated horses, and bondings are most notable among them. Even under free-range conditions in extensive territory, there is such group bonding that horses maintain visual contact with each other continually. Very modified social behaviour is seen in the domesticated horse's positive interaction with people. Such sociability varies considerably, but normally there is a relationship involving the positive association of the horse with mankind, termed socialization. Other interspecies affiliations can occur in remarkable forms between horses and dogs, goats and pet animals of various kinds, even chickens. Through the phenomenon of social facilitation, the goal of the majority of individuals in a group dominates and prevails generally. Well-being is often better developed in grouped animals. For example, horses in total isolation do not show the same stability in maintenance activity, such as ingestion, as shown within groups. It appears that optimum group size aids homeostasis in horses (Sondergaard and Ladewig, 2004).

Interactions at very close quarters depend on the position of the animals in the dominance order. Dominant and subordinate postures, as well as avoidance, are appropriately adopted. This stability of social relationships requires the following factors:

1. Permanent group membership.
2. Recognition between individual horses.
3. Established social positions.
4. Memory of social encounters that establish social status.
5. Possession of social versatility.

In their affiliative movements, horses often respond to the initiative of a lead animal by following. Horses show 'follow reactions' in various social circumstances involving changes of location. Such leadership, in socially stable groups of horses, is often provided by an older mare or gelding. Age is likely to affect leadership, and the status of the animal in the social hierarchy may not be a determinant factor. In fact, the lead role is often taken by horses from the middle of the group hierarchy.

Leadership may be shared but the follow order tends to be fairly similar from event to event. Types of leadership in grazing horses are subdivided into three categories as follows:

1. Leadership during movement to and from locations of eating, drinking, resting and sheltering.
2. Leadership in the initiation of grazing and resting phases.
3. Leadership in the group's grazing direction.

Since grazing essentially involves dispersive movement, followership becomes obscured. Aggregative movement, on the other hand, may have clear follow behaviour through social support of an initiator–leader.

In their communications among themselves, horses have clear understandings. They use a body language of subtle signals, feints, expressions, nips and postures. A mild nip with the bared incisor teeth on the shoulder of an associate affirms an alliance. Acceptance of this message in such a gesture might be shown by the other in a subdued squeal, with raised head and flattened ears. Showing the white of the eye to another indicates a readiness to defend position. Whinnying as vocal language is less in use than visual communication in which simple body signals are used. The wide eye warns while the flaring nostrils tell of adrenaline flowing. The eyes roll when a hostile attitude develops. In a relaxed facial expression, the ears are outward, the eyelids are relaxed, and the lower lip droops. When the face is set with muscles contracted, the eye protruding and ears twisted back, real anger is being expressed and the intent of an aggressive act, such as a vicious bite or kick, is being announced. Swinging the hindquarters at another is a serious threat. A 'two-barrelled' kick is often the next expression of dislike.

Social Facilitation

The goal of the majority seems to prevail so as to direct behavioural policy for a group. This group effect, depending on space, serves as a basis for the strategies of group behaviour (Rifa, 1990). Social facilitation in a herd or group may be a motivating force in the daily movements of horses, as in occasional running and marching from place to place. Social facilitation has the means to derive increased motive force from:

1. Allelomimetic pressure.
2. Common needs.
3. Cumulation of individuals' motivation.
4. Unified reactivity.
5. Synergism of maintenance acts, such as those of association, kinesis and exploration.

In addition, mass communication is apparently present, operating by discrete body action to arouse and intensify common activities in an assembly. Hypertrophied motivation develops from group effect or social facilitation in such a social subject as the horse. Evidently, in clearly established hierarchies, there is maximal group bonding and minimal aggression, creating the social stability that is a vital requirement in group welfare.

Settled Relationship

Settled relationships between horses often take the form of strong partnerships. These mutually supportive pairs, with their symbiotic tolerance, contribute to stability. Clearly the hierarchy is dependent upon mixed relationships and notably on basic, simple avoidance tactics. 'Dominance hierarchy' may be a misnomer for a social arrangement based on a mixture of social methods. Horse groups use organized tactics of stable social living that involve their own pacts and systems of pacts. One example of a group pact is the bachelor grouping among colts, as mentioned previously. A dominance relationship in a group pact is one in which one individual can inhibit the behaviour of another routinely. The order of the group is therefore the sum of all such inhibitory relationships. Dominant animals have more than likely been aggressive in the past to obtain their dominant positions; however, a dominant animal need not be aggressive subsequently in all social situations in order to maintain its position in the hierarchy. Quite simply, each horse's status is a known and constant factor to determine differences between animals.

Social relationships are the result of learning, with many different factors being involved in the formation of the relationship. Once learned, these relationships can persist for as long as the group remains a closed unit. Unsettled dominance relationships are usually found only in young horses. With maturity and experience, the social status of individuals in a relationship becomes fixed. There is a subsystem of preferred status within the dominance system, and this subsystem modifies the whole influence of the social structure, particularly in regard to the manner of interactions and the privilege of feeding. This explains why the theory of a dominance hierarchy in horses does not always fit the facts. The recognition of two social hierarchies (real and apparent) operating as one sheds light on horse sociology. In this system, a horse of low social rank becomes accepted as a preferred associate by one of high rank and then gains advantages through the relationship. Such advantages include easy access to provided food. This is an equine example of commensalism.

Avoidance Order

Horses generally have a clear unidirectional dominance order, which may not be linear from end to end. In this, 'a' might dominate 'b', and 'b' might dominate 'c', and 'c' might dominate 'a', giving an overall triangular dominance order. The group order can therefore be complex while quite stable. Social dominance is sometimes exerted actively by horses while grazing. However, subordinate horses deliberately avoid moving too close to dominant individuals, as the latter readily threaten nearby subordinates while eating. While social dominance is promptly exhibited in competition for supplementary feed given in a restricted place or at water troughs, subordinate horses are usually skilled in avoiding conflict.

Avoidance behaviour is the chief social tactic involved in maintaining social stability in a permanent herd of grazing horses. The 'avoidance order' is maintained chiefly through the behaviour of the subordinates. They perform the necessary acts of behaviour, mainly submissive and flight behaviour. In view of this, the avoidance order is a better measure of the social system than the 'aggression order'. Appropriate ethological methods of husbandry for horses, by use of adequate space in grazing, allow the proper operation of a social order and keep energy-wasting and stress-inducing aggression within groups of horses under control. Within systems that provide security of position at feeding and secondary space for resting, it is possible for a constantly settled avoidance order to exist continuously. Evidently, the generally accepted belief that dominance by itself establishes and operates social hierarchy is inadequate. The avoidance system in behaviour, which operates within the dominance system, is the vital component of the behavioural mechanism that generates social stability. Avoidance as a general strategy calls for specific behavioural tactics, and these tactics demand space for their effective operation.

The actions underlying an avoidance system must be prompt and effective enough to put the horse out of the range of an aggressor's space. In some situations of spatial restraint, an avoidance order can become unstable through inadequacy of tactical space. If the available area is too small to permit a subordinate horse to get outside the perimeter of an aggressor's individual social space at a critical moment, an avoidance tactic cannot operate. The operation of an avoidance system in the social behaviour of horses is the key to their social pax, in which there is acceptance of dominance.

Dominance does not have to be overt to be effective. A mature animal, very sure of its status at any time, can be placed in a strange group and be immune from the usual attentions given a newcomer. Such a horse employs a quiet authority, occasionally reinforced with a few discrete kicks or indignant squeals. A set of eye, ear, mouth, neck and head positions can compose a meaningful display and signal that a self-assertive individual has entered the herd. In the handling of assertive horses it is important that the human caretaker be dominant, particularly when the horse is to be given much human handling. The stallion asserts increased dominance with maturation and growth. For such an animal, dominance is best established at the appropriate time, usually early in life, when no punishment may be needed. Dominance, as a phenomenon, must therefore be appreciated, so that it can be manipulated.

Social Pony Grouping

Among ponies, most aggressive reactions occur when freshly mixed in one company. Much of the restless activities are exercises determining the status of each pony in the group. In a typical encounter between two ponies of different social status, one pony would act aggressively, reaching out to snap at the skin around the shoulders and neck of the adversary. If the adversary then recognizes that it is subordinate in the social hierarchy to the animal attacking it, its response would be one of quick avoidance. At this point the aggressive exchange between the two animals ceases, since its purpose has been fulfilled. A lot of minor aggressive acts are shown when one pony's 'individual space' has been violated by the sudden intrusion of another. Maintaining preferred partnerships eliminates much social aggressiveness for the 'preferred' individuals (Van Dierendonck et al., 2009).

When grazing in a group, ponies tend to space themselves out from each other as they seem to consider it important to have freedom from conflict when in the business of eating.

Ponies are very gregarious, enjoying the company of each other. Small groups tend to become closely compacted and move together, maintaining a private area around themselves. Although they act as a typical herding species, they show a marked preference for close contact with certain individuals in their group. Two ponies encountering each other for the first time show much mutual exploration (Fig. 13.7). This exploratory behaviour involves an investigation of the other's head, body and hindquarters by smelling. Bonds of friendship often become formed thereafter. At pasture, pairs of ponies spend long spells in mutual grooming. This form of grooming is shown in all age groups, though the pairs formed are usually matched for age and size.

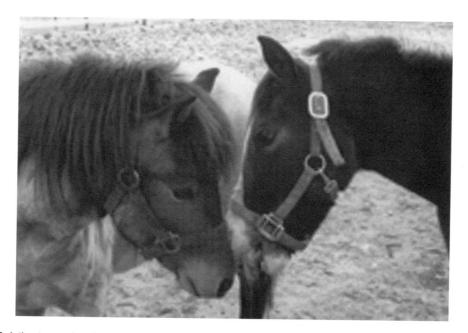

Fig. 13.7. Intimate nasal exchange between strangers. Photo: Melanie MacDonald.

The rich social ways of ponies and other horses living freely in groups is the natural life of the horse. Conventional horse husbandry takes much away from this animal, but the study of equine behaviour shows how husbandry can be imposed. Social interactions are evidently used in relative self-determination, and probably for this reason, horses held in social isolation do not always behave in the same way as others of their kind. It has been said, for example, that 'a horse confined on its own is in very bad company'. Solitary horses can all be considered to be in poor circumstances, as regards their social welfare. Society influenced their evolution (Hamilton, 1964b), and it remains as a basic need.

Equine association with mankind has been a long and successful relationship. The domestication of the horse has depended on this capacity for affinity. The bond between horse and user must be appropriately developed and maintained. This requires that the human supplies all the necessary protection against hunger, thirst, fear, discomfort, pain and environmental stress. Bonding is a highly qualitative association. The quality of contact must be recognized as the real nature of the social bond. Aversive social encounters are not conducive to bonding. However, in dealing with a fractious horse, carrying a riding crop or switch of some kind signals dominant intent and capability.

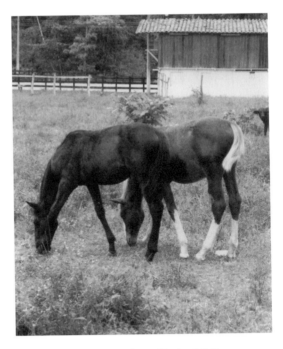

Fig. 13.8. Grazing associates. Photo: A.F. Fraser.

Welfare Addendum

The ethics of animal use compel animal husbandry to operate in good conscience. The horse's fundamental behavioural needs must be met. Two basic elements of need exist in the forms of social balance and environmental quality (Keeling and Gonyou, 2001). Behaviour of 'association' shows the extent of social activities in the total system of equine behaviour. Social needs cannot be met in confinement. Much freedom of movement and of association is required by horses if they are to function properly and naturally (Fig. 13.8). For this purpose they benefit greatly by being raised in a suitable natural environment. Young horses need the company of other horses to learn how to be completely equine. Humane handling from birth helps to make the young horse more amenable to firm handling later in life (Miller, 1992; Spier *et al.*, 2004).

Human–Animal Bond

It is now well recognized that a close relationship between a person and an animal can have significant beneficial effects on the health and the social well-being of both. The nature of this relationship has been termed the human–animal bond. While it is still somewhat mysterious, it appears that this bond is struck very readily by people who are able to make close physical contact with a friendly animal such as a horse. This contact uplifts the spirits of people who are not able, for any reason, to move widely in social circles. It is also observed that such people become more expressive after animal contact. In addition, the human–animal bond appears to make people more alert and more relaxed, and some of these effects show up in medical criteria, such as a reduction in blood pressure. The animal is also a beneficiary in this benign usage.

The human–animal bond is becoming recognized as a phenomenon that can be put to use in the interests of many people who require an extra stimulus, an extra interest or additional social factors in their lives. Organizations are established in many countries today in order to promote the human–animal bond. Such organizations have become established, for example, in the USA, Canada and several European countries. These organizations encourage various programmes such as the provision of horseback riding facilities for handicapped persons. The experiences of horse riding contribute to a sense of self-worth and provide some extra measure of self-confidence in people who may have lost this faculty as a result of the restricting circumstances of a handicap.

The horse is an excellent subject for human–animal bonding; it can reciprocate in the bond by giving equine service, such as in riding and in behaving agreeably. Looking after a pony creates a substantial duty for anyone with such an animal. Such duty is demanding in time, attention and thought. It provides both an opportunity to go outdoors with the horse and an opportunity for meeting others. Bringing a pony into open places acts as a most effective means of introduction to nature. For capable young persons seeking action, more demanding recreations with horses can fulfil the same purpose while also providing athletic exercise, as in cross-country riding and jumping.

14 Humane Control and Husbandry Welfare

Effective control is essential in all aspects of the horse's domesticated life. Without such control there can be no satisfactory care. The delivery of a horse's needs can only be carried out properly if the caregiver has control of the situation in which the horse is placed. Such control over a horse is, of course, limited to humane practices in all aspects of its husbandry. In horse care, it is a rule that any horse out of control has its well-being at risk.

The purpose of any form of restraint is to immobilize the horse for a short period of time so that some procedure considered necessary for its care can be carried out. Minimum discomfort to the horse and maximum safety to the operator are the criteria. These procedures should not be based on the infliction of pain upon the animal. It is emphasized, therefore, that such procedures are intended not to cause harm to the animal but to place it briefly in a simple state of mechanical disadvantage, in the interests of its own well-being. For example, a very young foal can be restrained by lifting it bodily with the arms encircling the fore- and hindquarters while it receives clinical attention.

Any control involving unnecessary pain and suffering is totally unethical and is now publicly unacceptable. Certain older practices such as casting a conscious horse with ropes and hobbles are no longer approved. Electric shock devices to try and stop crib-biting are other painful devices in training that are similarly unacceptable by an informed public. Harsh restraint by any means for any significant period is now regarded as cruelty.

Clearly there is need for a realistic recognition of the exercise of control that is humane and essentially beneficial to the horse on the one hand and control that is inhumane and detrimental to the well-being of the animal on the other hand (Sappington and Goldman, 1994). In this there is a need to have realism tempered with the understanding that if a form of control is of a doubtful nature, the horse should be given the benefit of the doubt.

The horse's nature should be borne in mind as a guiding light in such issues. Formerly, the first step towards control of an untamed horse was termed 'breaking', in which the objective was quick mastery over the animal's natural selfness. In principle this was done by roping the horse, forcibly putting on a bridle and bit, fixing on some harness and a girth, then firmly restraining the animal while it was directed in various ways within an enclosure. This enforcement was continued until the horse's resistance became diminished with fatigue.

The domesticated horse has to be taught comprehensively to accept all the controls imposed upon its life. Lessons are given in the form of training. It has to learn how to respond acceptably to a great variety of unnatural tasks and circumstances, including stable control (Brown et al., 1996; Harewood and McGowan, 2005; Visser et al., 2008). The instruction that is needed to implant all of this awareness in the horse's brain (or mind) calls for teacher aptitude. Without the aid of language for communication, or advanced intelligence for comprehension, there is much for the animal to absorb.

Training Principles

A view of behaviour as a dynamic form of mediation between the animal and its environment acknowledges that the animal makes continuous modifications to its conduct. Much of training is dependent on the modification process. A horse is required to perform numerous unnatural acts in the course of its association with man. It must learn to yield up its feet to the handler, even when it fears that its feet may be trapped. It must allow a weighty bulk on its back when fear signals an adversary landing on it. It must accept restraint passively when its fears warn it against ever yielding up its head or permitting the ensnarement of its body. It must accept confinement in a variety of poorly ventilated, dark, noisy areas when, as a plains creature, it likes the open spaces and a ridge to monitor sight and sound. It is asked to jump from sunlight into shadow without time to adapt to the light differential. It is asked for turns on the forehand, an unnatural movement for a horse, which, at liberty, turns on its hindquarters. Much of the animal's acceptance is based on trust. Many horse cultures utilize foalhood to teach the young horse to lead, stand tied and allow its hooves to be lifted and inspected. Williams *et al.* (2002) showed the beneficial effects of early training sessions on the reactions of foals at 1 month of age. However, at 3 months, no benefit was observed.

The recognition of the early ability to modify its behaviour has been used by trainers at the birth of a foal. The hours-old neonate is thoroughly handled to desensitize it to much of the potentially frightening visual, auditory, tactile and olfactory stimuli it will be exposed to in later life. Systematic, repetitive touching and rubbing of the neonate's body, orifices and feet, and moving to a different area of the body only when it shows acceptance of the current area, are employed as means of early training or conditioning. In a day or two, the foal can be exposed to a range of increasingly aversive sounds to allow it to become habituated to these for life. The evident result is a horse more amenable to training, handling and veterinary attention for the rest of its life. This handling of the neonate takes advantage of the knowledge that the immature animal is better equipped than the adult to absorb and retain social experiences. This is in accord with the theory of developmental plasticity (Bateson *et al.*, 2004). Good approaches focus upon preventing, or alleviating, adverse tension between trainer and foal. It is a recognition that cohesive behaviour is, in the horse's world, more important than dominance for alliance purposes. Environment can have an effect on health in later life (Gluckman *et al.*, 2005).

Training

The affiliative aspects of horse behaviour enhance the animal's ability to mimic, and trainers have long used allelomimetic tendencies to better instruct the horse. Some may train several yearlings at the same time to accustom them to seeing saddles on their companions as well as themselves. A horse designated for intricate reining patterns can be tied for several hours watching a seasoned performer before being introduced to the same procedure.

Housing in particular, has an influence on weanling horse behaviour. In a study by Heleski *et al.* (2002) it was found that stall-kept, isolated weanlings licked walls, chewed, kicked, pawed and had rearing bouts. Weaners in paddocked groups grazed and kept close to conspecifics. Their welfare was clearly better.

The young horse begins to test its limits around the age of 14 months. If it has not had an opportunity to be mannered by a herd, the testing of its human handler can be prolonged and rough. The young horse's natural tendency to follow and conform to its associates' direction is used in leading it out to explore. With good handling, the yearling soon learns to trust its handler. If startled, it will go towards them for reassurance rather than try to run. Early training under saddle or in long lines is done as much as possible in the outdoors. The horse's natural urge to explore, move forward, and retain its balance is encouraged as it is taken over undulating ground, across streams, and up and down steep banks and along trails.

Yearlings or 2-year-olds might be lightly backed and then wintered out until 2.5 years old or older. They can frequently be taken up in the spring to continue their training and sometimes show a better grasp of the previous year's lessons. Some trainers believe indoor schools inhibit boldness and forward movement, and make it more difficult to teach such gaits as the collected canter. For the novice horse, an outdoor beginning is best.

In training the 3-year-old, which is now a stronger and more exuberant animal, one must take account of the more developed mind and body. The horse may be asked to repeat and expand on its previous repertoire of weight-carrying or weight-drawing. Obedience and forward movement are encouraged, as is calmness of its mental attitude. Straight direction maintains the equal development of musculature.

At the age of 4, the horse is ready for introduction to serious work, such as short endurance rides, light hunting or draught work. Horses are not considered fully mature until the age of 5, though some may take longer in their development. It may be that mental capacity improves throughout the horse's lifespan.

A good trainer has practical or intuitive knowledge of horse behaviour. This gives the trainer the ability to understand a particular horse. The training of any horse is required to take place in a step by step progression. The first step is to evaluate the horse's temperament. To do this, the trainer should get to know the horse by studying it and watching it under various circumstances. If the trainer has a poor opinion of the horse, he or she should not proceed further. The first impression of a horse should indicate to its potential trainer whether the horse's temperament or its individuality is one that is appreciated. If appreciation develops, there is an excellent chance that the stages of training in a planned programme will be undertaken successfully.

Throughout the training programme, the horse's particular mental and physical limitations should be recognized. These limitations are very real and will vary from one horse to another. A good trainer teaches the horse to perform well within its physical and mental potential, but never attempts to force it beyond its limitations. Aversive confrontations between horse and trainer should be avoided at all costs, particularly in the early stages of training. If a good trainer observes that a horse does not respond enthusiastically or well to a given routine, that routine is ended promptly to avoid creating a bad experience for the animal. A good trainer uses a balance of discipline as well as reward in training, carried out in a rational manner and at the proper time. Rewards, such as vocal praise and reassuring patting with the hand in the vicinity of the shoulder, should be done immediately after a satisfactory lesson and when a new response is successfully learned. Any fractiousness in a novice horse may be due to fear, and this may take some time to pass. Delinquent activity in a horse should be countered by deliberately ignoring the horse for a period. Some horses go into a short period of depression if they are rebuked sternly by their regular attendant and user. Conflict and confusion are reduced or eliminated where the horse is induced to view its trainer as a senior partner, enlarging its equine world with as few artifices as possible.

A simple initiating method commonly employed with a young horse is to catch the animal, halter it and attempt to control it for a short period with the aid of the halter rope. This procedure is repeated at subsequent times, with intervening intervals of a few days. Three-day intervals have been found to be suitable for the horse to learn to accept this form of human control. This is not 'breaking', since the animal is given considerable time to adapt to the situation and modify its reactivity. All of this can be helped by promptly rewarding the horse with good food at the end of the haltering session. It is, of course, a time-consuming method. Haltering regularly from early foalhood obviates the need for such initial training and any attendant problems. The horse that enjoys lessons may whinny a greeting to its trainer at the approach of schooling time. This horse will learn faster and is safer than a horse that has had human presence forced upon it. The trainer assists the horse in learning, and the horse, in effect, educates itself. The right thing is made easy and the wrong thing difficult. A horse so taught rarely requires firm discipline. The trainer is constantly striving to communicate as clearly as possible with the animal (Waring, 2003).

Problems such as flightiness or lethargic behaviour are recognized early, and feeding and training schedules are adjusted accordingly. On the rare occasion when punishment is required, the behaviour should be identified as aggression, wilfulness or inappropriate playfulness, such as rearing and striking at the handler. Stallions are particularly ready to strike out with a foreleg. It should not be confused with an expression of discomfort or anticipated pain. Punishment such as a firm rebuke, a slap on the horse's chest or down its shoulder must be administered shortly and sharply at the moment the horse has acted wrongly. If punishment is prolonged, the horse is only encouraged to get away in flight.

Appropriate choice and use of a bit, curb, bridle, blinkers, etc. can be critical in the control of many horses. This is the realm of horsemanship and the reader is directed to publications on that broad area of expertise for more comprehensive information (McGreevy, 2004).

Ring-breaking

In the modern form of humane 'breaking' or taming of the totally untrained horse, the animal is placed in a wide ringed area that has high, solid sides. The breaker/trainer occupies the central area and carries a whip. In a manner that resembles lungeing, the horse is chased so that it runs around the inside perimeter of the circle. The trainer simply moves slightly towards the rear of the horse, implying a threat. In fact, the trainer does not leave the central area while constantly turning to face the location of the animal. Without touching the subject, the whip may be flourished to keep the horse running at a steady trot after it ceases to gallop. The horse's running is maintained, with an occasional change of direction, by the continuing show of pursuit being created by the trainer. The animal, in its flight, can only run close against the circular barrier and usually maintains its flight for an extended period.

In time, the stimulus loses its value and the horse may also experience some fatigue, ceasing to flee as a result. Running then stops and the horse is likely to move slowly towards the former threat in a tentative, exploratory manner. At this juncture, the suppressed horse also tolerates human approach and will probably permit cautious contact and handling. This does not constitute submission by the horse but is simply the social affinity that is in the equine nature. The duration of the circling procedure varies from about 0.5 h to as long as 2 h, depending on the horse's basic temperament and the time taken for the stimulus to lose its charge.

Although this ring-taming method seems unlike typical traditional ways of breaking-in, there are certain fundamental similarities. Essentially in both types the horse is faced with the frustration of human control that is inescapable and continuous until there is ultimately momentary compliance and acceptance of such control by the horse. In spite of fundamental factors in common, the method of ring-breaking appears to be the less agonistic means to accustom an untamed horse to human management, in the course of conditioning the animal to the general husbandry to follow (Marlborough and Knottenbelt, 2001).

Handling

Any form of restraint to immobilize or limit the movement of a horse in training and handling should only be in effect for a brief period of time and should be carried out by experienced handlers. Many horses are impatient. It deserves to be re-stated that the criteria in early handling are minimum discomfort to the horse and maximum safety for the person or persons handling the animal. No handling procedure should be based on the infliction of pain on the animal. The principal objective is to limit the horse's movement for its own well-being, while it is receiving some form of attention. In a paddock system, it is useful to have a catchment facility. Horses at pasture do not readily give up their freedom when an attempt is made to catch them in the middle of an open field.

Handling principles

Six principal rules in horse handling can be given as follows:

1. Special care should be taken when handling a horse in a narrow and confined space. When leading a horse into a box or a vehicle for example, sufficient time and opportunity should be given to the animal to allow it to accept the requirement.
2. Horses should be spoken to in a quiet and reassuring tone of voice as much as possible. Aversive handling is unwarranted. Horses can be reprimanded by appropriate voice without recourse to physical means.
3. The horse should be approached in the region of its shoulder, as it can see to the side and to the front most clearly. When the handler is familiar with the horse, the animal may be approached from the front, but the hand should be held out to allow the horse to sniff it and identify the handler.
4. Horses do not like to be handled in the region of the upper part of the head, the poll in particular. Similarly, most horses dislike being handled under the belly or over the lower flank region. It is advisable to place the hand on the side of the neck, followed by running the hand down the shoulder or along the back to the hindquarters, on the way down to the limbs. The legs and feet should be touched last in handling and grooming. To lift a hind leg, the handler should stand beside the leg, facing the rear, grasp the fetlock and draw it forward and upwards. The hoof is taken in the cupped other hand. While bent over and holding the hoof, a step is taken to the rear of the horse so that the cannon rests on the handler's thigh. The arm towards the horse is then put over the animal's hock so that the elbow helps to control the horse's leg. The upturned hind foot can then be held in both hands.
5. The signs of threat in a horse should be known and heeded as warning of the probable reaction of the animal. The handler, in turn, should give a clear signal of any intended handling procedure. Chronic biters can be muzzled if necessary when they are to be handled.
6. Always allow a mare to maintain visual contact with her young foal if it is separated from her during handling (McDonnell, 2002).

Any location where the horse is being restrained for examination or a special procedure should have good non-slip flooring. Examination places tend to become slippery with the excreta of a horse being examined and it is necessary to improve footing within the examination area with the addition of ash or sand. In the general handling of horses, appropriate use and choice of the bit and bridle are of critical importance. Horses should be made accustomed to this means of head control by appropriate training. This conditions them for the circumstances of handling. To control the head and hold the mouth open for the purpose of examining the teeth for example, the horse's tongue can be grasped and held outside the corner of the mouth. The tongue should not be pulled excessively, however.

In handling and controlling horses, it is necessary to apply knowledge of their natural mechanics of movement. The horse uses its head and neck as a way of resisting handling, and it is therefore essential for the head of the horse to be secured as a first step in the control of the animal. By raising the head, there can be effective control over any attempt by the horse to move forward. A common method of head control is to back the horse into a stall and cross-tie its halter to the two stall posts. In addition, control over the muzzle restrains the horse very effectively. Figure 14.1 illustrates a method of control using the 'Chifney' bit. The judicious application of a twitch for a brief period of time is a restraint measure frequently employed. However, twitching the upper lip of the horse should be done by someone who is trained, as excessive tightening of the twitch is not warranted or desirable. If the horse resists the application of the twitch once it has been appropriately tightened, the twitch should be removed and the animal restrained by some other means, such as raising a foreleg. This twitching method will be discussed further in a subsequent section.

Leg restraint

The limb movements of a horse require control in a variety of circumstances. Effective means of controlling kicking with the hindlimbs can be established by use of sideline or hobbles (see Fig. 14.2a and b). With this arrangement, a leather hobble or noose on a rope is placed around the fetlock region of each hind leg and the rope, secured to a collar, placed around the base of the neck. Minor forms of restraint are useful in simple procedures such as administering an intravenous injection or drawing a small blood sample. Blindfolds in the form of cloth can be applied over the eyes as another simple but very effective means of control, as they often have a subduing effect on a horse during handling.

The procedures of simple control include the following:

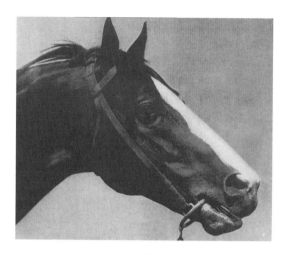

Fig. 14.1. Stallion controlled by 'Chifney' bit. This ring bit applies direct force, not weakened by joints, as on a snaffle bit. Photo: S. Hlatky.

(a)

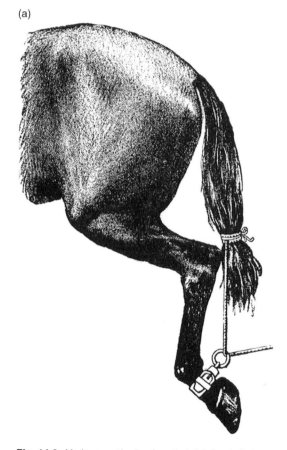

Fig. 14.2. Various methods of control. (a) Control of hind leg with rope tie. Drawing by D. Cody.

(b)

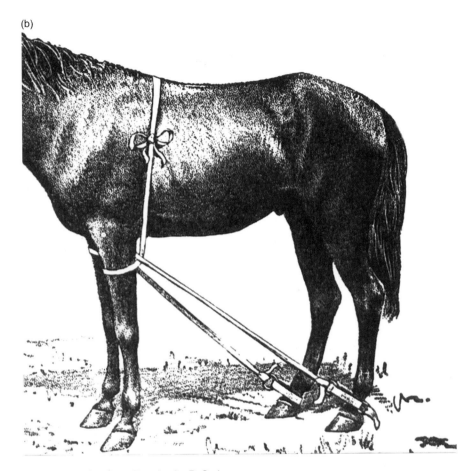

Fig. 14.2. *Continued.* (b) Sidelines. Drawing by D. Cody.

1. Holding up a forefoot with the knee flexed while the toe of the hoof is grasped by one hand while the bridle-rein is held with the other, or steadying oneself by catching hold of the mane with this hand. This is a precaution against the operator being kicked.

2. Strapping up a forelimb in the flexed position by means of a leather strap applied around the pastern and forearm, or tying them in this fashion with a piece of rope (Fig. 14.2c).

3. The forelimb may be held in the flexed position by means of a rope tied around the pastern and passed over the horse's withers.

4. Blinds completely covering the eyes. They often have a marked subduing effect on a restive horse during a minor procedure. A cloth fixed to the cheeks of the cavesson or head collar may be used instead of the regular blinds.

5. The side-stick and cradle can prevent the horse from biting or rubbing parts of its body that can be reached by the mouth (Fig. 14.2d and e).

There are numerous conventional ways of casting and fixing horses for surgery, but drugs are usually employed today for this purpose. The feet and limbs are then secured after the animal is fully anaesthetized.

Stocks

Stocks are sometimes used in the control of horses when they are subjected to veterinary examination or attention. Such stocks, if constructed of solid wood posts and side pieces, can be useful in protecting the horse and assistants working with it. Such procedures as rectal examination and

(c)

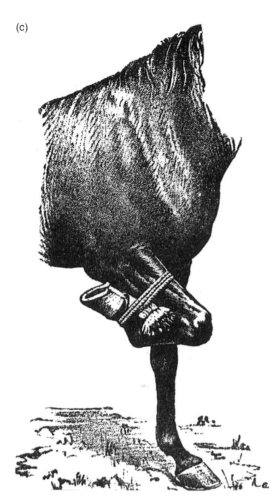

Fig. 14.2. *Continued.* (c) Control of foreleg with rope tie. Drawing by D. Cody.

clinical attention to the feet can be performed more effectively on a horse restrained within stocks. The stocks should be appropriate in size for the horse being examined, to ensure close restraint, permitting the least amount of movement. The stocks should not be made of moveable parts. In addition, the sides of the stocks should be capable of removal so the horse can be extracted from the stocks should it fall down in them. It is also essential that the side bars not be at a height that would permit the horse to kick them over and thereby entrap a leg. Some horses may have a tendency to panic when firmly restrained in stocks and must be gradually trained or conditioned to their use.

Management of Behaviour

Breed, temperament and the environment in which it was raised all affect the horse's behaviour under management. Horses that have been raised on free range or away from people will have a large flight distance and may panic and become agitated when a handler approaches within such a distance. Horses that have been raised in close confinement are usually more approachable and easier to handle. Very dense housing affects the time budget and social behaviour within a group, but crowding does not increase aggression. Group size and density have an effect on general social dynamics (Estevez *et al.*, 2007). Group size has greatest effect on the ability of individuals to learn from the given experience (Croney and Newberry, 2007). Awareness of the horse's flight distance and individual space requirements can reduce problems with baulking and alarm behaviour when it is to be subjected to handling and close control under unfamiliar circumstances. Anticipating a horse's reaction is undoubtedly the best means of exercising some control over its behaviour. This is particularly true when the handling of a temperamental or fractious horse is necessary for clinical or other such procedures.

In handling horses, the limitation of their vital space is used as a non-aversive method of initiating control. As far as possible, visual stimuli that stimulate flight, such as views through open doors, should be eliminated. Negative stimuli, intense sound, should not be able to reach collected horses. No sounds should come from a source that is in the direction that handled horses are required to go. Shouting represents disturbing sound and induces negative reactions ranging from avoidance to flight. Such reactions involve panic, which is an extreme fear reaction.

A runaway horse cannot be stopped by a person obstructing its path. At best it can be diverted into an enclosure, but some horses will run with abandon and at general risk. These are best directed towards open space. Horses in groups should only be moved by sufficient numbers of horse riders. If they are to be taken a significant distance or along a route with gates or exits, planning is required to organize the operation. Under difficult circumstances horses should be moved by lead-rein or hand-led individually.

A horse's behaviour can be controlled effectively in many ways, some of which are traditional, for example applying some modest amount of force to

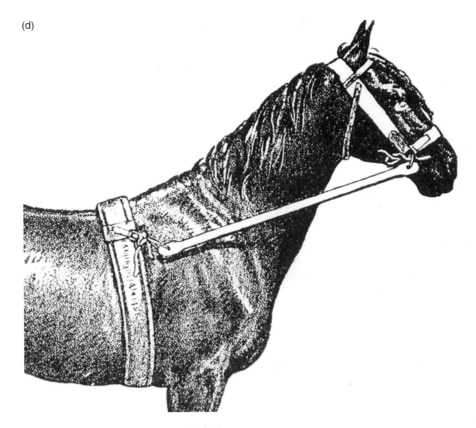

(d)

Fig. 14.2. *Continued.* (d) Sidestick. Drawing by D. Cody.

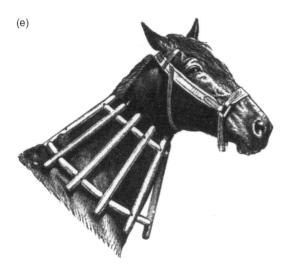

(e)

Fig. 14.2. *Continued.* (e) Cradle. Drawing by D. Cody.

a part of its body in such a way as to put the horse at a mechanical disadvantage. The head of the horse can be secured to effect overall control. Raising the head can sometimes restrain the general forward movement of ponies, although this is not so effective with the larger horse. Taking some form of tight control over the muzzle controls behaviour very effectively. A neck cradle or a sidestick can control the head very effectively.

Use of a twitch

Various methods of twitching horses make use of loops of rope or chain, which can be drawn or twisted tightly on the head region. A running noose can go over the poll and through the mouth (Fig. 14.3). It can pass between the upper incisors and the top lip or though the oral cavity, before being drawn tightly. The discomfort in this method

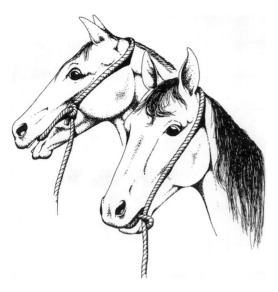

Fig. 14.3. Two methods of using a noose for head control. Drawing by D. Cody.

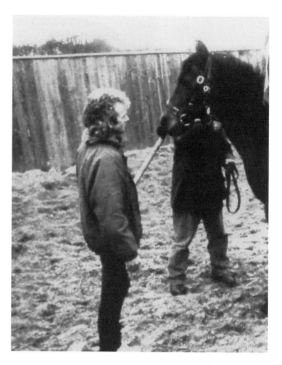

Fig. 14.4. Use of twitch for restraint. Photo: David Dugdale.

is obvious, as it is observed to upset some horses. The standard twitch is a loop on the end of a stout wooden shaft. The loop is put around the upper lip of the horse, and the handle, or shaft, is twisted to snare the lip firmly. The person applying the twitch must study the response of the horse very closely. The twitch should enclose an adequate portion of the lip. It is then quickly tightened until the horse shows the first sign of rigidity in the manner in which the head is held. Rotation of the shaft should cease at this point and the noose might be slightly slackened to the point where some head movement and reduced neck tension are shown. It can be slightly re-tightened to restore rigidity if the horse shows bodily movements (Fig. 14.4).

The theory is that the seizure of the lip causes the horse to freeze its posture, fixing its head and neck and keeping its body still. With its head tense, all of its body becomes immobilized. The fixation of the lip is considered to induce tonic immobility by reflex response to the sensation of head movement being momentarily arrested; short-term control over the horse is thus effected. The duration of this tonic immobility can be less than 5 min, but the state will not endure indefinitely. The response is not considered to be related to significant pain, although tolerable discomfort is undoubtedly present.

This control allows minor procedures to be carried out with safety. Such procedures commonly include close examination of any part of the body and rectal examination. Since all four feet remain planted on the ground, the hind feet cannot be easily lifted with a horse properly twitched. Certain horses react adversely to this control method but most respond satisfactorily. The noose should not be kept on for more than a few minutes. The circulation of the muzzle should be assisted by rubbing the lip when the twitch is removed. Twitching should only be performed by an experienced handler or done under expert supervision.

It must be emphasized that expertise is essential in the performance of this method of brief control for veterinary purposes. There has to be a precise amount of lip pressure to induce tonic immobility. The operator has to judge the exact amount of time and pressure, based on the horse's behaviour. The treatment facilitated by this control can contribute significantly to the subject's welfare. Experienced horses show no aversion to repeats of twitching.

Recumbent restraint

Drugs are more readily used today to assist in getting the horse to lie down. Resultant recumbency can be hazardous and should be under the direction and supervision of an experienced veterinarian. This method of control is usually employed out of necessity for major surgical operations, when total restraint is essential for success. Various veterinary procedures require the horse be put into a recumbent position. This ensures the safety of both the surgeon and the animal. The obsolete process of casting the conscious horse with ropes and hobbles was not only a source of stress and alarm to the animal but also exposed it to injury during the struggling and in the subsequent fall. The use of muscle-paralysing drugs for the purpose of casting the conscious horse is both inhumane and dangerous for the animal. The availability of modern drugs that induce very transient periods of unconsciousness enables this procedure to be performed in a way that should be safe and humane.

General anaesthesia, when required, should be induced in the horse in a well-padded enclosure or a stone-free, grassy paddock. Head protection for the horse is needed at this time. The unconscious, anaesthetized horse can be conveyed on a low trolley to the operating facility, where its limbs would then be covered and secured. Careful positioning of the horse is needed to prevent nerve or muscle damage from the pressure of recumbency arising from its own immobile weight. Prolonged static recumbency can lead to circulatory congestion and inadequate ventilation in the lower lung, and deficient circulation in the upper lung.

Pharmacological Control

Tranquillization

The use of drugs to influence or modify the behaviour of a horse is sometimes necessary to avoid excessive force. The range of modern chemical agents of varied pharmacological activities makes it possible to alter a horse's behaviour by tranquillization or sedation. Tranquillizers are commonly used when individual horses have to be subjected, for a period, to forms of total restraint or handling to which they are unaccustomed and that could induce a state of panic detrimental to their health. Tranquillizers produce psychological calming of anxiety without physiological depression or clouding of consciousness. They should not, however, be administered to horses if they are being transported.

It is usual to employ medications to control the horse for a limited period only. Certain narcotic preparations by themselves may be necessary for the control of severe pain, but they have no great need when restraint alone is required, since the horse's response to them can be very unpredictable. For example, narcotics in pain-free horses can produce increased activity, heightened apprehension or a state of excitement. The objective with medical restraint is to make the animal manageable in a standing position for veterinary procedures and obviate the need for the horse to be placed in a lying position.

For manageability, a tranquillizer has an anxiolytic effect, while sedatives diminish the perception of pain. Horses respond to sedatives and tranquillizers in variable ways. For example, they are still capable of kicking while in a stage of sedation or tranquillization and must therefore be handled carefully while under the effects of such drugs. In addition, they are capable of bolting food while recovering from a chemical restraint and this can lead to choking.

The phenothiazine drugs are good agents in controlling behaviour in the horse and generally have the effect of calming the animal or making it drowsy. In such states the subject can be more easily handled for certain exacting procedures. The chosen drug, such as valium or sedivet, will have the best effect when given intravenously. Acepromazine is a particularly common drug in this category, with a well-tried and true history of use.

Another drug of good effectiveness for suppressing anxiety and pain in the horse is xylazine (Rompun). It is effective in producing tranquillization and is sometimes combined with an additional drug, such as butorphanol (a narcotic analgesic), to enhance the sedative effects. This is administered intravenously and has a good margin of safety. It is sometimes combined with other drugs such as methadone, morphine or acepromazine for extra calming effects (Pavord and Pavord, 2002).

A further category of drugs sometimes used to sedate horses is the alpha-2 agonist group. This group includes detomidine and romifidine, and sometimes one of these may be combined with a tranquillizer to obtain optimal effectiveness. Anaesthesia, whether general, regional or local, is not warranted for behavioural modification and will not be addressed here. In summary, three well-used controlling drugs are considered below in more detail.

Acepromazine

It is frequently necessary to sedate horses to enable clinical and other procedures to be carried out easily and safely. Horses, however, are not good subjects for sedation. If they experience muscle weakness or ataxia they may panic in a violent manner. An improvement in the quality of sedation can be obtained by phenothiazine derivatives, which are utilized for both mood-altering and sedative actions. In horses, acepromazine is the most widely used of these agents. It has an elimination half-life of approximately 3 h in horses. It exerts a calming effect via intravenous or intramuscular administration. Obvious sedation is limited to about 60% of the subjects, and increasing the dose only increases the duration of effect. Even when apparent sedation is limited, the horse is easier to handle.

In male horses, effective sedation with phenothiazine derivatives is associated with protrusion of the flaccid penis from the prepuce; care must be taken to avoid physical damage to this organ. In the vast majority of animals the penis retracts spontaneously as sedation wears off, while in a very small proportion prolonged prolapse or extrusion occurs. Treatment of this complication is by manual massage, compression bandage and replacement in the prepuce, followed by suture of the prepucial orifice. Treatment must not be delayed, and it should be remembered that the sedated horse must be handled with caution, for the animal may be aroused by stimulation and when disturbed could respond with a very well-aimed kick.

Xylazine

Xylazine is a sedative agent suitable for horses. Intravenous administration is followed within 2 min by obvious effects. The horse's head is lowered, and the eyelids and lower lip droop. A horse may sway on its feet, cross its hind legs or knuckle on a foreleg. The horse will remain on its feet and show no panic. Sedation by intravenous injection is complete after about 5 min and lasts 30–60 min, depending on the dose. Intramuscular injection can give similar effects, with maximal sedation after 20 min. Despite the existence of analgesia, horses sedated with xylazine appear very sensitive to touch. Again, the well-sedated horse may react adversely.

Detomidine

Detomidine can be given intravenously or by intramuscular injection. It has some effect when injected subcutaneously. Since it is absorbed through mucous membranes, the latter property has been utilized by administering the drug on sugar lumps, for example. It can be administered more reliably by squirting under the tongue. This property of easy absorption across the mucous membranes can facilitate its application to a fractious or nervous horse. The pharmacological properties of detomidine are typical of those of an alpha-2-adrenoceptor agonist. The treated horse becomes relaxed and calm. The effects of detomidine can be reversed with atipamezole, but since only small doses of sedative are used reversal is unlikely to be necessary. A good feature of this drug is that it allows the horse to remain standing, even with a heavy dosage.

Welfare Husbandry

Much protection against illness can be given to horses by good husbandry. Preventive husbandry is applied welfare, if suitably implemented. Good rules of management that can contribute a great deal towards the prevention of illness in any horse facility are as follows:

1. Guard against overstocking. When horses are crowded together either indoors or outdoors, dormant illness can flare up and transmissible infections can become widespread and extensive. Injury is also more likely in crowded situations.

2. Maintain a high level of hygiene. This point cannot be overstressed. Cleanliness is needed at every level of care. Feed boxes and troughs must be kept free of old food. Buckets and drinking vessels must be hygienic. Grooming items have to be kept clean and periodically disinfected. Drains must be kept open and flushed regularly. Windows have to be clean and permit good ventilation. Dust must be controlled as much as possible. Premises must be kept rodent free. A hygienic environment should be the general objective in all aspects of stable management.

3. Turn out each horse in a stable on a daily basis. This should include wintertime, although severe weather such as a snowstorm, heavy rain or a driving cold wind would be exceptions. An outdoor facility should have a windbreak such as a section of boarding or natural shelter. Fresh air and free movement are health aids.

4. Protect from flies. In many situations and geographical locations, it is desirable to put horses indoors during daytime in the summer to protect them from the various flies that cause distress, skin disorders or viral infections, including sweet itch, anaemia and certain encephalitides. Mesh screens, vaporizers, fly paper and fine netting can be used to protect indoor horses from fly attacks at peak times and seasons of such risk. Smoke generators may be useful to clear stables of flies, even when horses are present, but this should only be done under continuous human supervision. Stables are fire hazards at all times.

5. Establish a close connection with a veterinary service. This is a most important requirement of management. It is a usual practice to call a veterinarian to treat a sick or injured horse or to administer vaccinations, but a better system of veterinary attendance can be arranged. The connection between management and veterinarian can be set out in a clear contractual arrangement. This could deal with routine horse care matters on a scheduled programme of visitations. The visits can be for a prescribed time, during which routine matters could be addressed. Matters such as pregnancy testing, nutrition review, teeth checking and floating, health checks, special examination, blood and faecal sampling, worming, vaccination and advice can be dealt with on a routine, preventive basis. A pre-set fee arrangement for such a visit, plus materials, could be understood by both parties and would assist in budgeting. Emergency visits would be reduced; however, any of these would be outside the contract.

Health control

A horse health and welfare programme could emerge from the system in item 5, and this could incorporate any new information of great value on an extensive range of health care topics. A health and welfare programme could provide assurance and guidance on matters of preventative medicine for the horse caregiver. The modern equine veterinarian can deliver a much more economically valuable service in such a scheme. This is usually impossible with urgent call-outs. Programmes of vaccination and worming can be tailored to the circumstances of a horse, in accordance with its known risks and regional circumstances (Pavord and Pavord, 2002).

Health and welfare programme

A modern and advisable system of horse care involves a health programme for a single horse or several under the same management. This operates by having veterinary input into horse husbandry to set out routine practices in order to maintain health through preventive medicine.

A most important part of infectious disease control is a vaccination programme. Proper vaccination gives horses a very good prospect of resisting common infections. Vaccination against the viruses of equine influenza and rhinopneumonitis plus the bacteria of tetanus and strangles are considered to be of basic importance. A veterinarian working in the area would best know of the need for additional vaccination. The full picture of disease prevalence in a given region is knowledge that a local veterinarian would likely have before others. Regional illnesses must always be considered when a horse is to be exposed to new contacts from different sources.

Effective vaccines are now available to protect against most of the serious, transmissible diseases of horses. Sometimes the immunity obtained by vaccination is of short duration and a re-vaccination is necessary. This is taken into account when a vaccination programme is planned. The most common and easily spread horse diseases are viral infections (Gore *et al.*, 2008). The movement of horses geographically spreads viruses to new populations. Young horses are usually most susceptible to such infections. Vaccination is essential for carriage horses.

A worming timetable is another very necessary component of a horse health programme. Parasite control involves regular worming of all the horses at the same time in a given facility. At a deeper level, the programme would also involve the faecal examination of any new horse and periodic faecal examinations of each resident horse to determine the type and amount of parasite infestation. Large strongyles (bloodworms) and roundworms are the most dangerous. Other internal parasites that can depress a horse's health include small strongyles, pinworms, tapeworms, stomach worms and bots. Modern broad-spectrum anthelmintics are available to kill such internal parasites, but they must be properly selected and accurately dosed. The programme's veterinarian would determine a schedule of regular worming, with occasional changing of the anthelmintic according to factors such as horse condition and the various types of parasites found on periodical faecal examinations.

Management can play a major part in parasite control, not only by pasture management but also by suitable segregation of animals. Newly weaned horses are very susceptible subjects and should be kept separate from other, older horses. Yearlings should be confined to the cleanest possible grazing and should receive the most frequent worming. Newcomers should be quarantined, as already recommended for infection control. Infection with microorganisms and infestation with internal and external parasites are two quite different states, but they have much in common; they plague horses and require control. Management can avoid known risks and give thought to a horse's circumstances at all times to help with such control. This can be termed preventative management. It is a modern concept in animal care and an economical objective. A standard in animal welfare is application of the five freedoms that should be afforded to livestock. Although it is a very idealistic and demanding concept, it is one that has been widely presented and well articulated. It is now present in both the public domain and the animal welfare orthodoxy, to be met in a set of desirable freedoms for horses.

The five freedoms

In livestock care, five freedoms are now accepted internationally as the welfare standard. They apply to horses now as the objectives sought in their humane care. These freedoms are as follows:

1. Freedom from fear and distress.
2. Freedom from pain, injury and disease.
3. Freedom from hunger and thirst.
4. Freedom from discomfort.
5. Freedom to express normal behaviour.

Good horse management provides these freedoms already, to the limit of reality. Occasionally there are circumstances beyond human control when management is unable to sustain some of these freedoms. In such cases, good management attempts to have them restored as quickly as possible. In the case of commercial transportation of horses in groups, it has to be said that all five freedoms of welfare can seldom be met at present. It rests with the transporter of a horse to aim at the full standard. Some horse owners do achieve the standard with their own animals, but some only partially manage to do so. In the long term, an endeavour must be made to bring the five freedoms into horse transportation generally. With regard to freedom number 5, some behavioural needs are only temporary or periodic. Other behavioural needs are continuous, such as reaction movements, stretching, resting and minor body shifting for comfort – these are all a part of item 5. In the context of husbandry welfare, this freedom is feasible.

Geriatric welfare

Beyond 25 years of age, a horse is extremely old, although many ponies reach this age group quite comfortably with moderate use. By this time they require comfortable control. Threats to health are numerous and a full programme of health service may be needed to keep the animal in a satisfactory state, free of suffering. Well-being can still coexist with age at this advanced level. Very old horses often have arthritis and cannot run for any significant distance. All health care principles apply in extreme old age. Because of the acute angle of the incisor profile, grazing may be adversely affected and extra rations of well-ground oats and dried lucerne or a good hay substitute will be needed to maintain what remains of health and well-being in this age group. In geriatric horse cases, old aches can recur. Chronic musculoskeletal lesions can become more debilitating in older horses. Due consideration to the likelihood of arthritis should be a part of their general care in such things as wide accommodation, rubber matting, outdoor resting and security from bullies. Euthanasia may be a necessary duty to pre-empt terminal suffering in old horses.

Chapter 14

15 Disordered Behaviour and Stress

From earlier times there has been recognition of various behavioural abnormalities in horses, known as stable vices. They are very genuine impairments, which reduce the horse's merit as well as the animal's well-being. These disorders in the subject's behaviour are pernicious and groups of them have certain characteristics in common. In particular, the manner of their display often has a stereotyped form or pattern. They are included in the category of 'stereotypies', as some of these abnormal actions are now called in ethology. Interest in this phenomenon has grown, in various disciplines of study and research, into an international debate (Wiepkema, 1987; Lawrence and Rushen, 1993; Kiley-Worthington, 1999; Bucklin, 2003; Jahiel, 2004).

The form of accommodation often imposed upon the horse represents immurement, or even solitary confinement. It is an old adage among thoughtful horse keepers that 'a horse on its own is in bad company'. Isolation is a stressor, which obviously contributes to disordered horse behaviour. Lack of diversionary quality in the environment is stressful. Horse keepers in the past were not sufficiently aware of the need for 'quality' within the equine environment. Attention was focused upon the nutritional and hygienic needs of the horse, but behavioural needs were unknown or neglected. In regard to causation, the stereotyped anomalies in horse behaviour evidently have a stress-related, hyperdopaminergic foundation. Horses appear to be able to tolerate stress up to a given level, which varies with individuals within the population. When a critical level of stressfulness is reached in an individual horse, some form of anomalous behaviour is likely to develop and serve as a lenitive treatment for its anguish. The company of another horse can help (Nagy et al., 2008), as well as feeding smaller meals (Cooper et al., 2005).

Signs of confinement distress, in addition to oral and ingestive disorders, which have some linkage, include weaving, head-nodding, stall-walking, pawing, self-mutilation, stall-kicking, crib-biting, wind-sucking, tongue-dragging and overdrinking. The list of different forms of anomalous actions in horses goes on further to include abnormal reactions. In full, 28 disorders are recognized now that more scientific attention has focused on dysfunctional forms of equine behaviour. These 28 conditions have all been summarized in four tables in this chapter. They are further described and discussed below in three main sections namely: disorders of oral and eating behaviour, abnormal actions in stabled horses, and abnormal reactions in horses. The various disorders were recognized by Mills et al. (2002).

Disorders of Oral and Eating Behaviour

Abnormal oral and ingestive activities are an important and complex category of disordered behaviour in horses. Manifestations of these disorders exist quite widely in the general horse population. Some have been well recognized historically. Most of the syndromes are associated with the joint circumstances of chronic restriction and isolation stress. Various types and varieties can be recognized with a common history of confinement and a lack of kinetic activity. The best known of these disorders is crib-biting with wind-sucking. This is a compound abnormality (Forrester, 1980; Keeling and Jensen, 2002).

Affected animals may display more than one form of abnormal oral–ingestive activity at different times (Houpt, 1987). Often a change of syndromes relates to an alteration in the animal's circumstances. This shows that the acquired maladaptive state can reveal itself in various ways. In spite of the variety of these disorders, it is notable that they occur in identical forms worldwide. This is due to their common underlying neural framework, plus the same changes in brain chemistry (excess or deficiency in neuro-transmitters).

Crib-biting

The 'cribber' or crib-biter performs its abnormal activity by grasping the edge of its stall or some other convenient fixture with the incisor teeth. The upper incisors are often used alone. The horse presses its teeth down and a swallowing movement occurs as a bolus of air is passed down into the stomach. A visibly enlarged and overdeveloped pharynx goes with the condition. Accompanying each effort of crib-biting there is usually a grunt.

Some horses may rest their teeth against any part of the crib or stall. The rim of any wooden ledge or a board can be used. In rare cases, the mouth may be placed against a knee or cannon of one or the other foreleg. Some horses that have been crib-biters may change to wind-suckers when control measures are attempted. Some wind-suckers can duly become crib-biters. Affected horses may engage in these activities when alone, while others will display it in the company of other horses. Some individuals exhibit it outdoors. A few affected animals may not show any sign of the disorder when under close observation, but most disregard the presence of humans. An affected horse might show its abnormality at work, but the majority of cribbers only show the condition when they are stabled. The upper incisors eventually become worn down, leaving the animal unable to graze properly. No physiological differences were found between cribbers, weaners and controls in a study by Clegg *et al.* (2008).

Wind-sucking

The behavioural disorder of wind-sucking or aerophagia often occurs in association with crib-biting. Wind-sucking can also occur alone. In both forms the abnormal ingestion of air is performed in the same strong, gulping fashion. Individual horses may have their own manner of regularly performing the activity, but the general method is similar in most affected horses. In pure wind-sucking, the horse nods its head and neck several times in preparation for the intake effort. Following this, the head is jerked up; the horse opens its mouth, takes in air, raises the floor of the mouth and contracts the musculature of the pharynx. The air is then very forcefully swallowed as the neck is flexed. The characteristic wind-sucking grunting sound is made as the horse expels a portion of the air. In some horses, the sound is made as they swallow the volume of air (Kiley-Worthington, 1999).

A very nervous, hyperactive horse kept in a stall much of the time with little exercise and grooming is a likely candidate for the disorder. Some athletic, wind-sucking, Thoroughbred families are thought to be predisposed to this disorder. This may not be inheritance, however; perhaps they simply have in common a low tolerance for stressful enclosure. By contrast, placid draught horses are less likely to wind-suck. The condition is chronic, and with persistent aerophagia the musculature of the throat enlarges due to hypertrophy from excessive use. Stomach dilation and an associated bloating may also occur. This can lead to gastrointestinal dysfunction and episodes of colic. Horses that practise aerophagia intensively over a long period eventually reduce their intake of feed and may scatter it during eating. The resultant nutritional deficiency causes poor physical condition. Good feeding practices can play a part in control (Hothersall and Nicol, 2009).

Bruxism

The abnormality of bruxism in the oral behaviour of horses was formerly unrecognized, although it is well known in human medicine as the dysfunctional habit of teeth grinding, often during sleep in the persons affected. It is usually taken to be stress related. Severe teeth grinding can be heard in some livestock when they are subjected to such stressors as being crated for the first time, but this by itself is not bruxism. As an anomalous condition, bruxism has to be an established habit. Among domestic animals, this condition is most obvious in stall-confined sows, where it has been variously termed as 'vacuous chewing', 'stereotypic sham chewing' and 'empty mouthing'. It is made evident in these sows by the regular accumulation of masses of frothy saliva along the edges of the mouth. Many such animals develop the 'thin sow syndrome'. Horses affected with bruxism do not show such signs, but they have comparable indicators of the anomaly, such as quidding and loss of condition. Quidding is a well-recognized sign of molar wear, in which partially chewed food, such as hay or grass, drops periodically from the horse's mouth. Treatment for quidding is filing or 'floating' the sharp outer molar edges of the worn upper teeth and the inner edges of the worn lower teeth. Severe cases of bruxism require this treatment to be repeated when the addiction again results in quidding. The habit may be initiated in stall confinement, but when it is established it persists in any environment.

Crib-whetting

Some horses in chronic confinement show disordered oral behaviour in which the body of the tongue is slowly, but repeatedly, drawn across the edge of the crib. The affected horse holds its tongue very firmly in this action so that the behaviour does not represent true licking. The repetitious nature of this disorder and the regular form of it make it stereotyped. As with other stereotyped syndromes, this condition is difficult to eliminate. A few cases improve, however, when given a salt lick.

Tongue-dragging

Tongue-dragging, tongue-over-the-bit and tongue-waving are basically modified forms of the same condition. The affected horse puts its tongue over the bit or out of the side of its mouth repeatedly (see Fig. 15.1). The activity may be shown by the horse during work, riding or in idleness in the stable. Although the condition is odd-looking, no physical dysfunction in the animal results from it. However, it is considered to be a commercial unsoundness. Riders object to it, but strapping the bit closer to the palate helps to keep better bit contact in the mouth during riding.

Wood-chewing

Abnormal chewing and eating of wood (lignophagia) is quite common in horses in restricted quarters or paddocks. Of all the oral–ingestive disorders in the horse, wood-chewing is the most common. It is not limited to indoor horses and is as frequent in horses in outdoor enclosures. Even in pastures, wood-chewing may take the form of severe de-barking of trees; limited paddock space per head of horse clearly aggravates the condition. Although wood-chewing horses do not usually ingest most of the wood they chew, they do ingest enough to risk splinter damage to the alimentary tract. Lack of cellulose roughage in the diet undoubtedly contributes to wood-chewing. Horses fed on concentrate diets with a low supply of roughage show the condition much more frequently than horses fed hay in abundance. A wood-chewer may chew half

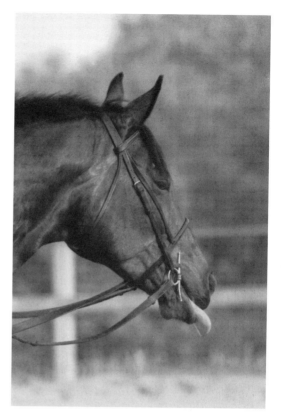

Fig. 15.1. Hanging tongue habit. Note eye expression. Photo: Melanie MacDonald.

a kilogram of wood a day. Wood-chewing can ultimately cause an intestinal obstruction (Green and Tong, 1988).

The true eating pattern of the horse is an almost continuous consumption of roughage. Its digestive tract is unsuited to rapid food processing. At pasture the horse will graze 70% of the day and night. Chewing coarse fibres takes extra time, thereby fulfilling the equine need for both chew time and fibre filling. Much roughage is needed by the horse's alimentary system for proper digestive fermentation. Unfortunately, modern horse care prefers refined diets, giving more grain and less hay. Hay is regarded as too bulky for storage space. The trend is to feed less hay and increase grain accordingly. All of this may satisfy the horse's need for energy, but it neglects the horse's basic need for fibre. Quality hay, such as lucerne, can be fed *ad libitum* to wood-chewers; in turn, they will show less of the disorder. The wood-chewing disorder can be diminished by the inclusion of sawdust in a high-concentrate diet when access to pasture is not possible.

Eating faeces

Ingestion of faeces (coprophagia) is typically a problem of confinement in adults. It is so often seen in foals under good management that it is considered normal in these animals while they are learning to chew and ingest roughage. Coprophagia in the adult horse, however, is a different matter.

In affected animals it is typically a problem of confinement in a box stall with insufficient roughage in the diet. Adult horses practising coprophagia are typically under chronic restrictions. They have often undergone a change in use or management and may have lost some attention. Affected animals consume their own faeces in substantial quantity. In some cases most of the faeces are regularly consumed. The condition can be controlled to the advantage of the animal by muzzling it. A horse with coprophagia should be removed to a tied stall or cross-tied in the box until the problem appears to be corrected. Roughage can be given *ad libitum*. In many cases, such a diet maintained for a period of at least 2 months is found to stop this behaviour.

Litter-eating

Horses confined on sawdust litter may eat their bedding, even after it has become soiled. Almost every horse in the confines of a stable can be observed to eat soiled litter on occasions, but with a litter-eating disorder this activity occurs habitually. The habit can develop in horses that are quite well fed. Several causes of litter-eating in horses have become recognized. Unbalanced rations, feeding at the wrong time of day, and heavy worm burdens have all been found to contribute to this condition. Horses at pasture graze most of the day; eating is clearly their chief occupation. Within stables this occupation is curtailed, and grain or compounded food is often consumed quickly. If such food is not followed up with the adequate provision of hay (for ingestive occupation as much as balanced nutrition), horses may seek other available cellulose materials to eat. A worm burden must be considered and treated in this condition. As in other allied forms of disordered eating behaviour, control calls for appreciation of potential needs, and these are clear in this case. Attention to this disorder of behaviour includes consideration of all aspects of the diet to ensure adequate quantity, quality and variety. Food should include salt licks and mixtures rich in minerals and vitamins. Fresh feed, such as greens or carrots, should be offered regularly. Feeding times should be observed on a precise timetable with late night and early morning being included in the feeding schedule.

Hair-eating

The disordered behaviour in horses of hair-eating (trichophagia) relates to the ingestion of hair, licked or chewed, from the bodies of associating animals. It occurs in conditions of husbandry in which horses are closely grouped. This allows the eating of tail hairs from associate horses, causing the development of hairballs in the large intestine. Hairballs can also be the result of excessive self-grooming at periods when the coat is being shed. Hair-eating is akin to wood-chewing. In aetiology, the therapy for both conditions is an increased supply of cellulose and fibrous roughage in the diet.

Soil-eating

Horses can develop the so-called 'depraved' disorder of eating soil, sand, or dirt (see Fig. 15.2). The affected horse licks at the soil, and when a portion of earth is dislodged, it is taken up by the teeth and eaten. The animal licks around its mouth and begins again to lick the soil. This becomes a habit, which can lead to alimentary dysfunction. The condition has sometimes been termed pica. It has been thought to be the result of mineral deficiency. Phosphorus and iron deficiencies are known, in some cases, to be responsible for soil-eating but other affected animals do not appear to have a nutritional deficiency. A simple desire for salt may be involved initially, before the disorder is established. Boredom and lack of movement appear again to be one of the causal circumstances. Excessive eating of sand or dirt can result in sand impaction of the horse's caecum and colon. Such impactions can have very serious clinical consequences. Soil becomes present in the faeces and may alter its colour.

This condition should take into account the possibility of a mineral deficiency. A supplementary ration of bone meal should therefore be provided to eliminate the possibility of phosphorous deficiency. In addition, affected animals can be examined for

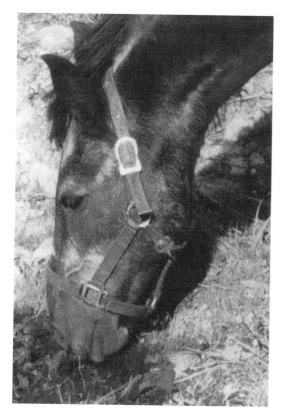

Fig. 15.2. Aged gelding licking and swallowing earth habitually. Photo: A.F. Fraser.

anaemia and worm burdens, where appropriate iron and anthelmintic treatment can be provided when indicated. As with other oral and ingestive behavioural disorders in the horse, enclosed animals should be given exercise and a good diet, consisting of high-quality hay *ad libitum* and a salt lick.

Bolting food

The disordered eating behaviours of overeating and rapid eating are forms of hyperphagia (bolting food) in some nervous horses fed in stalls. Many horses are extremely greedy and rapid eaters, but bolting takes this further. The bolting of food in some horses may cause choking. The food ingested by the bolter is not fully masticated and digestive disorders can result. Such horses may consume excessive quantities if they have access to an open feed bin containing concentrated rations. In turn, this could lead to a serious digestive illness with a fatal consequence.

The treatment of bolting involves the tactical feeding of affected horses. Spreading the grain in a thin layer in the trough and placing large, smooth stones in the bottom of the trough are methods used to make grain difficult to eat rapidly. Supplying the grain in feed several times during the day may help. Feeding hay prior to grain can also be of help in the partial control of the eating disorder. It may be impossible, however, to remove this condition entirely from the horse's behaviour.

Overdrinking

Overdrinking (polydipsia nervosa) is seen as an ingestive disorder in some horses that are isolated and confined in stalls with water supplied *ad libitum*. Some of these horses may consume up to 140 l daily, or about three to four times the normal quantity. This excessive consumption can be spread over a period of time or may be concentrated within a relatively short time of 2–3 h. An associated polyuria may be the disorder's first sign. The constant flushing of ingesta probably reduces the nutritional value of the ration. In some instances, polydipsia has been noted among overtrained horses.

Autopsies performed on horses that have died from gastric or intestinal volvulus sometimes show a significantly large volume of water in the part of the alimentary canal that has undergone the twist. In some veterinary opinions the sudden intake of an abnormally large quantity of water may allow a segment of the alimentary canal to become heavily loaded and liable to twist. Polydipsia does not appear to be a disorder that becomes fixed securely in the subject. It may lend itself to control by appropriate management, including the provision of rationed water and, as usual, more roughage. Since chronic boredom seems to be a contributing factor in this disorder, treatment includes an increase in freedom, exercise and companionship.

Tables 15.1 and 15.2 summarize the oral and ingestive disorders that have been discussed.

Abnormal Actions in Stabled Horses

It was once argued that a stress-induced behavioural disorder, such as stereotyped weaving, is a sign of adaptation to confinement stress. This interpretation, in terms of animal welfare, is illogical. Anyone who argues that repetitive, disordered behaviour is adaptive overlooks the fact that the

Table 15.1. Abnormal oral activities in horses.

Activity	Characteristics
Crib-biting	The affected individual typically grasps the edge of the manger of its stall with its incisor teeth. The upper incisors are often used alone to press down on the fixture. Air is then swallowed with a grunt. When the habit is well developed, the horse may bite down on any firm structure that it can grasp. The upper incisors may become worn down to the gum. The animal is then unable to graze.
Crib-whetting	The affected horse repeatedly draws the tongue slowly across the crib or manger in the stall. During this activity the horse holds the tongue in a firm and fixed manner that does not resemble normal licking.
Tongue-dragging	This condition is revealed when the horse is bridled and being ridden, or it may be performed in the stable. It rarely occurs when the affected horse is idle in a paddock. The tongue is displaced out of the side of the mouth. It is not an activity of great significance with regards to equine well-being.
Bruxism	A horse with this condition rubs its upper molars against the lower ones in a dysfunctional habit. The manner in which this is done is covert and usually goes unnoticed. In time, excessive wear occurs on the tables of all molars. This leaves the outer edges sharp on the upper molars, which are wider apart than the lower ones; the latter develop sharp edges against the tongue. Chewing becomes impaired and boluses of incompletely masticated hay or grass occasionally drop from the mouth.

Table 15.2. Abnormal ingestion in horses.

Abnormality	Characteristics
Wind-sucking	Persistent gulping of air with an accompanying grunt. May be associated with crib-biting or may occur in the form of air-swallowing without a biting action.
Wood-chewing	Regular and persistent biting, chewing and eating wood on fence tops, doorways of stables, bark of trees, etc. is seen mostly in horses kept fenced in or closed up. This often diminishes when fed roughage.
Eating faeces	Breaking up faecal piles and eating into the content is fairly common in young foals, especially eating the mare's dung. This is abnormal in an adult.
Litter-eating	Eating their own bedding, especially if it consists of wood particles or chaff. The litter may be clean or soiled.
Hair-eating	Chewing off and then eating the tail hairs of another horse. The eaten hair accumulates and remains in the gut.
Soil-eating	Persistent eating of quantities of earth or sand, depending on whatever is available, can result in the impaction of solid dirt in the caecum or colon. In some cases, a nutritional deficiency is suspected.
Bolting food	Eating quickly and greedily may be a regular occurrence or a single event of nervousness (e.g. trailer choke).
Overdrinking	Frequent drinking and excessive consumption of water will result in polyuria. This disorder may or may not relate to a disease process. Abnormal water intake can occur in confined horses with an *ad libitum* water supply.

causal factors of the disorder are probably still present. These and other behavioural disorders may or may not be attempts to achieve adaptation, but any adaptive level attained is inadequate if the disordered behaviour persists and there is no restoration of normality. At best, they might be lenitive additions. The full appreciation of disordered behaviour is a logical approach in the diagnosis of environmental stress, including stress in the stable. The various disorders of behaviour that indicate such stress in the horse's bodily actions are given below.

Chapter 15

Weaving

Long recognized as a 'stable vice', weaving is a behavioural disorder of horses that have nervous dispositions. The affected animal stands in one position but weaves from side to side or may rock back and forth. The main feature is swinging the head, neck and forequarters from side to side. Weight is taken alternatively on each forelimb. The forefeet usually remain on the stable floor during the behaviour, but in extreme cases each foot is raised in turn as the weight passes on to the other foot. It occurs most commonly in riding horses that have then been stabled in single stalls without adequate exercise after a phase of active use. The animal that has been 'programmed' for action is now totally deprived of it. This is not humane. The responsibility lies with the user and the owner of such a horse. Turning the horse into a paddock can provide daily freedom and exercise. Intense exercise can be beneficial and this can be supplied by lungeing. The use of a mechanical exerciser would be in order. If paddock space and a facility for exercise are not available, the custody of the horse should be surrendered. While it is possible to arrest the weaving by cross-tying the horse tightly in the stall, this procedure is counter-productive in the attempts to alleviate the inherent stress in the animal and is ultimately not an ethical procedure. Ideally, a weaver should be turned out into a spacious pasture. Returning the animal to nature, so to speak, is a fundamentally valid policy for such disordered behaviour, which indicates an evident state of spatial stress, in order to allow the animal to cope (Koolhaas et al., 1999). Making mirrors available so that the horse can view its reflection has been found to reduce weaving (McAfee et al., 2002).

Stall-walking

In stall-walking, the horse moves side to side or back and forward, turning sharply, in a repetitive, precise type of movement, which usually involves stepping actions of the forefeet. This may be sustained for such long periods that the continuous drain on the animal's energy becomes significant. In affected horses the physical condition deteriorates noticeably.

Stereotyped pacing is the essence of stall-walking. In this disordered behaviour the horse constantly paces or circles around its box. The behaviour is shown under conditions of minimal exercise, resulting in chronic confinement stress.

The condition resembles weaving with the stereotyped precision and repetition in which the horse performs its rhythmic movements. As distinct from weaving in a tied stall, the stall-walker makes use of the larger area afforded by a loose box. The greater space allows the affected horse to perform slightly more elaborate ambulatory actions than in weaving.

The quantity of work performed in stall-walking is often considerable. In many cases it leads to loss of weight through energy depletion. Since the amount of the area available to the horse is very limited, much spinal flexion is required in circling and turning. This can lead to painful back conditions, which can adversely affect the horse's performance and well-being when ridden or worked.

The abnormal action can be restrained by cross-tying the horse in a stall, but the basic problem is not solved by such control. This method cannot be recommended as humane therapy. On veterinary advice, however, this could be justified temporarily in some clinical circumstances, for example to ease any back pain from strain. The provision of adequate freedom and regular exercise for the horse, particularly the performance horse, is the rational and humane way for remedy in this form of disordered behaviour.

Pawing

It is normal behaviour for horses to paw at a recumbent foal or in such activities as clearing snow from herbage. Pawing becomes an abnormal activity when it is performed with vigour in a manner that is persistent and stereotyped. Minor episodes of pawing do occur very commonly and normally when horses are frustrated and evidently irritated while awaiting food. This pawing ceases when the horses are fed. Repetitive and enduring pawing, for a detectable clinical or other reason, is an abnormal action found in some stabled horses.

Continual pawing on the hard stable floor can result in various forms of leg strain and injury. Hooves become severely worn from the persistent digging action that pawing entails. The fact that the stable floor sometimes gets dug up in one spot is of minor consequence. This merely serves as a diagnostic sign of the disordered behaviour. This condition is difficult to eliminate in the stable since it is manifestly stable stress. It typically occurs in confined and isolated horses, as in others of this group of abnormalities. Regular periods of spacious freedom are a basic need. Turning the affected animal out to pasture in the company of other horses is the rational and humane way to deal with this abnormal state. A follow-up clinical examination would be justified to differentiate the condition from any associated disease. Subsequent hoof damage would require veterinary treatment.

Head-tossing/nodding

Horses can show a nodding of the head in a variety of circumstances, including various clinical conditions causing pain. Irritation in the mouth, ears or other parts of the body can cause a horse to engage in spells of head-tossing in the stable or while being ridden. A horse tilting its head frequently to one side often signifies pain from a dental condition. When head-tossing becomes frequent and stereotyped in manner, it can be identified as disordered behaviour. The activity should be studied from some distance for an extended period in order to determine if it conforms to stereotyped characteristics, such as exact regularity, precise repetition, continuing performance and the animal's apparent concentration on this one action. With eye closure, no evidence of pain would be included in the performance of head-tossing as an item of disordered behaviour.

The condition can often be seen in horses with their heads held over the closed, lower part of the box stall door as they are kept in idleness once eating is finished (see Fig. 15.3). This condition can increase in frequency until it becomes routine in the horse's actions. While being ridden the action creates difficulty for the rider for two reasons: the reins can be plucked from the rider's hands and the animal's concentration on the disorder can distract its attention from its way-of-going, including balance and the rider's aids. The disorder becomes a serious dysfunction in the horse's use.

Correction of head-tossing can be attempted by using lighter bits, fixing a standing martingale, reschooling the horse by lungeing and giving it a wide variety of exercises. The latter in particular can focus the horse's attention away from the abnormal action. Some affected horses can respond to these corrective attentions but some relapse or adopt a different stereotyped action. Boredom in the stable is a probable cause for initiating the condition. Once again, returning the horse to nature in a good-quality pasture can eventually eliminate the condition. As with weaving, the

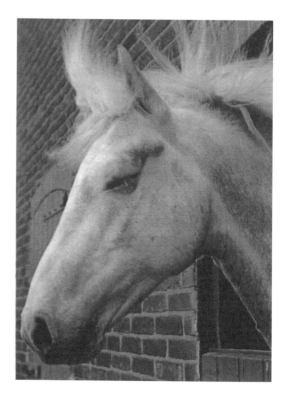

Fig. 15.3. Head nodding. Photo: A.F. Fraser.

provision of mirrors alleviates the disorder, as reported by McAfee *et al.* (2002).

Chronic standing

Chronic standing in horses kept stabled is by no means uncommon, particularly among older animals and among individuals of the very heavy breeds such as Belgians and Clydesdales. They can continue to stand in stalls, without lying down, for months on end. Some individuals never lie down in the stall. It can be speculated that the reason for chronic standing is the horse's fear of the consequences. However, it could simply be the case that the horse is physically unable to lie down in a confined stall through such orthopaedic conditions as spinal or limb joint pathology. A narrow stall can also induce the condition of chronic standing.

Remaining upright and still is a natural behavioural tactic of many large quadrupeds in times of uncertainty regarding potential intrusion into their space. Whether this phenomenon is in any way involved in chronic standing in horses is speculative.

However, it is a fact that some horses affected with this disorder of behaviour are perfectly capable of lying down and rising when they are at pasture or free range.

During times of heavy horse use, chronic standing in the stable was well recognized as a problem by workers on the streets or the farm. Some horsemen dealt with this matter by putting a resting fixture across the heel posts of the affected horse's stall for the animal to lean its rump on. One such fixture was a strong chain slung from post to post at the height of the horse's thighs, which was secured at night. At times the chain was inside a rubber sleeve for the horse's comfort, while at other times a heavy rope was used. Horses soon learned to lean heavily on such supports when they were resting or sleeping. As a means of dealing with this disorder today, a return to this old method can be considered. A large well-bedded box could also be beneficial in dealing with this condition, in which humane care is clearly required.

Tail-rubbing

In many instances of tail-rubbing, it is actually the horse's rump that is being rubbed. The action of tail-rubbing can be related to a parasitic condition. In addition, it is an element of maintenance behaviour: a normal action in the horse's own body care. Tail-rubbing is included here since persistent performance of this action can be shown by some horses without a clinical condition of parasitism, such as rectal helminth infestation, fungal disease or louse infestation of the tail head region. By itself, tail-rubbing is a non-specific action, also relating to certain hind leg diseases.

Little doubt exists that, parasitism aside, persistent, stereotyped tail-rubbing can occur as an item of abnormal body-based activity. Although it is not characteristically a stabled horse problem, it is placed among them because of its behavioural kinship with self-mutilation and pawing. It can, of course, be exhibited in the stable. More often, tail-rubbing is observed with the horse backing up to a tree, fence or wall, and pressing its rump against the upright surface while it rubs its tail and hindquarters rhythmically from side to side. Persistence of the action gives it a stereotyped appearance. The hairs on the tail against the dock become worn away, leaving a bristly look on the tail head; this sign characterizes the tail-rubber. Every case should be given a clinical examination and any

necessary curative therapy in order to differentiate between a clinical sign and a disorder of behaviour. Additional grooming would be appropriate in the latter state.

Self-mutilation

The condition of self-mutilation is a very dramatic event. The affected horse, appearing normal previously, suddenly becomes frenzied and attacks its own body by biting at its flanks. It may also rub itself furiously against the sides of the stall, including its neck and mane. Raw areas of skin, as well as flesh wounds, can develop. Occasionally, portions of the mane become removed. The affected horse may also make various sounds. The frenzied episode can continue for some time.

Affected horses are usually those that are permanently enclosed and isolated. Since this is commonly the lot of breeding stallions, the disorder seems to occur most often in these horses. Other horses, including mares, can also suffer the condition. Conceivably, the condition may be analogous to the sudden attack of widespread itching that can occur in human subjects. Any affected animal should be turned outdoors promptly to rescue it from itself. A wide pasture would be an ideal place for emergency accommodation. Emergency treatment with a sedative or tranquillizer may also be needed to end the condition. A return of this condition after one episode may not occur.

Humane treatment of confinement and isolation distress

The behavioural abnormalities – historically termed 'stable vices' – occurring in various forms as repetitive, compulsive activities in horses are symptomatic of dysphoria from enduring immurement. Many of these disorders in behaviour may or may not be reversible, but they can be diminished by humane care. Instead of attempting to treat the disorder exclusively, remedial measures should be applied to the circumstances that initially caused the effect. Horses affected with isolation distress should be given regular and adequate freedom of movement and the constant companionship of another animal. A small pony can be a good companion outdoors; however, it would not be suggested for a stallion.

Any harsh feature in the husbandry of cases of confinement or isolation distress, such as noise or rough handling, should be eliminated. Good nutrition, including salt licks and good-quality hay in proper quantities should also be constantly provided. The chronically established nature of most cases should be borne in mind while awaiting any reversal. Improvements may take years, but therapy by care should be maintained generously. Prophylactic measures simply add up to routine humane care, appropriate for this large, mobile and hungry, sentient and social animal. The following can be offered as a maxim: aloneness equals loneliness in the horse.

Humane care consistent with the horse's nature, is the only real hope for the prevention and treatment of these behavioural disorders. Various surgical insults to affected horses have been used and sundry technical methods have been employed in an effort to effect their control or elimination. These are unwarranted since the conditions are merely signs of maladjustment.

Some of these behavioural syndromes are more amenable to control than others. In general, if any control is effected by surgery or technology, there is likely to be a relapse, given time. The disorder is not the true problem; it falls within the causal circumstances. Treatment should be directed at their elimination through changed husbandry. Compensatory humane care should be provided to the affected horse for the remainder of its life. Modern bioethics would expect nothing less.

Table 15.3 summarizes the abnormal actions that have been discussed.

Abnormal Reactions in Horses

The various forms of abnormal reactions in horses constitute the third category of disordered equine behaviour. Several of these forms are hyperactive or fear-based states. All of these reactive abnormalities are well-known conditions in historical horse management (Youatt, 1858). They are now better recognized and understood as disorders of behaviour. Once regarded as vices, many can be better regarded as being the output of anomalous temperament.

When a horse is 'hyper', it presents a real handling problem. Hyper-reactions can be of a positive or negative nature. Both can be easily recognized by comparison with the widely known normality in horse reactions generally. The individual abnormal reactions dealt with here include aggressive approach, crowding, bolting, threatening, biting, kicking, shying, jibbing and baulking.

Table 15.3. Abnormal actions in stabled horses.

Action	Characteristics
Weaving	Affected horses stand in one position and weave from side to side in the stall. Some move back and forth, with the head, neck and forequarters swaying side to side rhythmically.
Stall-walking	Affected horse continuously walks side to side or in circles around a box stall. This is associated with deficient exercise or chronic confinement. The walking is precise, rhythmic and repetitive.
Pawing	Vigorous and persistent pawing at the stall floor in a stereotyped action, with the pawing directed at one spot. This is different from short spells of pawing when waiting to be fed.
Tail-rubbing	Persistent rubbing of the tail head in a side to side action of the hindquarters against a stable wall, tree or fence, etc. This action is also a sign of parasitism and needs differentiation.
Self-mutilation	Self-injury by vigorous biting of the flanks or excessive rubbing of the neck or body against an available structure. The action is typically intense and repetitive with vocalization.
Head-tossing	Usually occurs as continuous bobbing of the head up and down. This can occur in a stable or during riding as a stereotyped action. The tossing of the head is also shown in conditions of pain and requires differentiation.
Chronic standing	The subject will not lie down in the stall and there is no sign of soiling on the quarters in the morning. This can continue for many months. It can be taken as a sign of orthopaedic disease in some that are aged and/or infirm.

Aggressive approach

With this condition of temperament, horses have a habit of charging. An aggressive disposition is shown in the animal's tendency to rush forward, with mock threat, towards an approaching individual. The rushing terminates by the animal stopping at the objective. They may lunge forward with their teeth bared and their ears flattened back. This aggression appears to be shown more frequently towards humans if the horse has been socialized earlier with close human contact. The charging or lungeing reaction may be typical of the individual or may be shown only when the animal has been hormonally primed, as in some mares with young foals and mares with ovarian tumours.

Modified forms of this disorder are more common when horses are being fed. In this situation the affected horse approaches the feeder aggressively and the food must then be supplied in a hurry. Some of these subjects have known histories of food deprivation in their earlier lives, and even with continuous good feeding, the condition persists. Varying degrees of this disorder range from vigorous to mild (see Fig. 15.4).

Crowding

With this condition the horse habitually squeezes or 'crowds' an attendant person firmly against the wall of the stall. The disturbed behavioural feature of such an animal is that it responds bodily to an attendant's approach or presence with positive opposition when its individual space is breached. Appropriate resistance is in order. The disorder can be trained out of most cases by countering it aversively in the animal's interest, making it more of an acceptable individual while receiving increased in-stall attention in due course.

Bolting

Sudden galloping flight, unwarranted by circumstances, is the essence of bolting in the domesticated horse. Its occurrence in human custody is manifested in a hyperkinetic form. These features make it a behavioural disorder when it is characteristic of a given animal. A bolting subject typically displays a sudden aversion to events or stimuli that impose no real threat to it. The mobile alarm reaction is not rational in its general

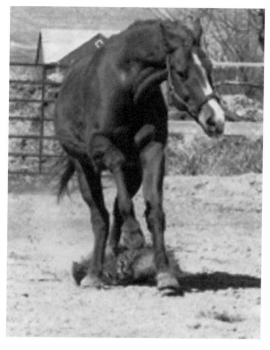

Fig. 15.4. A state of tracassie or exhibited annoyance. Note: (i) head extended and tilted; (ii) ears turned back; (iii) watching with one eye; (iv) mane bristling; (v) jaw clenched; and (vi) advancing aggressively. Photo: Melanie MacDonald.

performance. This form of flight can stimulate corresponding flight in associating horses through a natural 'group-effect'.

This disorder of behaviour is dangerous, both to the horse and to its handler. While being ridden or harnessed to a vehicle, the consequences of a bolting episode can be a disastrous accident with some casualty. Since it is evidently a feature of the subject's temperament, its elimination from the animal's behaviour might never be certain. Adequate training and good experience, however, can make the animal settle into its customary use. As elements of temperament are heritable, a horse with this disorder would not be a breeder's choice.

Threatening

A threatening attitude is a display of the horse's inherent temperament and constitutes a form of disordered behaviour. Like many of the other forms, it is a very undesirable characteristic in a horse in regular use. The subject with this disposition can be assumed to have a nervous temperament: temperament being its general nature and disposition, its periodic attitude. The latter is the source of its abnormal reactive behaviour and is a pathological degree of assertion.

The subject's typical display of threat includes a static posture: there is muscular tension; the head is extended to the target of its aggression; the ears are laid back; and the white sclera of the eyeball is shown under the pressure of the facial expression. This is the state known physiologically as 'fight or flight' and it naturally incorporates the body's physiological changes that are involved with the phenomenon, including increased blood flow to the voluntary muscles. The threat display will dissolve without a response from the person involved.

Once again, as it is a factor of temperament, the removal of a threatening attitude from the horse's habitual behaviour might only be gentled-out with good experience over a long period of time using humane care.

Biting

Habitual, aggressive biting by a horse is clearly disordered behaviour in domesticated circumstances. The disorder occurs most commonly among stallions, young horses and horses with confinement distress. Biting is in the form of a quick initial response to being approached or held. The horse grasps the individual with its incisor teeth for a moment. The bite is generally strong, while minor bites are in the form of nips. The bite is aggressively directed, and a warning sign of an intended bite may or may not be clearly shown. The signs of biting intent, when shown, include laying the ears back, retracting the lips and baring the teeth. Again, this is a pathological degree of assertiveness.

Chronic biters have their disorder rooted in their temperaments. Biting can be brought under some degree of control by negative conditioning. Basically, this requires that punishment be supplied to the subject immediately when it bites or shows a clear attempt to do so. Vocal punishment does not carry sufficient force. Devices to supply an electric shock to the horse's muzzle are said to be effective. A sharp pinprick to the horse's muzzle each time it bites or attempts to bite can control the action in time. Such conditioning is essentially intended to improve the horse's behaviour. Carrying a riding crop or a long stick can be helpful in showing the person's authority to the horse.

Kicking

Many horses kick, as it is in their nature to do so. This is the horse's natural method of self-defence or self-assertion. Any horse showing abnormal kicking activity, however, must be recognized as having disordered behaviour. This disorder is considered to be derived from a hyper-reactive temperament. Hyper-reactivity in general appears to have a hereditary foundation. This, of course, creates the great difficulty in all attempts to remove such reactions from the affected horse's behaviour (McCall, 1988).

Striking out with one forelimb, without rearing, is a feature of kicking shown by stallions. If this is done frequently and readily, it is considered abnormal behaviour in the common circumstances of horse husbandry. Animals with this disorder may perform it on initial approach or they may do it after being held for an extended period.

One hindlimb can be used in kicking out backwards or to one side, with some precision. This kick can reach back to target another animal or a person up to 1 m (3 ft) away. A hindlimb kick can be forward then back, in the style of a 'cow-kick'. Both hindlimbs can kick back together, with an extended reach of 1.5 m (5 ft). Such double kicks can be sudden, high and explosive (see Fig. 15.5). Treatment of the kicking horse calls more for avoidance by personnel than direct intervention. Awareness of this equine potential brings with it appropriate caution in horse users. The best thing to give a potential kicker is a wide berth at its rear.

Shying

Many an unschooled horse will shy when startled. This is not so much a disorder as a lack of equine education. Shying becomes an abnormality in behaviour when it is shown readily by an individual horse, almost as an idiosyncrasy. Basically it is an equine form of intense alarm reaction. Underlying factors may be temperament, a history of bad experience, inexperience, uncertainty, fear or poor eyesight. Regardless of contributing factors, habitual shying is not normal. It should be distinguished from rearing, which is a normal display of assertion.

The act of shying takes place as follows: the horse throws up its head, rises up, vocalizes and

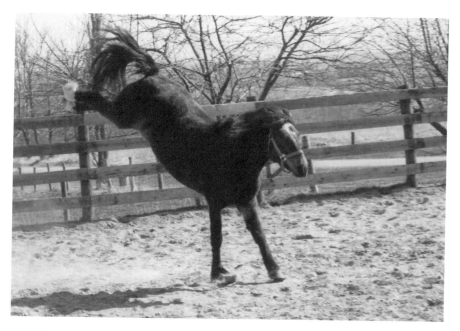

Fig. 15.5. High kicking. Photo: Melanie MacDonald.

turns away from the apparent cause of its alarm. If the reaction goes no further than this, the horse may stand and tremble. It is believed that shying is usually a reaction to suddenly perceived visual impacts, such as flashing light, fluttering items or the sudden appearance of another animal in close proximity to it. Shyers have a high level of fear in their constitution (Lansade *et al.*, 2008). This can be replaced with self-confidence through appropriate schooling. The use of blinkers on the bridle can be helpful, particularly when the horse is in full harness. This cuts down on the horse's peripheral vision, which is its main alarm receptor. Some horses will always be timid; restricting the vision of these nervous animals with blinkers, visors and hoods, for example, when the animals are in use is being humane to them. An unblinkered, timid horse can shy away from an aggressive competitor in the heat of racing.

Jibbing

In jibbing, the horse suddenly refuses to continue forward when being led, ridden or in vehicular use. In this form of reaction to its use, the jibber is akin to the baulker. These are probably two forms of the same disorder, the difference being a slight degree.

The baulker, described next, has the disorder in a more advanced stage.

The jibbing horse shows a temporary arrest in its use, but given a short stoppage without punishment, the horse might be backed up and then urged forward if given a slight and temporary alteration in course. The condition is essentially one of stubbornness. The equine nature contains such a factor, but it is normally obscured by this creature's willingness to suppress its own interest to those of humankind's uses. Jibbing is a minor character flaw in a horse, although it could worsen into baulking. Unfortunately, it sometimes does.

Baulking

In baulking, the horse completely arrests its motion while in use. It refuses to move in any direction, forward, backwards or to either side. This reaction against its use is increased in a horse with this form of behavioural disorder. In baulking, the horse assumes an enduring tonic state of antagonism to any further usage. When no further work or use follows this curtailment, the baulking behaviour of the horse is reinforced. This, however, may not be the factor involved in the course of this condition. Speculation as to the possible origins of the condition includes temperament, pain, fear, overuse and mental dysfunction. Regardless of its origin, the disorder tends to progress to a state in which the animal totally refuses to move in the face of encouragement, neither physical nor psychological, such as strong pushing or food offerings. No type of management has any effect at this stage. Severe force is not only cruel, it is also ineffective. It has been reported from logging operations that some have been killed in this state. If the baulker is left unattended, it may not move of its own volition for hours.

Once the condition is well established, the horse is probably beyond re-training and beyond further use. Any syllabus for re-training would need to be extensive, psychological and eclectic. Ironically, if the animal is returned to nature, so to speak, by putting it out to pasture with other horses, its behaviour is seen to be perfectly normal in all respects. Evidently, the subject's abnormal reaction is directed only against the insult of its domesticated use.

Table 15.4 summarizes the abnormal reactions that have been discussed.

In order to arrive at a synthesis of matters relating to disturbed horse behaviour, it can be postulated that a network of physiological features normally support equine well-being. Should this well-being network become stressed, the result can be disturbed behaviour in forms that typically remain as chronic anomalies. These often appear to be addictive in nature. A well-being network in the horse can be defined here as a composite, non-volitional, interrelated system of CNS-operated perceptor, releaser, messenger, transmitter and receptor linkages directly affecting and moderating visceral, muscular, circulatory and emotional functions (Mason, 1991; Mason et al., 2007). A network of such linkages involves the limbic, hormonal and autonomic systems. There are secondary effects on immune and behavioural functions when network operation is significantly disturbed.

When exploration is thwarted, acts of self-mutilation occur. Common to many abnormalities in the behaviour of confined animals, self-stimulatory acts apparently flourish in conditions of such frustration. These activities are often mouth-based and in many cases involve abnormal chewing. Evidently, sensory reception originating in the mouth region is a major source of stimulation. Some acts of abnormal swallowing in certain anomalies also appear to have self-stimulus value. Abnormal swaying motions may also activate self-directed stimulation. Self-stimulation is implicit in forms of self-directed behaviour, serving in a lenitive role.

Table 15.4. Abnormal reactions in horses.

Reaction	Characteristics
Aggressive approach	Typically the horse reacts aggressively to intrusion into its 'individual space' or 'visual field' with a threat charge. Some cases may show aggressive approach at feeding.
Crowding	The horse deliberately squeezes or 'crowds' a person against the stall when it is approached. This habit can be a very fixed reaction, even against a known person.
Bolting	The horse shows excessive alarm with slight stimulus and will take the opportunity to run away out of control.
Threatening	The horse readily shows a threat display when approached. The display is a 'fight or flight' reaction, with the animal showing the white of the eye and a raised head.
Biting	A fixed habit of biting, snapping or nipping in an 'antisocial' way when approached closely. This is a sign of a bad temperament and some horses have to be muzzled.
Kicking	Striking aggressively with one or both hind feet. No warning sign may be given. Stallions may also kick forward with a forefoot. This is also associated with a bad temperament.
Shying	The individual has a tendency to react readily to avoid novel items or situations by raising the head and turning away sharply from the source of fright. To be distinguished from rearing. Can be a sight problem.
Jibbing	The horse arrests its forward movement, throws up its head and refuses to go on. The period of arrest may be short. It may yield to urging or being blindfolded briefly.
Baulking	The subject effectively freezes in harness and refuses to move regardless of coaxing, urging or punishment.

Equine Stress

In this text, stress is regarded basically as an endogenous response to particular stressors in the horse's ongoing ambience. The condition of stress, as it affects the horse, has been addressed frequently in the text. A concluding overview of equine stress is given here, now that various features of this factor have been specified. The definition of equine stress, which has been used as a guide throughout the text, is the one given in the glossary. Equine stress is identified here as a state of overstrained control systems, resulting from noxious stimulation, in which the state reduces the animal's fitness. Fitness, as a term, is used in this particular context as being fitness for living. It is therefore analogous to well-being. This concept shows the inverse relationship between stress and well-being (Gibbs, 1986a; Zayan and Dantzer, 1990; Moberg and Mench, 2000).

In recognizing environmental sources of stress and strain in a horse's living, it is important to acknowledge that certain circumstances may be noxious for one horse and may not be so for another. When a horse manages to cope, given potentially noxious factors, this is regarded as adaptation (Cooper and Albentosa, 2005). If an animal fails to cope with such factors, its loss of fitness for living is evidence of disturbance to the animal's regulatory network; that is to say simply that the subject is suffering from stress. Stress is therefore an inner dysfunction. However, it has manifold signs or expression and has differing types. All of these variables make stress a very complex condition. Such complexity has resulted in much controversy in the past about its identification in animals. The topic is more settled now; its jigsaw pieces have been, for the most part, put in place with the helpful workings of disputation. Neurophysiology has also contributed significantly. A fairly clear picture of animal stress has emerged along the lines given here. In the horse, stress has its clearest impact on well-being. Stressors cause severe disturbance to the vulnerable features of an individual animal.

A system of sympathetic nerves issues arousal from the spinal cord to the body to adapt to emergencies. Continuing overactivation of this sympathetic division of the autonomic nervous system through disturbances to life duly establishes stress, with its physical, medical and psychological characteristics (Axelrod, 1984). Some individuals may cope with stressful factors better than others; however, this should not be counted upon when horses are subjected unavoidably to stressful circumstances, such as their transportation. Suffering is rooted in severe disturbance in the state of living or significantly suppressed well-being. It can emanate in behaviour, either actively or passively. Maladjustment to its given circumstances is usually seen in a stressed or suffering horse's conduct. Partly in recognition of the capacity of the horse to suffer, codes of practice have now been defined for this animal. Many horses require more health care, veterinary monitoring and humane conditions of transportation.

At fundamental levels, the biochemistry, physiology, psychology and pathology of stress show it to be a biological phenomenon of boundless intricacy (Gibbs, 1986a,b). Nevertheless, its clinical existence in animals and here in the horse require that an effort be made to give it a realistic scanning in keeping with its occurrence as a clinical entity. In accord with medical convention, the main types of equine stress can be classified as acute, subacute and chronic.

The acute type generally has association with major trauma. It may be regarded also as a primary type when it is related to sudden illness of a severe nature. The duration of such stress is variable. It may resolve in convalescence or it may be lifelong in its effect, as in heart muscle damage (cardiomyopathy).

The subacute category is typically associated with inhumane experience. If it endures, its effects are most likely to be on the horse's temperament, making it a more difficult subject to handle. It may be an animal that is of an unsettled nature and this may be long lasting.

The chronic type of stress is typically the outcome of an accumulation of episodes of loneliness, boredom, restriction, neglect or insufficiency of attention. It may also be the result of repetitious discomfort or pain. The stereotyped forms of anomalous action patterns clearly belong in this category. Disordered behaviour that resembles addiction is of this type.

In all of these three categories or types of equine stress, the animal's well-being is impaired and, with this, its performance, its usefulness and its constitutional soundness are all diminished. However, many cases respond to continuous humane care in due course. Conceivably, humane care is the only satisfactory treatment for equine stress of any type. Table 15.5 illustrates the three categories.

Table 15.5. Equine stress features.

Principal stress types	Factors of husbandry and experience	Some consequential conditions	Resultant well-being defects
Acute (primary and traumatic)	Ingestive faults, surgery or injury, traumatic transport, over-exhaustion	Colic, dehydration, nerve damage, wounds, lameness, cardio-myopathy	Mortalities, morbidity, weight loss, infectious flare-ups via depression of immunity, wellness dysfunction, reduction in physical performance, reactivity and training
Subacute (collateral)	Episodes of alarm, frequent fear, inhumane handling	Fractiousness, temperamental flaws	
Chronic (cumulative)	Enduring confinement, boredom, deficient exercise, COPD, lasting lameness, back problems, dental problems	Addictive behavioural disorders, unresponsiveness, loss of usability	

Humane treatment of confinement and isolation stress

Many of the disorders in behaviour associated with confinement and isolation may or may not be reversible, but they can be diminished by humane care. Instead of attempting to treat the behavioural element of the disorder exclusively, remedial measures should be applied to the circumstances that initially caused the effect. As mentioned previously, horses affected with isolation stress should be given regular and adequate freedom of movement and the constant companionship of another horse.

Any harsh feature in the husbandry of cases of confinement or isolation stress, such as noise or rough handling, should be eliminated. The chronically established nature of most cases should be borne in mind while awaiting any reversal. Improvements may take years, but therapy by care should be maintained generously. The animal's immune system will have been adversely affected and a high level of health is needed (Kelley, 1980).

Perception is largely satisfied with variation in environmental stimuli. This is the first feature commonly lost to the animal in restrictive systems of husbandry. Under circumstances of very close and chronic confinement, exploratory behaviour soon diminishes. The reduction in exploratory acts and the inherent tendency to explore is likely to lack outlet in an environment of minimal variety. This creates the actions characterized by repetitive self-stimulating behaviour, which has functional consequences (Dantzer and Mittleman, 1993).

Some of these behavioural syndromes are more amenable to control than others (Moberg, 1985). In general, if any control is affected by surgery or technology, there is likely to be a relapse, given time. The stressful causal circumstances are the true problem, and not the disorder. Treatment should be directed at their elimination through changed husbandry (McGreevy *et al.*, 1995).

Autonomic nerve network in stress

As previously indicated, the two divisions of the autonomic nervous system are largely antagonistic in their functions. The parasympathetic division is chiefly concerned with the basic control of the internal organs. The sympathetic division can exercise a dominant effect, particularly under stressful conditions, as when the sympathetic nerves accelerate the heart. The chemistry of this requires brief mention since it is featured in the biology of stress (Moberg and Mench, 2000).

The parasympathetic nerves have acetylcholine as a neurotransmitter to relax blood vessels, stimulate gastric juices and tone some musculature. Only sympathetic connections go to the medulla of the adrenal gland (which produces adrenaline), sweat glands, skin and the capillaries of voluntary muscles. Noradrenaline is a sympathetic transmitter and has its derivation in the transmitter dopamine. It should be noted that neurotransmission utilizes significant amounts of calcium and potassium, perhaps more so under stress. The sympathetic nerves react to stressors. In stress, noradrenaline serves to stimulate the secretion of adrenaline into the bloodstream. Adrenaline is thus an emergency hormone, going to all parts of the body and stimulating major bodily action.

Disturbed physiology in the limbic, hormonal and neural autonomic network influences certain hormones (Mason, 1975) and transmitter substances such as adrenaline and dopamine, respectively. Severe or chronic imbalance in this elaborate network underpins stress and numerous equine behavioural anomalies (Bachmann et al., 2003). Many of the latter relate to excess dopamine activity (hyperdopaminergic). Stability in this network is of such fundamental importance in horse wellbeing that it could be regarded as a seat of stress.

Clinical Behavioural Expressions

Clinical behaviour in the horse contains certain major features and conditions, notably pain, suffering and depression (McEwen, 2001). These are indicated by behavioural features such as posture, overactivity, underactivity and altered ingestion or excretion.

Pain

Horses experiencing pain show periods of restlessness. They may hold uneaten food in the mouth, for example. During pain, the horse has an anxious look, with dilated pupils and glassy eyes. Its respiration and pulse rates are increased, while flared nostrils, profuse sweating and a rigid stance are commonly observed. The ears may be laid back tightly. In prolonged pain, the horse's behaviour may change from restlessness to depression, in which the head is lowered. In pain associated with bone damage, the limbs may be placed in unusual positions with a reluctance to move. The head and neck can be seen as stiff. With abdominal pain or colic, the horse will look around at its abdomen. It may also bite or kick at its belly. It may get up and lie down frequently, walk in circles or roll. A horse with colic will sometimes paw at its bedding and gather it under its body. When near collapse, a horse in pain may stand very still, rigid and unmoving. The gums will show mucosal cyanosis and prolonged capillary filling time. Horses in pain generally show reluctance to be handled. The key overall signs are anxious appearance, restlessness, biting at the seat of pain, fixed position and general depression (Soulsby and Morton, 2001).

A horse with intra-abdominal pain may show tail-swishing, but this sign on its own may not always relate to pain. If the tail hairs are fanned or fluffed out in swishing, this may only be a sign of transient annoyance. The annoyance may, however, amount to anger and notice should be taken of this likelihood. The fluffing of tail hair is the manifestation of piloerection resulting from stimulation of pilomotor nerves by the sympathetic nervous system. A definitive distinction must therefore be made between the periodic tail-swishing in serious pain and the brief temperamental fanning form (pain versus temper) (Wall, 1992).

Suffering

In addition to painful association, suffering is a component of more amorphous conditions, such as stress or distress, as they pertain to the mental state of the subject in such conditions that appear to create anguish (Fraser, 1990). The nature of anguish in animals is intangible, although substantial subjective evidence attests to its existence. Animals can suffer in very real ways, with which we can identify. The clinical arrest of behavioural homeostasis is assumed to be linked with suffering (Peterson et al., 1991).

Recognition of equine suffering clearly requires appropriate experience and medical knowledge of horse behaviour and health. In clinical veterinary work, levels of suffering are implicitly understood. The eight chief clinical–behavioural manifestations, in an order that approximates diminishing degrees of disturbance to the affected subject, are collapse, arresting pain, agitation, depression, anorexia, inactivity, self-disuse and behavioural anomalies (Radostits et al., 2000).

Suffering is also a component of more ambiguous conditions such as stress or distress. Distressful circumstances of husbandry can disturb the animal beyond its ability to adapt to them. Suffering can therefore result from psychological insults, independently of a physical cause. Certain acute behavioural signs, such as intensive vocalizations and struggling and trembling, are clear evidence of a reactive variety of suffering. In addition, chronic forms such as passively depressed behaviour (e.g. 'souring') and stereotyped behaviour (e.g. 'vices') can occur as states of suffering. The latter varieties of suffering can therefore be classified as psychological. Forms of stereotyped behaviour are widely assumed to indicate such suffering. Suffering and well-being are opposite states, either tolerated or enjoyed by the horse's constitution. It is a valid clinico-behavioural rule that the development of either state displaces the other. The imbalance between these two endogenous states demands the recognition of both states in behavioural manifestations (Wiepkema *et al.*, 1983; Wiepkema, 1985).

Frequency can also measure high incidences of irregular acts (such as agitations or stereotypies) and changes in ongoing behaviour. Agitated states of behaviour in animals can clearly be seen as forms of suffering. Agitated behaviour can be the result of psychological distress or it may be a manifestation of pain, as, for example, in the condition of colic. Features that are responses to pain include inactivity such as is seen in head-pressing (Fig. 15.6), a tucked-up posture, restlessness, rigid limbs, fixed expression, self-inflicted bites, reduced ingestion and abnormal vocalization (Dallman, 2001). These clinical criteria, together with other unexplainable behaviour such as panic biting, suddenly increased appetite, postural change and altered or modified activity, must be considered in conjunction with the nature of any disease process present (Flecknell, 2001).

Depression

Among the observed signs of many clinical conditions in domestic animals, mention is made of

depression in standard veterinary literature (Beaver, 1994). Animal depression is defined by Blood and Studdert (1988) as: 'decreased interest in surroundings…decreased response to external stimuli'. The depressed animal's activity is likely to be derived from aversive stimulation rather than through spontaneous relationships with the environment. In depression, the suffering animal shows a marked depletion of the behavioural repertoire characteristic of the normal animal. The principal features of maintenance behaviour such as trophic activities and restorative functions, together with collateral social behaviour, become significantly diminished, adding to the picture of suffering in the depressed state. Loss of maintenance homeostasis appears to be an essential criterion of that general aspect of animal illness referred to as depression in clinical terms. The established concept of adjunctive depression in animal illness recognizes the behaviour of the animal as globally changed rather than regionally modified. In this, the main significant measure is behavioural frequency. It shows most often in the reduced frequency of maintenance activities.

Dysphoria

Explicit is the fact that behavioural anomalies are products of a faulty relationship with the immediate environment. Implicitly, these activities have neurological bases that are closely akin to certain normal actions such as biting, deglutition and rhythmic motion inherent in normal kinetics. These two points imply that a neurological disturbance has developed from the experience of an ambient disconnection. Quite simply, the subjects have not been in harmony with their accommodation over a period of time and adopt anomalous behavioural expressions as some manner of coping.

The overall implication is that the affected subject has suffered a state of continuing unrest, of emotional unease and of enduring a placement that is unsuited to its natural motivations. Such significant emotional unease has the contemporary term 'dysphoria' (Pryse-Phillips, 2009), the antithesis of euphoria. That it should result in behaviour that expresses this is no surprise. All other states of emotion have their expressions in equine behaviour, including disturbed emotions, such as in separations of mare and foal, and in aggression (Fig. 15.7), hunger and anger, for example.

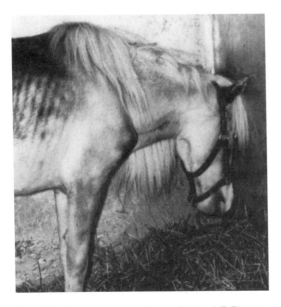

Fig. 15.6. Head pressing in illness. Photo: A.F. Fraser.

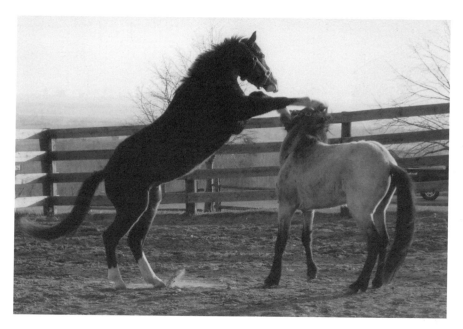

Fig. 15.7. Aggressive action. Photo: Melanie MacDonald.

The term dysphoria was used in Chapter 1, where it was mentioned as a likely consequence of curbing movement in this animal, which clearly has its inherited capacity for kinetic life in a free or wild state. It appears that some products or signs of this dysphoria have now been described in this chapter, making this state the probable root cause of these stereotyped forms of behaviour in the horse. A dysphoric state would not coexist with thorough well-being. In activities such as racing or eventing, its probable existence is therefore of significance. In critical horse use, well-being is a fundamental need.

Welfare Addenda

For horses, constant confinement without a visual field and with restriction of activity can have adverse effects. While a horse's physical condition may be preserved in the stable, its emotional condition is likely to be adversely affected by chronic restriction. In many cases, if the restrictive husbandry is constant, the animal's natural activities become redirected, so to speak, into anomalous action patterns. To put this more simply, restriction affects behaviour and creates bad habits that become ingrained. In constant close confinement,

horses can suffer the affective dysfunctions that have been described, together with hormonal changes (Gibbs, 1986b). The typical dysfunctions usually occur in mouthing, marking time and reacting, but affective states can also appear in adverse features of temperament or disposition. These symptoms of Equine Immurement Dysphoria (EID) resist elimination by corrective management. As a mental disorder, EID is a condition that cannot be rationally treated by curbing its behavioural symptoms. These become addicted items of behaviour. They are not usually removed permanently, even if the primary condition of EID is relieved by naturalistic, liberal husbandry.

A traditional form of restriction used on horses was in the form of 'breaking-in' for human use, where taming the horse was achieved forcibly. The term says much about the animal's affected spirit. Today, there is increasing awareness of the alternative method of inducing compliance in the horse by humane manipulation of the animal's nature. Compliant horses seem to perform better on the trail or the track. A test of compliance shows how easily the horse can be caught at pasture. Paradoxically, submissive horses tend to avoid capture.

Evidently, the equine condition is somewhat enigmatic and this causes some gap in human

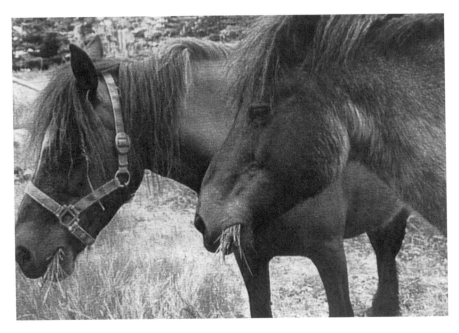

Fig. 15.8. A friendship pair, sharing eating space. Photo: A.F. Fraser.

understanding of the animal. While modern knowledge on the horse's nature has advanced, it still has a long way to go if it can ever be complete. In the meantime, comprehending the horse in many ways brings realizations of its sensibility and vulnerability. Those findings and our ethics give it the right of humane care in appropriate ways, to establish a general state of well-being for this ultimate athlete in human servitude.

No longer can the horse be viewed as a 'beast of burden' in developed countries. No longer can the horse be regarded merely as a periodic plaything or a recreational item. It is deserving of some natural time of its own, some quality of equine existence. The seemingly modest concession of a 'right' for humane care involves revision in all aspects of equine attention. One concept that could be helpful in the provision of rational horse care is in the recognition that the horse has a set of fixed behavioural traits that, collectively, give it a specific life culture. Recognition of this holistic, genetically based culture provides better awareness. The horse is an alien in human culture, having developed its range of speciological traits before humankind existed. One exemplary trait is the formation of close friendships with shared well-being (Fig. 15.8).

16 Equine Culture and Protection

Considering horse behaviour holistically, it is possible to recognize amorphous characteristics that are of the equine essence. They provide horses with their dynamic commonality and show that there is a given equine culture behind their modality. It is a culture that guides their conduct, in the form of certain major strategies for living. While recognizing their great biological heritage, mankind may also recognize a need to protect it. For their natural methods of living in human culture, they merit protection from this culture in several ways.

A unity of perception is needed to see the quintessential image of the horse. All around the world, horses are alike in their various ways of living. Their common strategies and tactics were evidently well established in their distant past, when they lived in a man-free world. Long before they spread themselves far from their original niche, it is clear that they had arrived at the set of fundamental characteristics that make them a successful species, fit for survival in the face of the world's great variables. The countless mutations thrust upon them by the vagaries of nature were put to their harsh test of realistic value in life. Better equine function was the acid test for every genetic novelty that was sprung upon some distinct breeder in the population.

Equine Culture

Over millions of years, the genetic process of infinite mutational trials and errors must have created the horse as seized by man a mere 5500 years ago. Long before then, primitive horses mixed with their mutual betters, which were both pre-potent breeders and potent parents. This added their improvements to the population of horses at large.

Serendipity visited the ancient horses with mutational discoveries that helped them to prevail and proliferate. The single hoof, the mobility, the competent neonate and the great physique were the result of mutational dice-throwing. The streamlined

body mass gave it the aesthetic and athletic property that is unique to the horse. The long, slender limbs are ideal levers for a larger-bodied creature that lives by mobility and has spectacular kinetics always in reserve. The cup-shaped, horny hooves on the ends of strong-jointed limbs are a natural gift for an animal destined to cover any surface that the world has to offer. Every textbook on horse anatomy contains descriptions of the physical attributes special to this subject, all exemplifying the horse's long physical evolution, which utilized the ungulate template.

The modern horse's progenitor was a little primitive ungulate that had its niche on the fringe of Siberia. It had to travel from valley to valley in search of food, and at times may have had to travel long distances. Today's horse's behavioural mosaic has its broad configuration from its functions in its long prehistoric existence (Clutton-Brock, 1999). The physique dictated the dynamic. The latter, in time, required better musculature. These muscles at work needed rich oxygen. A capacious chest held the apparatus adequate for extra bodily oxygenation. General mass is the result of these correlated factors. The mass needed the long levers of limbs to shift position actively. Standing on tiptoe was of extra help in progression, allowing the horse to run at speed. Sprinting brought security, and this security improved the prospects of survival for those that were well fitted with all of these features. Survival created populations and these generated societies. The societies developed ways of individual living within them. Behavioural elaborations flourished in such ambience.

The totality of its behaviour gives the horse its ethos, which is, at once, bucolic and galvanic. The composition of this ethos is tangible, while clouding the comprehensive details behind its expression. The horse has an elegant image of physical presence with manageable power in a shy, friendly and permissive nature. It has no method for living at the expense of others. It does not use intense aggression in its life and does not possess anatomical weapons such as horns or protruding tusks. If attacked, it can either fight by biting or kicking, or take flight with its capacity for strong running, if there is enough space in its surroundings. The horse shows a love of space in its natural ways, and its natural ways are becoming appreciated (Roberts, 1996).

Clearly, the objective of the horse is essentially one of self-preservation, through caution, compliance and conservation, balanced by association, assertion and spatiality. These are the horse's general strategies for living and constitute its manifest equine culture. The tactics that implement this animal's culture are abundant. They have been covered in the preceding chapters and are listed below as encoded tactics, since they are clearly in the equine genes. Many of these tactics are involved in more than a single strategy; their whole behavioural mixture being the inherited culture that maintains this singular species.

Tactical Instructions

1. Acquire an intimate partner.
2. Socialize and establish general friendships in the herd system.
3. Maintain a bubble of personal individual space.
4. Feed selectively and frequently, and occasionally consume some ligneous matter if hungry.
5. Move constantly with others in a grazing direction.
6. Rest and drowse in suitable styles and positions of comfort.
7. Sleep deeply, in short sessions, only when lying flat out in sufficient space.
8. Move often and utilize all natural forms of locomotion routinely.
9. Attend to sensations in the integument by grooming and sheltering.
10. Maintain all-round visibility against entrapment or other danger.
11. Adapt to all pressing circumstances by modified action.
12. Accept care and food for conforming to required functions.
13. Use reaction withdrawal or avoidance in challenges.
14. Use play to activate self and social events.
15. Chase inferior intruders from regular territory.

16. Drink water in large quantities on a few occasions daily.
17. Excrete at random unless a pattern of locations can be established.
18. Use close grouping, sheltering and shading in fly disturbance.
19. Prepare to mate only when internally impelled and externally stimulated.
20. Accept a newborn as an extension of self while freshly impelled.
21. Comply with attendance-seeking from new progeny.
22. Leave the location of restraint when possible.
23. Wander in freedom, explore, seek, investigate open space.
24. Check possible associates in nose-to-nose exchange.
25. Flee at maximum speed in fearful circumstances.
26. Adopt any lenitive habit to cope with frustration of chronic confinement.
27. Utilize experience to resolve problem situations.
28. Investigate environmental limits and features.
29. Kick/bite in self-defence.
30. Use nipping for tactile assertions and grooming.

The inherent strategies are general; the tactics are specific. These 30 items are traits that are inherent in horses, lodged in equine genetics. Their management is possible but their total eradication by discipline or selected breeding is impossible. Realization of this fact is of fundamental importance in welfare concepts. Forms of husbandry that fail to take these natural traits into account as behavioural features to be tolerated or managed humanely act counter to basic welfare. In general, methods, intended or not, that prevent the operation of most of these actions where they are appropriate are not in the interests of welfare (Webster, 1994).

A notable item is 26. When it has been induced, it cannot be reduced effectively by negative reinforcement without addressing the cause. The aetiology of behaviour in this item is complex. It lies in the frustrations of several items listed (items 8, 10, 14, 22, 23 and 28) and, in particular, enduring immurement. Even if the affected subject of lenitive activity is put into a system of extensive husbandry, the habitual activities enacted as palliatives during the horse's incarceration may persist in the open environment. The neurological damage may not be reversible. Cribbing and wind-sucking in particular are usually continued outdoors, often in times of some excitement. Such a horse's well-being is evidently destroyed permanently. The equine forms of stereotyped behaviour are psychological disorders. That they are induced by dysphoria (Pryse-Phillips, 2009) appears to be a valid hypothesis.

Caution

The exercise of caution by the horse is practised through investigation, exploration and curiosity. This aspect of the equine culture is serviced by items 10, 23, 25 and 28. These are among the most influential traits in the equine culture. Investigation can be brought readily into operation when circumstances demand it. By this means, relevant and useful experience is gained through it. Although it is of a non-specific nature, being largely empirical, the role of investigation in learning is considerable. In a state of heightened awareness induced by the stimulus of new circumstances, the animal investigates and acquires experiences. Trial-and-error activity is of particular value in gaining experience as the animal grows and matures. Trial-and-error actions usually bring improvement in performance. Examples of this can be most clearly seen in the behaviour of the long-legged and very short-sighted newborn foal. The foal's rising attempts, which begin soon after birth, involve coordination, balance, effort and change. Several failures to stand up usually occur, with the foal falling back down each time. With successive trials improvements occur and soon the foal is able to rise to a fixed, partly upright posture. Once the ability to rise and stand is achieved, the trial-and-error process of rising from a lying position is complete.

Exploration and investigation extend the field of the individual; the purpose of such behaviour is therefore one of self-interest. Investigations are made to acquire further resources and security. Horses show a strong motivation to explore and investigate their environments. Only when the environment has become very familiar to them does the exploratory behaviour subside; it reappears in an animal's behaviour when there is any change in its surroundings. Investigation can be reproduced with intensity should an alteration in the environment occur. This reserve of exploratory behaviour allows the animal to direct its attentions suitably when the environment changes. A desire to explore maintains a potential for activities that focus the sense of the animal upon additions, changes, salient features and novelties in its close environment. Social relationships and hierarchies, in all equine groups, have been determined essentially through investigation to explore. While this stems principally from perceptive needs, it is also generated by other, even less tangible needs such as determination of status.

Empirical interactions are evidently used in relative self-determination, and this is probably the reason why horses raised in a confined environment do not usually develop behaviourally in the same way as those who enjoy early social contact with their own kind. Exploratory behaviour becomes significantly suppressed in many illnesses, thus curiosity is a very healthy sign. The exploratory trait in horse behaviour can be outlined simply as a sensory need. First, there is a need in the animal for the perception of environmental factors that will feed its aroused senses. Secondly, the receipt of sensory feedback from the environment satisfies the original need.

Sensory exploration

The senses of sight, hearing, smell, taste and touch supply the perceptive need of the animal, but even all of these combined may not meet the collective need in a situation of restrictive confinement when the sensory composition is inadequate. It is a general sensory impression, taken from the totality of sensory composition, which is the perceptive need in social animals such as the horse. Exploration secures stimulation from perceptible external factors, and stimulation is the excitation process in the perceiving animal. The quantity of stimuli provides quality in the satisfaction obtained. Horses must determine their own characteristics, abilities, limitations and social status, and they expend much activity investigating these factors. They do this through social exploration and constant empirical interactions with their animate and inanimate environments. They test their powers of dominance with others in encounters of petty aggression. They can learn of their general physical power by pushing. Through play they can also determine their powers of flight, attack and defence. The fundamental need of self-determination, or self-identity, is one which is closely allied to inquisitiveness.

A perceptive need in the horse is met with variation in environmental stimuli. This is the first feature commonly lost to the animal in restrictive systems of husbandry. Under circumstances of very close and chronic confinement, exploratory acts are reduced and the inherent tendency to explore is likely to lack outlet in an environment of minimal variety. This creates the actions characterized by repetitive self-stimulation behaviour.

Horses will explore any new field they are released into and pay most initial attention to the field boundaries. They are likely to follow the boundary before exploring the interior of their enclosure. This is in accord with items 8, 10, 23 and 28. As previously mentioned, when released into small pastures that permit overall vision, a group will disperse quickly and adopt the extensive spacing characteristics of grazing. In a very large pasture, several days or weeks may elapse before its entirety has been explored by each of the horses within it.

One of the main features of exploratory behaviour in the horse is that it occurs only as long as the emotions of fear or apprehension are not present. The animal's curiosity is normally aroused when it sees an unfamiliar object or hears an unknown noise, but what may induce exploratory behaviour in one animal may very often be ignored by another. Older animals, being more acquainted with the objects and sounds of their environment, are less curious than young animals. When curiosity is first aroused, the animal approaches with its nostrils quivering and sniffing. The size and nature of the object in which the animal has become interested determines the speed of approach. The horse sniffs the object and may lick it or even chew it. This kind of exploratory behaviour is often induced by the sight of familiar objects in an unfamiliar context.

Association

Another prominent facet of horse culture is a consistent engagement with social traits. These are listed as items 1, 2, 5, 14, 18, 20 and 21. In addition, the sundry features of the horse's social behaviour have been given in Chapter 13. The overall social component of the equine culture can be seen as a prominent force in life. The horse is commonly regarded as a fairly sociable animal, but its social standard merits fuller appreciation. Its social drive is seen to be strong when all social features are put together and viewed as a singular facet of the culture of the species. Benign social interchanges are commonplace between horses accustomed to one another (items 4, 6, 7, 9, 12, 16 and 18). The horse's

sociability deserves to be elevated to a level of general amicability.

The normal extent of the horse's amity is not limited to its own kind or to mankind, as it is with the dog, but has a comprehensive nature. The horse's capacity for relationships is of a broad dimension. In this respect the horse is a socially unique animal. Furthermore, the quality of its association with chosen affiliates of its own kind is analogous to close friendship. Such friendships are not occasional phenomena but are routine types of association that occur in every congregation of horses. Dogs, cats and goats are acceptable surrogates.

To prevent a horse from having a close relationship is social deprivation. Such an arrangement falls short of an adequate level of welfare. Although this animal readily develops tolerable associations with a wide range of other species, the fullness of a social connection can best be achieved with the company of its own kind. The existence of social needs in a horse is a fact that may not have been appreciated previously to the extent that is apparent now. Clearly it is a salient facet of equine culture that calls for attentive husbandry. Wherever the justification for good welfare is recognized, there should be no isolated horse.

Spatiality

The variety of traits relating to spatial activity is listed as items 3, 18, 22 and 28. Spatial behaviour as an ethological category is also addressed in Chapter 8. Viewed as a unified body of equine function, spatiality emerges as another major dynamic in the equine ethos. The horse's affinity for spaciousness is a feature that dominates other environmental concerns, such as a bed area or a walled, sheltered enclosure with an overhead cover.

Horses use space for social conduct, foraging and grazing. They also utilize space for their kinetic habits and territorial practices. Open space equates with freedom in this animal, in spite of its domestication. It remains free-loving, as deducible from its choice of habitat when liberated from custody. Feral horses in many locations around the world are further evidence of an inherent equine desire for free space, within which they can live in the essential equine manner.

Use of extensive space can save the horse from the heavy burden of helminth infestation, which is the common health problem of horses housed in limited space. In addition, horses on open space do more travelling, in the course of which their hooves are trimmed down by chipping and friction. Extended space usually provides more variety of grasses and plants, with a wider range of trace elements. This affords added nutritional insurance for the roaming horse.

The domesticated horse in regular use cannot be granted unlimited space for its nutrition or its natural lifestyle of its freedom, although this is not what is required for its welfare. The horse will be in better circumstances if it has a companion in a hectare or two of good-quality grazing, and is in receipt of daily inspection and frequent, appropriate attention from a dedicated care-giver. On the other hand, the horse without regular release into sufficient space to enact spatial practices, including running, rolling, out-looking and cropping grasses, is not living in a generous amount of welfare. It may or may not have the ability to cope. At the extreme end of limited space, strict confinement of a horse is totally at variance with equine culture. Such a form of custody for a healthy horse is the cost of its domestication (Price, 2002).

Assertion

Although the well-trained horse is normally a compliant subject in its customary use, and although horses of normal mentality are never aggressive to any significant degree, this animal's nature contains some features of assertiveness. The traits relating to this behavioural property are given in the list of encoded tactics numbered 3, 15, 19, 29 and 30. Chapter 14 deals with methods of controlling this form of behaviour in handling circumstances likely to prove an assertive response. The descriptions relating to reactivity are relevant to this feature as well.

In the course of the horse being handled aversively, there is likely to be resistance in a firm reaction. Although customarily compliant, most horses will not tolerate aversive manipulation beyond a certain limit. At a given point, an animal in such circumstances will assert itself by refusal to accept the manipulation further. Most horses have limits of tolerance, and assertiveness quickly develops when such limits are reached.

Assertive actions vary with individuals and circumstances. Commonly, horses held by a lead rope and reacting to some procedure will raise their heads and pull back strongly in an attempt to break away. If they succeed in their attempt, they run away; if not, they continue to pull back, making it difficult for the handler to retain a hold on the horse. Providing that the horse is not frightened further, it may cease to struggle after a short period of time. In similar circumstances, some stallions will strike out at the handler with a forefoot and may succeed in raking a hoof down the handler's body. Again, in a situation of this kind, the horse may act aggressively, laying its ears back and extending its head and neck while attempting to bite the handler about the shoulders or chest. Such an attack obviously has to be repelled. This can be done by frightening the animal with shouting and shaking the lead rein or rope at the horse's face. No physical punishment is necessary.

An assertive action by a loose horse towards an adversary or a handler is often performed by turning the hindquarters towards the object of assertion and kicking back with both hind feet. If the target is beyond reach the action continues, with the horse shuffling backwards, aiming its rump at the object of its disaffection. Often, when a double-legged kick is delivered, it is not as forceful or as far-reaching as a kick with one hind leg; this by no means is a rule of horse-kicking. The double-legged kick can sometimes be very high and very forceful. A softer double-legged kick is the type used socially; they are common amongst social scuffles taking place in a group of horses. They usually occur in order to re-assert a social dominance that had been asserted previously. In this instance the dominant horse kicks the other horse on the side of its chest or belly. This action is intended as a message as opposed to a real injury.

In other situations with a caste clash at close quarters, the superior horse asserts its dominance by biting the other in a nipping manner. Once again, it is the delivery of a message or a reminder that is taking place and not the expression of pure aggression. These inflicted signals are seldom returned. The fact emerging from the total sum of socially assertive interchanges among horses is that there exists a type of caste system in the culture of horses. It is created and maintained only within groups, by the degree of assertiveness in the nature of each individual in the given group. Frequently, a friendship between a high-caste and a lower-caste animal alters the social order, making it more complicated.

Conservation

Self-conservation is a clear motive in many equine performances. Traits relating to this feature are provided in the list of encoded tactics and numbered 4, 6, 7, 9, 12, 16 and 18. Chapter 9 also presents a detailed account of restful behaviour, which is the main form of self-conservation in horses. Lounging and loafing are two terms for the same type of resting, which can be performed standing or lying upright. Such loafing in a group is normally taken by several at one time for lengthy sessions. The upright position permits watchfulness. It appears to be a commandment among horses that they should never be caught napping – in a literal sense.

When going uphill with a haulage weight or a rider, the horse does not seek to stop until it has reached the top of the hill. If permitted, it may stop there for a while before moving on. This type of tactical resting is useful for the animal to restore energy, not only to continue but also to put some back into reserve. The great amount of resting taken by horses in the conscious state indicates that conservation of energy is practised opportunistically and well beyond the current needs, evidently in order to maintain an energy reserve. Such a reserve might be for an emergency, such as flight or perhaps fight. Long-term survival demands such a plan, and the horse, with nearly eight million years behind it, has shown itself to be a good survivor – all the while using the speciological tactics of its culture. No doubt there is great evolutionary merit for an animal living on tip-toe in giving a high priority to energy conservation in its glycogen-loaded muscle mass.

With its kinetic power, the horse utilizes its energy resources at a great rate when in full motion. This power is typically turned on in an instant, even in the midst of grazing hungrily. Additional oxygen is then in demand, and so the running horse's response becomes forced breathing. If it was an oral breather (like the canine runner) and had grass in its mouth, it would probably choke and possibly die. The horse, being exclusively nasal in its breathing, has no such problem. With its great glycogen reserves as its savings in its massive musculature, it is always prepared to get on the road to survival.

Compliance

As a special strategy for adaptive capability, compliance with its circumstances serves the horse very well in domestication, just as it did during its wild days, when it adapted completely to variable environments, including climates, terrains and variable foods. It managed to travel on frozen rock, lush plains, hot sand and wet swamp. It could ingest by grazing, cropping and browsing, and live in frigid temperatures and in burning heat. The horse still has such capabilities, of course. In the list of encoded tactics, items numbered 5, 11, 12, 20 and 21 relate to this feature of compliance.

This property is amorphous and relates to some stoic attitude in the horse's culture as much as it does to a range of anatomical and physiological features. For example, the horse can commit its working endeavours with equal readiness at the behest of many different handlers, drivers and riders. It can continue to function without any change in performance in different locations, accommodations and styles of usage. It can deliver its best efforts in traces, in shafts and under saddle.

The full extent of a horse's readiness to comply with a given role is evident in the way that it will carry a rider at the gallop, if demanded, until it collapses. A horse can exert itself in some given demanding task until its heartbeats cease. Horses in older wars ran to their deaths in compliance with their circumstances. Similar examples of total compliance under domestication could be of infinite numbers in human service around the world. This compliance is from an animal culture like no other. To afford good welfare to a horse is a major ethical duty in our current civilization. If for no other reason, horse welfare is a modest attempt to deal with a debt to a species of animal that can never be fully repaid.

Equine Protection

Protection

Recognition of the horse's manner of living brings out the fact that this is an animal with an array of sensuous and cognitive properties in addition to its physical powers. Its biological composition is a compound of great qualities that have allowed mankind to use it to achieve much. Such realities bring obligations to the fore, relating to contemporary values in society. In fact, this drives attention to the point where this monograph began, namely the emergence of ethics in horse husbandry. Such ethics are not simply niceties of care but are civilized standards and guidelines for protection of life and prevention of suffering in an animal with significant sensory faculties.

Human medicine has developed such a field, termed bioethics, and it is timely for animal medicine and ethological science to enter an analogous field, with regard to horses in this instance.

Equine bioethics

Within human custody, the horse is no longer totally at the mercy of the natural elements; it is instead at the mercy of domestication. In human employment its protection depends largely on the concepts of the employers towards it. Such concepts are customarily based on tradition and may function in the interest of the employer alone or, in other cases, in the interests of both. In either event, the scale of conceptual merit is varied. The horse may be viewed as a living machine, an item of capital, a servant, an indentured labourer, a sports colleague or a friend. Its level of welfare may relate to its place on such a scale of appreciation. A rational standard can be determined by bioethics based upon evidence from ethology applied to the domesticated, utilized horse and upon veterinary science.

A body of bioethical guidances will establish a code. Such a bioethical code for horses will recognize as its basic principle the overall protection of the horse in its various uses. It will therefore support good standards in horse use and specify factors that can oppose equine well-being, not by edicts or legislation but by denoting humane practices that realistically benefit horses as they cope with use. Its purpose would be more positive than negative to achieve results within the horse industry. The foundation of such an equine bioethical code can emerge from a summarized overview of equine difficulties that require the protective intervention of welfare.

Horse welfare is a compound discipline, with relevance to animal science and veterinary medicine. In addition to these two parent subjects, horse welfare has relationships with several applied areas of scientific animal study. These include animal management, animal care and applied ethology. As a result of these five related disciplines, horse welfare can be recognized as being based on a rational policy using applied collateral sciences. The World Veterinary Association endorses this view and also the definition of animal welfare given in *Baillière's Veterinary Dictionary* by Blood and Studdert (1988) as follows: 'Maintaining appropriate standards of accommodation, feeding and general care, the prevention and treatment of disease and the assurance of freedom from harassment and unnecessary discomfort and pain.'

Horse welfare takes the form of services that act upon the animal externally. In contrast, both well-being and suffering are endogenous states within the animal. Welfare and well-being are not synonymous here. The distinction lies clearly in the definition of well-being as follow: 'A state or condition of physical and psychological harmony between the organism and its surroundings. The most reliable indicators of well-being are good health and manifestation of normal behavioural repertoire' (Hurnik *et al.*, 1985). A horse with well-being is usually in a suitable environment. An unsuitable environment may cause a horse to make significant adjustments in its behaviour. Horses in monotonous and restricting environments seek out opportunities for exercise and stimulation. Most applied ethologists now accept that restriction of movement, 'boredom', thwarting of action, stressful stimuli and deficiencies of the environment lead to abnormal forms of behaviour. These are signs of affective suffering (Panksepp, 1998). They show up as forms of highly repetitive, stereotyped actions and have been thoroughly studied as a behavioural group (Mason, 1993; Mason and Rushen, 2008). No realistic control of these states is evident once they are established. They also undermine cognition (Hausberger *et al.*, 2007).

The veterinary bioethical code is to control or prevent unnecessary suffering among animals. It is an allied objective to promote well-being in animals dependent on mankind for their care. Both suffering and psychological well-being can be regarded as being endogenous ethological conditions, since their manifestations are behavioural to a considerable extent. Although general well-being refers to both physical and psychological aspects (these two are normally interwoven), the existence of psychological well-being is revealed in behavioural signs, particularly those which indicate active fine-tuning of the animal, such as volitional conduct in the form of grooming, play, stretching, sleeping and sociability.

The horse, as a sentient animal, carries with it an affective (psychological) factor that determines attitude and is revealed in its conduct. Healthy animals usually have a positive demeanour. This is portrayed in their specific components of behaviour. Animal illnesses, diseases and injuries, however, usually become apparent through behavioural signals of suffering (Dawkins, 2004). These signals include unusual actions, locomotor changes, reduced activity, changes in appetite and sundry alterations in attitude and general behaviour (Dallman, 2001). Such clinical signs are forms of body language and they are used for diagnostic purposes when cases of illness and injury are being examined. Signals of conduct are therefore the means to comprehend the affective or psychological status of an animal and to estimate whether this status is bad or good, clinical or normal (Bracher *et al.*, 1998; Bagley, 2005). The theory of EID is that it is a mental disorder resulting from frustration of the horse's inherited, instinctive impulses relating to free-ranging behaviour and that it is manifested in anomalous action patterns of stereotyped character. This theory is based on a synthesis of the closely related factors linking cause and effect.

Suffering and stress protection

The most respected of the anthropomorphic tenets is that animals can and do suffer. They are often seen to suffer, chiefly from their own diseases, from injurious accidents and from cruelty. The principal obligation of veterinarians is the relief of animal suffering as it mainly relates to clinical problems, but suffering goes beyond the clinical boundaries. Suffering has various definitions but is essentially the extended experience of negative feelings from pain, through malaise, frustration, depression and fear.

Some suffering is a product of stress. It should be emphasized that the term 'stress', as used in a veterinary context, refers not to any single parameter or set of bodily reactions but to a heterogeneous assortment of phenomena (D. Fraser *et al.*, 1975). Stress has a considerable variety of meanings in physiology, psychology and human medicine and in common usage. It is still used by veterinarians and agriculturalists in practical discussions on a host of husbandry problems. In a veterinary context, the term stress is used when there is a profound physiological change in an animal's condition, generally leading to a disease state and loss of well-being (Kelley, 1980).

Certain behavioural manifestations are unequivocal evidence of suffering through being outward expressions of mental states in clinical conditions accompanied by pain, distress or fear. Intense vocalizations, struggling, trembling, passively depressed behaviour and agitated behaviour certainly reflect states of suffering. If physiopathological correlates are absent, evidence of suffering may relate to stress (Broom and Johnson, 1993, 2000; Broom and Kirkden, 2004; Broom, 2006).

Suffering requires clarification as a veterinary term. Although it can occur independently of any physical cause, animal suffering is usually an adjunct to a clinical condition or insult. It is now regarded as being the affective (mental) component of this condition (Fraser and Quine, 1989). Affective suffering and psychological well-being are directly opposed states, either endured or enjoyed by the animal. It is a clinico-behavioural rule that these states displace each other as behavioural manifestations. The maintenance of a state of well-being in a horse is a means of protecting it from suffering and stress.

With the increasing recognition that stress in animals is a component factor in the aetiology of numerous animal diseases, it is recognized that these too might be preventable through exercising some control over the stressful circumstances to which they may be exposed. The general well-being of animals used materialistically should be assured by adequate standards of welfare. The recreational use of horses is now their major field of activity. The propriety of such use has a rational foundation. Many veterinarians become professionally involved in such organized activities as showing horses, horse racing and horse riding. Their role includes monitoring and administering to the well-being of the animals involved. In addition, horses are used increasingly to assist people with handicaps. The welfare of these animals involves veterinary attention from time to time, and the practitioner is required to appreciate the philosophy of the service and any rational or irrational concerns in the public regarding such use.

As companion animals, horses can enter a human–animal bond. Special links between people and animals are now universally accepted as a natural phenomenon. The relationship in pair-bond associations are now recognized to be a form of symbiosis or 'mutualism'. Horses in this service have found a fortunate new role, for which they are well suited, given good matching (Podberscek, 2006).

Code of Equine Care

A bioethical rationale can be seen in horse use, which incorporates a code of care in keeping with the inherent manner of living in this animal. Such a code could consist of four cornerstones of equine care as follows:

1. Regular spatial freedom with exercise.
2. Companionship of an equine associate.
3. Good-quality nutrition suitably rationed.
4. Complete physical and health care.

This code of care, completed with practical and technical details, could protect the horse from many of the sources of distress to which its nature is vulnerable in the alien culture of our civilization.

Glossary of Terms

Abnormal behaviour: Behaviour that deviates from a defined, comparable norm. The norm may be a behavioural form typical for a given genotype, age group, sex, type of use, housing condition, husbandry system, etc.

Action pattern: A series of connected behavioural actions having consistent form and sequence typical of the species. Action patterns typical of lower species are often designated as modal action patterns or fixed action patterns.

Adaptation: The evolutionary process of becoming better adjusted to the environment through genetic change. Adaptation is also used to refer to short-term changes in sensitivity to stimulation, e.g. sensory adaptation.

Adaptive behaviour: A behavioural change to suit the circumstances.

Aeration: Inflation of the lung with air. When the horse is lying flat on one side for a while, there is inadequate aeration or ventilation of the lower lung. Aeration is seriously impaired in COPD (see **Chronic obstructive pulmonary disease**).

Aerophagia: Pathological and excessive swallowing of air: a behavioural dysfunction in horses (also called wind-sucking).

Affective: Emotional factors in behaviour.

Aggression: Any purposeful action of a horse towards another with the actual or potential result of harming it, dominating it or depriving it of resources.

Aggressive behaviour: Actions with the tendency to initiate a vigorous conflict.

Agitation: Non-directed emotional activity or extremely restless behaviour.

Agonistic behaviour: (1) Any activity indicative of social conflict, such as threat, attack and fight, or escape, avoidance and subordination. (2) Any behaviour associated with conflict or fighting between two individuals.

Air hunger: Inadequate oxygenation of the body, e.g. when the horse has run close to its physiological limit, it extends its head in an attempt to get more air by reaching forward.

Airs-above-the-ground: High kicks, leaps, bounds and athletic exercises, as performed by the Lippizaner stallions.

Animal care: A system of husbandry for animals secured individually or in groups in places which specify high standards of environment, feeding, hygiene, health, protection and appropriate handling under technical monitoring.

Anomalous behaviour: (1) Irregular behaviour. (2) Behaviour that is a variant of a normal activity but displayed abnormally, e.g. excessive self-grooming or locomotor stereotypies.

Anorexia: Abnormal lack of ingestive behaviour, e.g. in severe illness with a depressed state.

Appetitive behaviour: Behaviour manifested during the initial phase of an activity that indicates a desire to attain a certain goal, e.g. searching for food.

Applied ethology: The study of animal behaviour conducted primarily for practical application or for understanding the utilized species: the horse in this instance.

Aversion stimulus: A noxious or painful stimulus to the horse, such as whip use.

Aversion therapy: Treatment of a compulsive form of behaviour by associating the behaviour with an electric shock or other aversion stimulation, e.g. applying a shock to the horse when it crib-bites (it often fails).

Avoidance: Non-involvement with aggressive challenge by positioning.

Barren environment: An environment of insufficient complexity for a horse's sensory needs, e.g. a stable stall without a visual field.

Baulking: Frequent, stubborn refusal to go forward.

Behavioural action: Any observable factor, particularly a singular action that is an integral part of a complex behavioural pattern, e.g. strutting before elevation in the entire jumping pattern.

Behavioural category: A class of behavioural activities, usually based on some essential or fundamental function, e.g. maintenance and reproduction.

Behavioural disorder: Manifestation of behaviour that differs from that of a typical healthy horse, thus indicating disease, injury, stress or inability to adjust to the environment, e.g. head pressing. Behavioural disorders may be temporary or chronic.

Behavioural display: Any behaviour that has or may have communicative function, e.g. oestrous display.

Behavioural pattern: An organized sequence of behavioural actions having a specific design, e.g. early activity of the newborn foal.

Binocular vision: Vision in which images of the same object(s) are projected on the retinas of both eyes simultaneously, e.g. good forward vision.

Biostimulation: Stimulation of reproductive functions in mares by the presence and behaviour of an associating stallion.

Boredom: A state of weariness and diminished attention, outwardly similar to symptoms of fatigue, caused by lack of environmental complexity. Considered as a factor in the aetiology of some forms of stereotyped behaviour, e.g. crib-biting.

Bruxism: Habitual grinding or clenching of the teeth, leading to the formation of sharp edges on the molars. In the horse, frequent clenching alone acts to sharpen the outer (cheek) edges of the upper molars and inner (tongue) edges of the lower molars because of the off-set surfaces (tables) of these opposing rows of grinding teeth.

Bullying: Persistent aggression by one or several horses towards one or more horses of lower rank. If allowed to continue, it can lead to serious deprivation, injury or exhaustion and emaciation in extreme cases. Bullying actions typically include threatening, pushing, and biting and kicking another horse.

Chronic obstructive pulmonary disease (COPD): Allergic, spasmodic constriction of pulmonary airways, persisting over a long period of time and causing broken-windedness in horses.

Circadian: Referring to cyclic rhythm, corresponding closely to a 24-h interval.

Clinical behaviour: Behaviour indicative of disease or injury, e.g. colic.

Cognition: A process of perception, reasoning and development of expectations, e.g. anticipation of events.

Colic: Any condition characterized by abdominal pain.

Colt: A young uncastrated male horse.

Comfort movement: Any movement performed to temporarily relieve stiffness or integumentary irritation, e.g. stretching, scratching, shifting position, shaking, rubbing.

Commensalism: A partnership in which only one horse gains advantages, e.g. the one with preferred associate status.

Competition: (1) The direct struggle between individuals for a limited supply of resources or environmental necessities. (2) The common striving for living requirements, such as food, space or shelter, by two or more individuals.

Competitive behaviour: Behaviour manifested to attain adequate or preferential use of a limited resource, e.g. food, space, sexual partner, high social rank, etc.

Condition: The general health and soundness of a horse or the amount of flesh or finish on it.

Conditioning: (1) Preparing a horse for certain circumstances with aversive potential by exposing it progressively to stimulations of the circumstances. Supplying some treatment to a horse to enable it to cope with imminent challenges to its well-being. (2) This occurs when a reflex behaviour is modified by specific experience.

Conduction (of neural impulse): The transmission of an excitatory signal from a neuron to a target cell or cells.

Confinement housing: A housing system where a horse is seriously restricted in ambulation for an extended time, e.g. stall confinement.

Congenital: Existing from birth (with or without inheritance).

Consummatory act: An act that constitutes the termination of a given behavioural pattern.

Contactual behaviour: Maintenance of bodily contact. Examples are the close association of the young foal and mother, the intimate partnerships in pair bonds and the tending bond with the stallion and oestrous mare.

Cope: The ability of the horse to deal with demanding circumstances.

Coprophagia: Eating dung. Occurs normally in young foals and abnormally as an ingestive disorder in adults.

Core area: A territorial location heavily used for grazing and associating.

Crate: A restraining compartment that keeps the horse standing up but prevents the animal from turning around, kicking out or leaving the crate. Also termed stocks.

Cribbing: Frequent biting on boards, posts and other structural surfaces used for confinement. Assumed to be indicative variously of boredom, pain or nutritional deficiency. In horses, the term cribbing may also include swallowing of air through the open mouth when biting on an object (also called crib-biting or wind-sucking).

Critical period: The infantile and maternal phases when the subject is most sensitive to specific environmental features and experiences.

Crowding: An unusually high spatial density of animals, which may cause discomfort to some or all animals in the group but not always serious deprivation or injury. Reduced individual distance zones, for the most part, may be maintained.

Dam: The female parent.

Defecation: Elimination of faeces from the body.

Defensive behaviour: Behaviour performed to prevent or neutralize a real or perceived aversive stimulus. According to the circumstances, such behaviour may encompass aggression, avoidance or signs of appeasement and subordination.

Depression: In a behavioural sense, a state of severe emotional dejection and atrophied behaviour occurring in various clinical disorders (stuporous depression).

Deprivation: Removal of needed substances (feed deprivation, water deprivation), perceptual isolation from things desired (social isolation) or prevention of the performance of necessary behaviours (sleep deprivation, exercise deprivation).

Disorientation: Failure of an animal to acquire and keep a proper spatial orientation in its own surroundings, e.g. some neonatal foals fail in their teat-seeking attempts.

Displacement activity: (1) An activity belonging to an instinct other than the one activated. (2) An activity performed by an animal that is in a state of frustration, e.g. self-grooming when flight is blocked.

Distress: An emotional state of a subject resulting from excessive fear, loss of companion or object with which it has a strong psychological bond, physical discomfort, food and/or water deprivation, pain, etc. Compare: **Suffering**.

Diurnal: Pertaining to daylight hours or recurring daily, e.g. grazing or feeding times.

Dominance: (1) An individual animal is said to be dominant over another when it has priority in feeding and sexual behaviour, and when it is superior in aggressiveness and in group control. (2) Dominance status is indicated by superiority in fighting ability of one individual over others.

Drowsing: Being in a somnolent state characterized by reduced attention, eye closure, muscular relaxation and immobility.

Dysphoria: A state of unease, mental discomfort, maladjustment.

Ecology: The study of the relationships between animals and their environment.

Eliminative behaviour: (1) Behaviour involved in the expulsion of faeces or urine from the body or dwelling place. (2) Patterns of behaviour connected with evacuation of faeces and urine, e.g. stallions excreting at set locations.

Emotional behaviour: Behaviour that indicates a high level of excitation to cope with a disturbing situation.

Empathy: The ability to understand or assess feelings of other beings.

Empirical: Based on experience of trial and error, e.g. teat-seeking by the foal.

Environment: The total sum of non-genetic factors that interact with the genotype of a horse.

Epigenesis: The development of the individual through early growing stages in a set order.

Epimeletic behaviour: The provision, in behavioural terms, of care or attention, includes suckling in particular.

Epistaxis: Bleeding from the nose, e.g. heavy nosebleeding in Thoroughbred horses while racing.

Equine Immurement Dysphoria (EID): A distraught/disordered mental state that occurs in some horses kept in close confinement (walled-in). Its main symptoms are repetitive, compulsive, patterned, limited actions such as ledge-biting, air-gulping, head-nodding, jaw-clamping, forebody swaying and short paradings in a box stall. Other effects of EID include a reduction in comfort movements (e.g. less alteration of hind limb flexion) and diminished reactivity (e.g. poor attentiveness).

Et-epimeletic behaviour: Care-seeking behaviour in the young foal when soliciting maternal attendance.

Ethics: Responsible standards of moral conduct.

Ethogram: (1) A record of behavioural activities. (2) An inventory of behaviour patterns typical of an animal or a species.

Ethology: The study of the behaviour of animals.

Ethostasis: The repression, through environmental controls, of major items of natural behaviour.

Euthanasia: A painless killing without fear, anxiety or pain on the part of the subjected horse (by derivation, it means easy death).

Experience: Retention of knowledge or information from previous events in the life of a horse.

Extensive husbandry: An animal care system characterized by low spatial density of animals, in which animals spend considerable amounts of time outdoors and obtain much of their feed by grazing or foraging. Such a system is often labour intensive and has a low level of mechanization.

Extensor muscle: A muscle that extends or straightens out a part of the body.

Fight: An aggressive social interaction involving interchange of forceful and/or potentially harmful actions, generally through some means of physical contact, e.g. fights between colts.

Filly: A young female horse.

Flexion: Bending movement of a body part or limb of a horse that reduces the inner angle of a joint or joints, e.g. bending the knees while going over a jump.

Flight: An escape response, e.g. a runaway horse that will not be stopped.

Flight distance: The radius of an area surrounding a horse that, if breached by intrusion, provokes a reaction.

Flight reaction: A characteristic escape reaction, specific for a particular enemy and surroundings, occurring as soon as the intruder approaches.

Foal: Infant horse of either sex.

Frustration: A state of emotion that is produced when a horse is blocked in its attempts to achieve a goal. Behavioural symptoms of frustration vary among horses and may include elevated levels of pacing, grooming, pawing, vocalization and aggression.

Gelding: A castrated male horse.

Gestation: The period of intrauterine development of a mammal.

Goal: A commodity or condition capable of reducing or eliminating motivation when attained. An incentive.

Grooming: An act of integumentary care, e.g. biting, scraping, etc. Grooming is subdivided into: (i) self-grooming: a horse grooms itself; (ii) allogrooming: one horse grooms another; and (iii) mutual grooming: two horses grooming each other simultaneously.

Group structure: The internal arrangement of a group, such as age differentiation, sexual composition and social subdivision.

Habit: A persistent pattern of behaviour that has been acquired.

Habitat: The surroundings and conditions in which horses live.

Habituation: The permanent weakening of a response as a result of repeated stimulation unaccompanied by reinforcement. This is regarded as distinct from fatigue.

Harem: A social group of mares for breeding, under the control of one stallion.

Health: A relative state of physical, psychological and social well-being.

Herd: A socially coordinated group of horses, in a husbandry sense. A herd is a group of horses in one managerial unit.

Hierarchy: Any social rank or order established through direct combat, threat, passive submission, avoidance, tolerance or some combination of these behavioural methods.

Home range: The locality whereby an individual(s) conducts all its principal functions.

Homeostasis: A state of psychophysiological balance within an animal by means of vital control mechanisms of maintenance.

Homologous behaviour: Behaviour in different species that is similar in form, for example see **Pandiculation**.

Hyperphagia: Consumption of an excessive quantity of food; can occur, for example, after recovery from sedation.

Hyperventilation: Excessive flow of air into and out of the lungs, resulting in reduced carbon dioxide levels in the blood. Antonym: hypoventilation.

Hypothermia: Abnormally low body temperature (chilling).

Idling: Being stationary for extended periods of time while apparently not engaged in any other activity, such as true sleep. Daily idling occurs normally in horses.

Immure: Enclose within walls, imprison.

Imprinting: Very rapid learning in foals to approach and follow their adjacent mares. Imprinting occurs in foals during an early critical period in their lives.

Indoor housing: A housing system in which a horse is kept predominantly or continuously inside buildings. Modern indoor housing facilities generally include mechanized systems for water delivery.

Ingestive behaviour: (1) Actions by which an animal takes substances into the body by swallowing. (2) Behaviour concerned with the selection and consumption of food and drink.

Intelligence: Ability of a horse to learn to cope with new situations and deal effectively with its environmental circumstances.

Investigative behaviour: Behaviour of a horse that involves inspection of an object or surroundings.

Kinesis: Bodily movement, notably locomotion using the limbs.

Kinetic: Pertaining to locomotion.

Laminitis: Inflammation of the sensitive laminae, the 'quick' of the hoof.

Leadership: (1) The ability of an individual to control or direct the behaviour of the members of a group. (2) A special form of facilitation, in which one animal sets the pace of group activity or initiates changes in it.

Learned behaviour: Any action performed as a result of, or influenced by, experience.

Learning: The process that produces adaptive change in an individual's behaviour as the result of experience. In horses, it is especially the outcome of training.

Lenitive: Soothing means.

Libido: Used synonymously with male sex drive.

Linear hierarchy: An occasional type of social hierarchy formed as a straight ranking line of dominance–subordinate relationships in a small horse group. The highest-ranking animal dominates all, the second highest all but the first, the third highest all but the first two, etc., down to the most subordinate horse.

Locomotor: Relating to performance of significant motion.

Loose housing: A housing system where animals are not restricted in ambulation within a large pen or similar enclosure.

Maintenance behaviour: Any behaviour through which a horse sustains its own physiological equilibrium by use of resources. In a broader sense, this term refers to activities required for essential physical and psychological comfort and well-being.

Maladaptive behaviour: Any behaviour that directly or indirectly diminishes well-being or leads to health problems or causes dysfunction of any kind.

Maladjustment: Failure to be comfortable with circumstances. See **Dysphoria**.

Malnutrition: A state of extended inadequate nutrition caused by deficient or unbalanced diet.

Mare: An adult female horse.

Morbidity: A state of sickness or suffering a severe disease.

Moribund behaviour: Behaviour an animal performs when it is dying.

Motivation: The urge to perform a given behavioural function. Motivation arises when some neural controlling mechanism stimulates an appropriate activity for the well-being of the subject.

Motive state: The behavioural manifestations of a given state of motivation, e.g. threat postures indicating the physiological condition of fight or flight.

Motor activity: A function resulting from the excitation of the musculoskeletal system.

Mutilation of self: The process of biting, tearing or otherwise damaging normal, healthy parts of the horse's own body.

Normal behaviour: Behaviour that qualitatively and quantitatively does not deviate from regular or stabilized form. Commonly interpreted as behaviour of an animal that is healthy and free from a pathological condition.

Noxious: Unpleasant, painful, harmful or injurious.

Noxious stimulus: A stimulus that is unpleasant or harmful, e.g. hot branding or docking a foal without anaesthesia.

Odour: Sensation caused by chemical stimulation of receptors in the mucous membranes of the nasal cavities.

Oestrus: Temporary and recurring state of sexual receptivity in fillies and mares. Occurring in coordination with ovulation. Behavioural signs of oestrus, which may vary between mares, typically include increased motor activity, higher excitability, reduction in feeding time, more frequent urination, presenting towards males with a tolerance of bodily contact. The most reliable sign of oestrus is standing for the stallion. The usual duration of oestrus is 3–7 days in mares.

Pain symptom: Any sign or behavioural display indicative of distinct discomfort due to the experience of pain, such as lack of or reduced eye movement, puckered eyelids, dilated nostrils, ears pulled back (horse), head turning towards affected part of the body, distress vocalization, abnormal postures, frequently changing body position, pawing with the feet, head pushing towards the wall, etc.

Pair bond: A continuing and physically close relationship between two horses.

Pairing: A voluntary affinitive relationship between two individuals. Typical pair formations can be observed temporarily between sexual partners, and between horses of the same age maturing together.

Pandiculation: General outstretching as an action pattern.

Parturition: The process of giving birth.

Pasture: Land with growing plants suitable for grazing.

Pheromone: A substance secreted by one individual and received by a second individual of the same species, releasing a specific reaction of behaviour, e.g. oestrous mare's sexual odour detectable by a stallion.

Phonation: Expression by sound, e.g. the whinny.

Photoperiodicity: Regular, cyclic alternation between periods of light and darkness. Especially featured in seasonal changes of sunshine periods.

Pica: Abnormal appetite for unusual and often inappropriate feed, e.g. dirt, hair, faeces, etc.

Play behaviour: A set of activities experienced as pleasurable in themselves by the performing organism. Play behaviour is frequently social in nature and may imitate serious situations but without experiencing serious consequences.

Polydipsia nervosa: Excessive drinking of water beyond physiological needs, e.g. excess water intake in horses as a stable vice.

Preconditioning: Preparation of an animal(s) to cope with changes in environment (social and/or physical). This preparation may involve exposure to novel feeds, familiarization with different environments, handling, transporting, working, etc.

Predation: A form of interspecies relationship in which the attacker (predator) kills and eats the victim (prey).

Reflex: An innate and simple bodily/behavioural response involving the central nervous system and occurring immediately after the stimulus that evokes it.

REM: Rapid eye movement: a deep stage of sleep during which the eyeballs make rapid, flickering movements beneath closed eyelids.

Responsiveness: The capacity of a subject to respond to given stimulation. It may be measured by some assessment of response latency.

Resting: A behavioural state characterized by cessation or reduction of movement and lowered expenditure of bodily energy, in order to avoid or recover from exhaustion. It is often accompanied by a lowered level of alertness in the horse.

Restraint: Any technique used to temporarily discourage or prevent unwanted movement. Restraint is used for examination, surgery, convalescence, breeding and safe handling.

Reward training: A type of operant conditioning in which a reward (positive reinforcer) is directly contingent on the desired performance of the subject. According to the training objectives, the performance resulting in reward may be either a produced response or a withheld natural response. It may be as simple as patting the horse.

Saltation: A sudden, spontaneous act of leaping, running, or dancing. A sudden transition in movement.

Seasonal breeding: Breeding that occurs exclusively and regularly during a certain part of the year when certain conditions of the light/dark ratio per day stimulate reproductive physiology.

Sensitization: The process of becoming more responsive to a given stimulus with practice or a number of trials.

Sentience: Capacity for sensing or feeling.

Sociability: The tendency to seek and maintain the company of peers. This term is sometimes used inaccurately to refer to an animal's attachment to humans.

Social acceptance: A positive or at least neutral attitude towards other individuals or groups.

Social adaptation: Conforming fully with behavioural standards of a given social environment.

Social behaviour: (1) Activities directed towards and influenced by other members of a social unit. (2) The reciprocal interactions of two or more animals and the resulting modifications of individual action systems. (3) Any behaviour caused by or affecting another animal, usually one of the same species.

Social dominance: Ascendancy of an individual over another individual(s).

Social facilitation: (1) A phenomenon in which the behaviour of some organisms has a positive influence on the desire and ability of their social partners to perform such behaviour. (2) Synchrony of certain activities; increases under the influence of group effects.

Social hierarchy: The rank order of individuals in some social unit according to their dominance–subordinate relationships. Synonym: social rank order.

Social organization: (1) Any more or less stabilized system of intra- and/or interspecies social relationships. (2) An aggregation of individuals into a fairly well-integrated and self-consistent group in which the unity is based upon the interdependence of the separate individuals.

Social releaser: Any specific or complex feature of an organism eliciting an instinctive activity in another individual of the same or another species.

Social role: A pattern of behaviour that an individual is reinforced to adopt as a member of a group.

Social status: The position attained by an individual in its social group, dependent on interaction between this individual and other members of the group. Synonym: social hierarchy status.

Social subordinance: Acceptance of the ascendancy of another individual(s).

Social tolerance: The ability to accept the proximity of other subjects when using some common resource.

Socialization: A process of mutual familiarization between subjects, which, if successful, leads to full social integration and relatively stable social arrangement, e.g. 'preferred associate' status in some horse groups.

Society: A group of individuals organized in some socially cohesive assembly.

Standardbred: A breed of horse, originating with individuals meeting a standard speed in trotting.

Stereotyped behaviour: Behaviour repeated in a very constant way. The term generally is used to refer to behaviour that develops as a consequence of a problem situation, such as extended social isolation or a low level of environmental complexity, for example.

Stimulus: Any property of the body's environment that evokes a response, e.g. vocal commands for start or stop.

Stocks: See **Crate**.

Stress: The psychophysiological consequences of challenging, tense or noxious situations. The endogenous result of aversive, exogenous factors.

Stress symptom: Any sign or behavioural display indicative of the presence of a stressor. The most common symptoms are increased excitability, reduced appetite, displacement activities, stereotypic movements, reduced coordination of locomotion, lethargy and, in an extreme case, death of the horse, e.g. from extreme exertion.

Stressor: Any stress-inducing agent, e.g. physical injury, fear-provoking stimulus, etc.

Stretching: A muscular activity characterized by brief, forceful extension of limbs and/or other parts of the body. Stretching is considered to be a comfort movement (see **Pandiculation**).

Suffering: The state of a horse enduring a noxious experience, injury, disease condition, infirmity or severe deprivation.

Symptom: Subjective evidence concerning the abnormal health condition of a horse, e.g. a limp.

Syndrome: A set of signs that occur together and usually reliably indicate the occurrence of a specific disease or behavioural or physical disorder in the horse, e.g. coughing, lassitude.

Tenesmus: Continual straining to evacuate the terminal bowel.

Tensor muscle: A muscle that tightens or stretches a body part.

Thigmotaxis/thigmotrophism: Behaviour revealing an intent to make and maintain close bodily contact with an associate animal, e.g. a foal with its dam.

Threat: Indication of intent to harm directed towards a specific adversary(s). Functionally, threat provides an opportunity for the threatened individual(s) to resolve the situation by escape or avoidance.

Threat signal: Any indication of threat. Such signals may include aggressive fight movements, striking out with a foreleg, foot stamping and an approach to the limit of the opponent's individual distance zone.

Tonic immobility: (1) A state of locomotor inertia shown particularly in an unwillingness to make responses that involve complex, coordinated bodily movements. (2) An apparent absence of coordinated responses in an animal without an associated physical impairment.

Tracasserie: A state of annoyance with anger.

Training: The acquisition phase of a conditioning process. The term training is also used for progressive conditioning, e.g. behaviour-shaping in equine dressage or physical exercise to improve some aspect of performance (for racing, for example).

Trial-and-error learning: A type of learning whereby an animal progressively adopts actions that are most successful for a given purpose, e.g. teat-seeking by a foal.

Ungulate: An animal with hooves.

Unnecessary suffering: Any suffering that is not essential for vital needs.

Valgus: An outward displacement of the lower leg and hoof from the midline.

Varus: An inward displacement of the lower leg from the midline, e.g. 'knock knees'.

Visual acuity: Capacity for distinguishing visual detail.

Visual field: The complete area, including all objects in it, visible to the eye at any given time.

Vocalization: Production of sounds by the vibration of vocal cords in the larynx. The sounds may be modified by the structures of the oral or nasal cavity.

Volition: Cognitive process that deals with decision making and voluntary pursuit of objectives.

Welfare: The provision of care and services for the animal's well-being (in this text).

Well-being: A state of good physical and psychological condition exhibiting harmony between the horse and its surroundings. The most reliable indicators of well-being are good condition and health, combined with manifestations of normal behavioural repertoires.

References

Ahmed, S.A. and Schurig, G.G. (2007) The immune system (Section X). In: Cunningham, J.G. and Klein, B.G. (eds) *Veterinary Physiology*. Saunders Elsevier, Amsterdam.

Appleby, M.C. and Hughes, B.O. (eds) (1997) *Animal Welfare*. CAB International, Wallingford, UK.

Appleby, M.C., Cussen, V., Garces, L., Lambert, L.A. and Turner, J. (eds) (2008) *Long Distance Transport and Welfare of Farm Animals*. CAB International, Wallingford, UK.

Asa, C.S. (1986) Sexual behaviour of mares. In: Crowell-Davis, S.L. and Houpt, K.A. (eds) *Veterinary Clinics of North America: Equine Practice*, Vol. 2. W.B. Saunders, Philadelphia, Pennsylvania, pp. 519–534.

Asa, C.S., Goldfoot, D.A. and Ginther, O.J. (1979) Sociosexual behaviour and ovulatory cycle of ponies (*Equus caballus*) observed in harem groups. *Hormone Behaviour* 13, 49–65.

Axelrod, J. (1984) The relationship between the stress hormones, catecholamines, ACTH and glucocorticoids. In: Usdin, E., Kvetnansky, R. and Axelrod, R. (eds) *Stress: the Role of Catecholamines and other Neurotransmitters*, Vol. 1. Gordon and Breach, New York, pp. 3–13.

Bachmann, J., Bernasconi, P., Herrmann, R., Weishaupt, M.A. and Stauffacher, M. (2003) Behavioural and physiological responses to an acute stressor in crib-biting and control horses. *Applied Animal Behaviour Science* 82, 297–311.

Back, W. and Clayton, H.M. (eds) (2001) *Equine Locomotion*. W.B. Saunders, London.

Bagley, D.V.M. (2005) *Fundamentals of Veterinary Clinical Neurology*. Blackwell, Ames, Iowa.

Balcombe, J. (2009) Animal pleasure and its moral significance. *Applied Animal Behaviour Science* 118, 208–216.

Barry, E. (2001) Inter-limb coordination. In: Back, W. and Clayton, H.M. (eds) *Equine Locomotion*. W.B. Saunders, London, pp. 77–94.

Bateson, P. (2003) The promise of behavioural biology. *Animal Behaviour* 65, 11–17.

Bateson, P. and Horn, G. (1994) Imprinting and recognition memory: a neural net model. *Animal Behaviour* 48, 695–715.

Bateson, P., Barker, D., Clutton-Brock, T., Deb, D., D'Udine, G., Foley, R.A., Gluckman, P., Godfrey, L.K., Kirkwood, T., Marazon Larh, M., McNamara, J., Metcalfe, N.B., Moneghan, P., Spencer, H.G. and Sutton, S.E. (2004) Development plasticity and human health. *Nature* 430, 419–421.

Beaver, B.V. (1994) *The Veterinarian's Encyclopedia of Animal Behaviour*. Iowa State University Press, Ames, Iowa.

Beech, J. (1985) Neonatal equine disease. *Veterinary Clinics of North America: Equine Practice* 1, 1.

Bertone, J.J. (1994) Emergency treatment in the adult horse. *Veterinary Clinics of North America: Equine Practice* 10, 489–728.

Block, M.L., Volpe, L.C. and Hayse, M.J. (1981) Saliva as a chemical cue in the development of social behaviour. *Science, New York* 211, 1062–1064.

Blood, D.C. and Studdert, V.P. (1988) *Baillière's Comprehensive Veterinary Dictionary*. Bailliere Tindall, London.

Booth, D.W. and Signoret, J.P. (1992) Olfaction and reproduction in ungulates. In: Milligan, S.R. (ed.) *Oxford Reviews of Reproductive Biology*, Vol. 14. Oxford University Press, Oxford, pp. 263–301.

Bracher, V., McDonnell, S., Stahler, T. and Green, R. (1998) Equine clinical behaviour. *Equine Veterinary Education* Suppl. 27.

Broad, K.D., Mimmack, M.L., Keverne, E.B. and Kendrick, K.M. (2002) Increased BDNF and trk-B mRNA expression in cortical and limbic regions following formation of a social recognition memory. *European Journal of Neuroscience* 16, 2166–2174.

Brooks, C.M (1981) The autonomic nervous system, molder and integrator of function. Review of a concept. *Brazilian Journal of Medical Biological Research* 14, 151–160.

Broom, D.M. (2000) Welfare assessment and problem areas during handling and transport. In: Grandin, T. (ed.) *Livestock Handling and Transport*, 2nd edn. CAB International, Wallingford, UK, pp. 43–61.

Broom, D.M. (2005) The effects of land transport on animal welfare. *Revue Scientifique Technicale Office Internationale des Epizoöties* 24, 683–691.

Broom, D.M. (2006) Behaviour and welfare in relation to pathology. *Applied Animal Behaviour Science* 97, 71–83.

Broom, D.M. and Fraser, A.F. (2007) *Domestic Animal Behaviour and Welfare*, 4th edn. CAB International, Wallingford, UK.

Broom, D.M. and Johnson, K.G. (1993) *Stress and Animal Welfare*. Chapman and Hall, London.

Broom, D.M. and Johnson, K.G. (2000) *Stress and Animal Welfare*. Kluwer, Dordrecht, the Netherlands.

Broom, D.M. and Kirkden, R.D. (2004) Welfare, stress, behaviour and pathophysiology. In: Dunlop, R.H. and Malbert, C.H. (eds) *Veterinary Pathophysiology*. Blackwell, Ames, Iowa, pp. 337–369.

Brown, J.H., Polliner, S. and Powel-Smith, V. (1996) *Horse and Stable Management Incorporating Horse Care*, 3rd edn. Blackwell Science Ltd, Oxford.

Brownstein, M., Russel, J.T. and Gainer, H. (1980) Synthesis, transport and release of posterior pituitary hormones. *Science, New York* 207, 373–378.

Bruner, J.S., Jolly, A. and Sylva, K. (eds) (1974) *Play: its Role in Development and Evolution*. Penguin, Harmondsworth, UK.

Bucklin, G. (2003) *What Your Horse Wants You to Know*. Wiley Publishing, Oxford.

Budiansky, S. (1997) *The Nature of Horses*. The Free Press, New York, pp. 211–234.

Caanitz, H., O'Leary, L., Houpt, K., Petersson, K. and Hintz, H. (1991) Effect of exercise on equine behaviour. *Applied Animal Behaviour Science* 31, 1–12.

Canadian Agri-Food Research Council (1998) *Recommended Code of Practice for the Care and Handling of Farm Animals. Horses.* Heritage House, Ottawa, Ontario.

Cannon, W.B. (1953) *Bodily Changes in Pain, Hunger, Fear and Rage*. Charles T. Brandford Company, Boston, Massachusetts.

Christiansen, S.B. and Forkman, B. (2007) Assessment of animal welfare in a veterinary context – a call for ethologists. *Applied Animal Behaviour Science* 106, 203–220.

Clegg, P.D., Blake, D.L., Conwell, R.C., Hainisch, E., Newton, S.A., Post, E.M., Senior, M.J., Taylor, S.L. and Wise, A.G. (2001) Anatomy and physiology. In: Coumbe, K.M. (ed.) *The Equine Veterinary Nursing Manual*. Blackwell Science Ltd, Oxford, pp. 25–73.

Clegg, H.A., Buckley, P., Friend, M.A. and McGreevy, P.D. (2008) The ethological and physio logical characteristics of cribbing and weaning horses. *Applied Animal Behaviour Science* 109, 68–76.

Clutton-Brock, J. (1999) *A Natural History of Domesticated Mammals*. Cambridge University Press, Cambridge, UK.

Clutton-Brock, T.H. (1991) *The Evaluation of Parental Care*. Princeton University Press, Princeton, New Jersey.

Colgan, P. (1989) *Animal Motivation*. Chapman and Hall, London.

Collery, L. (1969) The sexual and social behaviour of the Connemara pony. *British Veterinary Journal* 125, 151–152.

Cooper, J.J. and Albentosa, M.J. (2005) Behavioural adaptation in the domestic horse: potential role of apparently abnormal responses including stereotypic behaviour. *Livestock Production Science* 92, 177–182.

Cooper, J.J., McCall, N., Johnson, S. and Davidson, H.P.B. (2005) The short term effects of increasing meal frequency on stereotypic behaviour of stabled horses. *Applied Animal Behaviour Science* 90, 351–364.

Coumbe, K.M. (2001) (ed.) *The Equine Veterinary Nursing Manual*. Blackwell Science Ltd, Oxford.

Courouce, A. (2000) Comparison of some responses to exercise on the track and the treadmill in French Trotters. *The Veterinary Journal* 159, 57–63.

Croney, C.C. and Newberry, R.C. (2007) Group size and cognitive processes. *Applied Animal Behaviour Science* 103, 215–228.

Cunha, T. (1991) *Horse Feeding and Nutrition*, 2nd edn. Academic Press, New York.

Cunningham, J.G. and Klein, B.G. (2007) Neurophysiology (Section II). In: Cunningham,

J.G. and Klein, B.G. (eds) *Veterinary Physiology*. Saunders Elsevier, Amsterdam.

Cymbaluk, N. (2002) About vaccines. In: *Equine Ranching* (spring issue). North American Equine Ranching Information Council, Kentucky and Saskatchewan, p. 17.

Dallman, M.F. (2001) Stress and sickness decrease food intake and body weight. In: Broom, D.M. (ed.) *Coping with Challenge: Welfare in Animals Including Humans*. Dahlem University Press, Berlin, pp. 300–316.

Dantzer, R. and Mittleman, G. (1993) Functional consequences of behavioural stereotypy. In: Lawrence, A.B. and Rushen, J. (eds) *Stereotypic Animal Behaviour*. CAB International, Wallingford, UK, pp. 147–172.

Davidson, A.P. and Stabenfeldt, G.H. (2007) Reproduction and lactation (Section VI). In: Cunningham, J.G. and Klein, B.G. (eds) *Veterinary Physiology*. Saunders Elsevier, Amsterdam.

Davies-Morel, M.C.G. (2000) *Equine Reproductive Physiology, Breeding and Stud Management*. CAB International, Wallingford, UK.

Dawkins, M.S. (2004) Using behaviour to assess welfare. *Animal Welfare* 13, 53–57.

de Mazieres, F.C. (1993) Grooming at a preferred site reduces heart rate in horses. *Animal Behaviour* 46, 1191–1194.

Domjam, M. (1998) *The Principles of Learning and Behaviour*, 4th edn. Brooks/Cole, London.

Dyce, K.M., Sack, W.O. and Wensing, C.J.G. (1996) *Textbook of Veterinary Anatomy*, 2nd edn. Saunders, Philadelphia, Pennsylvania.

EFSA AHAW (2004) *The Welfare of Animals During Transport*. Available at: http://www.efsa. europa.eu/EFSA/efsa_locale-1178620753812_1 178620785233.htm (accessed 23 November 2009).

Estevez, I., Anderson, I.-L. and Naevdal, E. (2007) Group size, density and social dynamics in farm animals. *Applied Animal Behaviour Science* 103, 185–204.

EUSC AHAW (EU Scientific Committee on Animal Health and Animal Welfare) (2002) *The Welfare of Animals during Transport* (details for horses, pigs, sheep and cattle). Available at: http://ec. europa.eu/food/fs/sc/scah/out71_en.pdf (accessed 23 November 2009).

Fagen, R.M. (1976) Exercise, play and physical training in animals. *Perspectives in Ethology* 2, 189–219.

Fagen, R. (1981) *Animal Play Behaviour*. Oxford University Press, New York.

Ferguson, M.J. and Borgh, J.A. (2004) Liking is for doing: the effects of goal pursuit on automatic evaluation. *Journal of Personality and Social Biology* 87, 557–572.

Flannigan, G. and Stookey, J.M. (2002) Day-time budgets of pregnant mares housed in tie-stalls: a comparison of draft versus light mares. *Applied Animal Behaviour Science* 78, 125–143.

Flecknell, P. (2001) Recognition and assessment of pain in animals. In: Soulsby, Lord and Norton, D. (eds) *Pain. Its Nature and Management in Man and Animals*. International Congress and Symposium Series 246, pp. 63–68.

Forkman, B.A. (2002) Learning and cognition. In: Jensen, P. (ed.) *The Ethology of Domestic Animals*. CAB International, Wallingford, UK, pp. 51–64.

Forkman, B., Blokhuis, H.J., Broom, D.M., Kaiser, S., Koolhaas, J.M., Levine, S., Mendl, M., Plotsky, P.M. and Schedlowski, M. (2001) Key sources of variability in coping. In: Broom, D.M. (ed.) *Coping with Challenge: Welfare in Animals Including Humans*. Dahlem University Press, Berlin, pp. 249–270.

Forrester, R.C. (1980) Stereotypes and the behavioural regulation of motivational state. *Applied Animal Ethology* 6, 386–387.

Francis-Smith, K. (1979) Studies on the feeding and social behaviour of domestic horses. PhD thesis, University of Edinburgh, UK.

Fraser, A.F. (1977) Foetal kinesis and a condition of foetal inertia in equine and bovine subjects. *Applied Animal Ethology* 3, 89–90.

Fraser, A.F. (1989) Detection of norms in the behaviour of the newborn foal. *Animal Behaviour Society, 25th Anniversary Meeting*, Kentucky, p.175 (Abstract).

Fraser, A.F. (1990) Analysis of suffering. In: Rollin, B. (ed.) *The Experimental Animal in Biomedical Research*, Vol. I. CRC Press, Boca Raton, Florida, pp. 217–229.

Fraser, A.F. (1992) *The Behaviour of the Horse*. CAB International, Wallingford, UK.

Fraser, A.F. (1995) Horses. In: Rollin, B. (ed.) *The Experimental Animal in Biomedical Research*, Vol. II. *Care, Husbandry and Well-being. An Overview by Species*. CRC Press, Boca Raton, Florida, pp. 5–166.

Fraser, A.F. (2008a) Early days in applied ethology. *Veterinary Heritage* 31(1), 17–18.

Fraser, A.F. (2008b) Veterinarians and animal welfare – a comment. *The Canadian Veterinary Journal* 49(1), 8.

Fraser, A.F. and Broom, D.M. (1990) *Farm Animal Behaviour and Welfare*, 3rd edn. Bailliere Tindall, London.

Fraser, A.F. and Quine, J.P. (1989) Veterinary examination of suffering as a behaviour linked condition. *Applied Animal Behaviour Science* 23, 353–364.

Fraser, A.F., Hastie, H., Callicott, D. and Brownlie, S. (1975) An exploratory ultrasonic study on quantitative foetal kinesis in the horse. *Applied Animal Ethology* 1, 395–404.

Fraser, D. (2009a) Animal ethics and animal welfare science: bridging the two cultures. *Applied Animal Behaviour Science* 65, 181–189.

Fraser, D. (2009b) Animal behaviour, animal welfare and the scientific study of affect. *Applied Animal Behaviour Science* 118, 108–117.

Fraser, D., Ritchie, D. and Fraser, A.F. (1975) The term 'stress' in a veterinary context. *British Veterinary Journal* 131, 653–662.

Freeman, D.W. and Slusher, S.H. (2002) Nursing foal management. *Equine Ranching* (spring issue). North American Equine Ranching Information Council, Kentucky and Saskatchewan, pp. 10–13.

Friend, T.H. (2000) Dehydration, stress, and water consumption of horses during long-distance commercial transport. *Journal of Animal Science* 78, 2568–2580.

Freire, R., Clegg, H.A., Buckley, P., Freund, M.A. and McGreevy, P.D. (2009) The effects of two different amounts of dietary grain on the digestibility of the diet and behaviour of intensively managed horses. *Applied Animal Behaviour Science* 117, 69–73.

FVE (Federation of Veterinarians of Europe) (2001) *Transport of Live Animals*. FVE Position Paper. FVE, Brussels.

Gerros, T.C. (2002) Foal emergencies. *Equine Ranching* (spring issue). North American Equine Ranching Information Council, Kentucky and Saskatchewan, pp. 32–34.

Gibbs, D.M. (1986a) Dissociation of oxytocin, vasopressin and corticotrophin secretion during different types of stress. *Life Science* 35, 487–491.

Gibbs, D.M. (1986b) Vasopressin and oxytocin: hypothalamic modulators of the stress response: a review. *Psychoneuroendocrinology* 11, 131–140.

Giraldeau, L.-A. and Caraco, T. (2000) *Social Foraging Theory*. Princeton University Press, Princeton, New Jersey.

Gluckman, P.D., Hanson, M.A., Spencer, H.G. and Bateson, P. (2005) Environmental influences during development and their later consequences for health and disease: implications for the interpretation of empirical studies. *Proceedings of the Royal Society of London Series B: Biological Sciences* 272, 671–677.

Goodship, A.E. and Birch, H.L. (2001) Exercise effects on the skeletal issues. In: Back, W. and Clayton, H.M. (eds) *Equine Locomotion*. W.B. Saunders, London, pp. 227–250.

Goodwin, D., Davidson, H.P.B. and Harris, P. (2005) Sensory varieties in concentrate diets for stabled horses: effects on behaviour and selection. *Applied Animal Behaviour Science* 90, 337–349.

Gore, T., Gore, P. and Griffin, J.M.L. (2008) *Horse Owner's Veterinary Handbook*, 3rd edn. Wiley Publishing Inc., Hoboken, New Jersey.

Grandin, T. (ed.) (2007) *Livestock Handling and Transport*, 3rd edn. CABI International, Wallingford, UK.

Green, P. and Tong, J.M.J. (1988) Small intestinal obstruction associated with wood chewing in horses. *Veterinary Record* 123, 196–198.

Gregory, N.G. (2004) Sickness and disease. In: *Physiology and Behaviour of Animal Suffering*. Blackwell, Oxford, pp. 183–192.

Grinberg, A., Leyland, M., Pomroy, W.E., Roe, W., Learmonth, J.J. and Oliver, M. (2003) Identification of *Cryptosporidium parvum* 'cattle' genotype from a severe outbreak of neonatal foal diarrhea. *Veterinary Record* 153, 628–631.

Hall, S.L. (1998) Object play by adult animals. In: Bekoff, M. and Byers, J.A. (eds) *Animal Play: Evolutionary, Comparative and Ecological Perspectives*. Cambridge University Press, Cambridge, UK, pp. 455–460.

Hamilton, W.D. (1964a) The genetical evolution of social behaviour II. *Journal of Theoretical Biology* 7, 1–16.

Hamilton, W.D. (1964b) The genetical evolution of social behaviour II. *Journal of Theoretical Biology* 7, 17–32.

Hanggi, E.B. (1999a) Categorization learning in horses. *Journal of Comparative Psychology* 113, 1–10.

Hanggi, E.B. (1999b) Interocular transfer of learning in horses. *Journal of Equine Veterinary Science* 19, 518–523.

Harewood, E.J. and McGowan, C.A. (2005) Behavioural and physiological responses to stabling in naïve horses. *Journal of Equine Veterinary Science* 25, 157–169.

Hausberger, M., Gautier, E., Muller, C. and Jego, P. (2007) Lower learning abilities in stereotypic horses. *Applied Animal Behaviour Science* 107, 299–306.

Heidemann, S.R. (2007) The cell (Section I). In: Cunningham, J.G. and Klein, B.G. (eds) *Veterinary Physiology*. Saunders Elsevier, Amsterdam.

Heimer, L. (1978) Limbic mechanism. In: Livingston, K.E. and Hornykiewicz, G. (eds) *The Continuing Evolution of the Limbic System Concept*. Plenum Press, New York, pp. 95–187.

Heleski, C.R., Shelle, A.C., Nielsen, B.D. and Zanella, A.F. (2002) Influence of housing on weaning horse behaviour and subsequent welfare. *Applied Animal Behaviour Science* 78, 291–302.

Herdt, T.H. (2007) Gastrointestinal physiology and metabolism (Section IV). In: Cunningham, J.G. and Klein, B.G. (eds) *Veterinary Physiology*. Saunders Elsevier, Amsterdam.

Hickman, J. (1987) *Horse Management*, 2nd edn. Academic Press, London and New York.

Hockman, C.H. and Bieger, D. (1976) *Chemical Transmission in the Mammalian Central Nervous System*. University Park Press, London.

Hogan, J.A. (2005) Motivation. In: Bolhuis, J.J. and Giraldeau, L.A. (eds) *The Behaviour of Animals*. Blackwell, Malden, Maryland, pp. 41–70.

Home, J.A. (1977) Factors relating to energy conservation during sleep in mammals. *Physiological Psychology* 5, 403–408.

Horn, G. (1985) *Memory, Imprinting and the Brain*. Oxford University Press, Oxford.

Hothersall, B. and Nicol, C. (2009) Role of diet and feeding on normal and stereotypic behaviours in horses. *Veterinary Clinics of North America: Equine Practice* 25, 167–181.

Houpt, K.A. (1987) Abnormal behaviour. In: Price, E.O. (ed.) *The Veterinary Clinics of North America*, Vol. 3. *Farm Animal Behaviour*. Saunders, Philadelphia, Pennsylvania, pp. 357–367.

Houpt, K.A. (1991) *Domestic Animal Behaviour for Veterinarians and Animal Scientists*, 2nd edn. Iowa State University Press, Ames, Iowa.

Houpt, K.A. (2002) Formation and dissolution of the mare–foal bond. *Applied Animal Behaviour Science* 78, 319–328.

Houpt, K.A. and Olm, D. (1984) Foal rejection: a review of 23 cases. *Equine Practice* 6(7), 38–40.

Houpt, K.A. and Wolski, T.R. (1982) *Domestic Animal Behaviour for Veterinarians and Animal Scientists*. Iowa State University Press, Ames, Iowa.

Houpt, K.A., Eggleston, A., Kumkle, K. and Houpt, T.R. (2000) Effect of water restriction on equine behaviour and physiology. *Equine Veterinary Journal* 32, 341–344.

Hoyt, D.F. and Taylor, C.R. (1981) Gait and the energies of locomotion in horses. *Nature, London* 292, 239–240.

Hubbal, A., Martin, J.E., Lang, B.D.E., Giorgio, R. and Knowles, C.H. (2009) On the organization of olfactory and vomeronasal cortices. *Progress in Neurobiology* 87, 21–30.

Hurnik, J.F., Webster, A.B. and Siegel, P.B. (1985) *Dictionary of Farm Animal Behaviour*. University of Guelph, Guelph, Ontario.

Ingolfsdottir, H.B. and Sigurjonsdottir, H. (2008) The benefits of high rank in the wintertime – a study of the Icelandic horse. *Applied Animal Behaviour Science* 114, 485–491.

Insel, T.R. (1992) Oxytocin – a neuropeptide for affilation: evidence from behavioural, receptor autoradiographic and comparative studies. *Psychoneuroendocrinology* 17, 3–35.

Isaacson, R.L. (1982) *The Limbic System*, 2nd edn. Plenum Press, New York.

Jahiel, J. (2004) *The Horse Behaviour Problem Solver*. Storey Publishing, North Adams, Massachusetts.

Jean, S., Halley, J., Hannigan, D. and Leveille, R. (1999) Thoracic trauma in newborn foals. *Equine Veterinary Journal* 31, 149–152.

Jensen, P. (ed.) (2002) The study of animal behaviour and its applications. In: *The Ethology of Domestic Animals: an Introductory Text*. CAB International, Wallingford, UK, pp. 3–11.

Jones, R.B. and Faure, J.M. (1984) The technique of jumping a steeplechase fence by competing event-horses. *Applied Animal Ethology* 7, 15–24.

Jones, S. (2001) *Darwin's Ghost. The Origin of Species Updated*. Anchor Canada, Random House of Canada Ltd, Toronto.

Kandel, E.R. and Schwartz, J.H. (eds) (1981) *Principles of Neural Science*. Elsevier, Amsterdam.

Katcher, A.H. and Wilkins, G.G. (2000) The centaur's lessons: therapeutic education through care of animals and nature study. In: Fine, A. (ed.) *Handbook on Animal-assisted Therapy: Theoretical Foundations and Guidelines for Practice*. Academic Press, San Diego, California, pp. 153–177.

Kaur, C. and Ling, E.A. (2009) Periventricular white matter damage in the hypoxic neonatal brain. *Progressive Neurobiology* 87, 264–280.

Keeling, L. and Gonyou, H. (eds) (2001) *Social Behaviour in Farm Animals*. CAB International, Wallingford, UK.

Keeling, L. and Jensen, P. (2002) Behavioural disturbances, stress and welfare. In: Jensen, P. (ed.) *The Ethology of Domestic Animals*. CAB International, Wallingford, UK, pp. 79–98.

Keiper, R.R. and Berger, J. (1982) Refuge-seeking and pest avoidance by feral horses in desert and island environments. *Applied Animal Ethology* 90, 111–120.

Kelley, K.W. (1980) Stress and immune function. A bibliographic review. *Annales de Recherches Vétérinaires* 11, 445–478.

Kiley-Worthington, M. (1999) *The Behaviour of Horses*. J.A. Allen & Co. Ltd, London.

Kilgour, R. and Dalton, C. (1984) *Livestock Behaviour: a Practical Guide*. Granada, London.

Knottenbelt, D.C., LeBlanc, M.M. and Pascoe, R.R. (2001) *Handbook of Equine Stud Medicine*. W.B. Saunders, Philadelphia, Pennsylvania.

Koolhaas, J.M., Korte, S.M., de Boer, S.F., Van der Vegt, B.J., Van Reenen, C.G. and Hopster, H. (1999) Coping styles in animals: current status in behaviour and stress-physiology. *Neuroscience Biobehavioral Review* 23, 925–935.

Koterba, A.M., Drummond, W.H. and Kosch, P.C. (1990a) *Clinical Neonatology*. Lea and Febiger, Philadelphia, Pennsylvania.

Koterba, A.M., Drummond, W.H. and Kosch, P.C. (1990b) *Equine Clinical Neonatology*. Lea and Febiger, London.

Langley, G. (1990) *Understanding Horses*. Trafalgar Square Publishing, North Pomfret, Vermont.

Lansade, L., Bouissue, M.F. and Erhard, H.W. (2008) Fearfulness in horses: a temperamental trait, stable across time and situations. *Applied Animal Behaviour Science* 115, 182–200.

Lawrence, A.B. and Rushen, J. (eds) (1993) *Stereotypic Animal Behaviour – Fundamentals and Applications to Welfare*. CAB International, Wallingford, UK.

Lawrence, E.A. (1998) Human and horse medicine among some Native American groups. *Agriculture and Human Values* 15, 133–138.

Leach, D.H. and Ormrod, K. (1984) The technique of jumping a steeplechase fence by competing event-horses. *Applied Animal Ethology* 12, 15–24.

Lehner, P.N. (1996) *Handbook of Ethological Methods*, 2nd edn. Cambridge University Press, Cambridge, UK.

Ligout, S., Bouissou, M.F. and Boiviu, X. (2008) Comparison of the effects of two different handling methods on the subsequent behaviour of Anglo-Arabian foals towards humans and handling. *Applied Animal Behaviour Science* 113, 175–188.

Lloyd, A.S., Martin, J.E., Bornett-Gauci, H.L.I. and Wilkinson, R.G. (2008) Horse personality: variation between breeds. *Applied Animal Behaviour Science* 112, 369–383.

Lorenz, K. (1965) *Evolution and Modification of Behaviour*. University of Chicago Press, Chicago, Illinois.

Madigan, J.F. (1991) *Manual of Equine Neonatal Medicine*, 2nd edn. Live Oak Publishing, Woodland, California.

Mair, T., Love, S., Schumacher, J. and Watson, E. (1998) *Equine Medicine, Surgery and Reproduction*. Saunders, London.

Malyshenko, N.M. (1982) The role of corticosteroids in the genesis of fear and aggressive reactions. *Zh Vssh Nerva Deiat Im I P Pavlova* 32, 144–151.

Mark, R. and Whibney, H. (2003) *Life Lessons from a Ranch Horse*. Johnson Books, Boulder, Colorado.

Marlborough, L.C. and Knottenbelt, D.C. (2001) Basic management. In: Coumbe, K.M. (ed.) *The Equine Veterinary Nursing Manual*. Blackwell Science Ltd, Oxford, pp. 1–24.

Martin, P. and Bateson, P. (2007) *Measuring Behaviour*, 2nd edn. Cambridge University Press, Cambridge, UK.

Mason, G.J. (1991) Stereotypies: a critical review. *Animal Behaviour* 41, 1015–1037.

Mason, G.J. (1993) Forms of stereotypic behaviour. In: Lawrence, A.B. and Rushen, J. (eds) *Stereotypic Animal Behaviour*. CAB International, Wallingford, UK.

Mason, G. and Rushen, J. (eds) (2008) *Stereotypic Animal Behaviour: Fundamentals and Applications to Welfare*. CAB International, Wallingford, UK.

Mason, G.J., Clubb, R., Latham, N. and Vickery, S. (2007) Why and how should we use environmental enrichment to tackle stereotypic behaviour? *Applied Animal Behaviour Science* 102, 163–188.

Mason, J.W. (1975) Emotion as reflected in patterns of endocrine integrations. In: Levi, L. (ed.) *Emotions – their Parameters and Measurements*. Raven, New York, pp. 233–251.

McAfee, L.M., Mills, D.S. and Cooper, J.J. (2002) The use of mirrors for the control of stereotypic behaviour in the stabled horse. *Applied Animal Behaviour Science* 78, 159–173.

McCall, J. (1988) *Influencing Horse Behaviour*. Alpine Publications, Loveland, Colorado.

McDonnell, S.M. (1989) Spontaneous erection and masturbation in equids. *Proceedings of the 35th Annual Convention*. American Association of Equine Practitioners, Boston, Massachusetts, pp. 567–580.

McDonnell, S. (1999) *Understanding Horse Behaviour*. Eclipse Press, Lexington, Kentucky.

McDonnell, S.M. (2002) Behaviour of horses. In: Jensen, P. (ed.) *The Ethology of Domestic Animals: an Introductory Text*. CAB International, Wallingford, UK, pp. 119–129.

McEwen, B.S. (2001) Protective and damaging effects of stress mediators: lessons learned from the immune system and brain. In: Broom, D.M. (ed.) *Coping with Challenge: Welfare in Animals Including Humans*. Dahlem University Press, Berlin, pp. 229–246.

McGreevy, P. (2004) *Equine Behaviour*. Saunders, Edinburgh.

McGreevy, P.D. and Thomson, P.C. (2006) Differences in motor laterality between breeds of performance horse. *Applied Animal Behaviour Science* 99, 183–190.

McGreevy, P.D., Cripps, P.J., French, N.P., Green, L.E. and Nicol, C.J. (1995) Management factors associated with stereotypic and redirected behaviour in the thoroughbred horse. *Equine Veterinary Journal* 27, 86–91.

McGrogan, C., Hutchison, M.D. and King, J.E. (2008) Dimensions of horse personality based on owner and trainer supplied personality traits. *Applied Animal Behaviour Science* 113, 206–214.

Meredith, M. (1999) Vomero-nasal organ. In: Knobil, E. and Neill, J.D. (eds) *Encyclopedia of Reproduction*, Vol. 4. Elsevier, Amsterdam, pp. 1004–1014.

Meyer, H. (1987) Nutrition of the equine athlete. In: Gillespie, J.R. and Robinson, N.E. (eds) *Equine Exercise Physiology*, Vol. 2, 2nd edn. KEEP Publication, Davis, California, pp. 645–673.

Miller, R.M. (1991) Imprint training the newborn foal. In: Royer, M.G. (ed.) *Proceedings of the 36th Annual Convention of the American Association of Equine Practitioners*. Lexington, Kentucky, 2–5 December 1990, pp. 661–666.

Miller, R. (1992) *Imprint Training*. The Lyons Press, Guilford, Delaware.

Mills, N.J. (1991) Mound making in azoturia cases. *Veterinary Record* 128, 215.

Mills, D.S., Alston, R.D., Rogers, V. and Longford, N.T. (2002) Factors associated with the prevalence of stereotypic behaviour amongst thoroughbred horses passing through auctioneer sales. *Applied Animal Behaviour Science* 78, 115–124.

Minero, M., Tossi, M.V., Canali, E. and Wemesfelder, F. (2009) Quantitative and qualitative assessment of the response of foals to the presence of an unfamiliar human. *Applied Animal Behaviour Science* 116, 74–81.

Moberg, G.P. (1985) Biological response to stress: key to assessment of animal well-being? In: Moberg, G.P. (ed.) *Animal Stress*. American Physiology Society, Bethesda, Maryland, pp. 27–49.

Moberg, G. and Mench, J.A. (2000) *The Biology of Animal Sress: Basic Principles and Implications for Animal Welfare*. CAB International, Wallingford, UK.

Morresey, R.R. (2005) Prenatal and perinatal indicators of neonatal viability. *Clinical Techniques in Equine Practice* 4, 238–249.

Munroe, G. (1999) Subconjunctival hemorrhages in neonatal Thoroughbred foals. *Veterinary Record* 146, 579–584.

Munroe, G. (2000a) Study of the hyaloid apparatus in the neonatal thoroughbred foal. *Veterinary Record* 146, 579–584.

Munroe, G. (2000b) Survey of retinal hemorrhages in neonatal thoroughbred foals. *Veterinary Record* 146, 95–101.

Nagy, K., Schrott, A. and Kabai, P. (2008) Possible influence of neighbours on stereotypic behaviours of horses. *Applied Animal Behaviour Science* 111, 321–328.

Nelson, R.J. (2000) *An Introduction to Behaviour and Endocrinology*, 2nd edn. Sinauer Associates, Sunderland, Massachusetts.

Nicol, C.J. and Badnell-Waters, A.J. (2005) Suckling behaviour in domestic foals and the development of abnormal oral behaviour. *Animal Behaviour* 70, 21–29.

Nicol, C.J., Badnell-Waters, A.J., Bice, R., Kelland, A., Wilson, A.D. and Harris, P.A. (2005) The effects of diet and weaning method on the behaviour of young horses. *Applied Animal Behaviour Science* 95, 205–221.

NRC (1989) *Nutrient Requirements of Horses*, 5th edn. National Academic Press, Washington, DC.

O'Connor, M. (1987) Management procedures to prevent outbreaks of diarrhea in foals. *Journal of Equine Veterinary Science* 7, 316–317.

Odberg, F.O. and Francis-Smith, K. (1976) A study on eliminative and grazing behaviour – the use of the field by captive horses. *Equine Veterinary Journal* 8, 147–149.

Odberg, F.O. and Francis-Smith, K. (1977) Studies on the formation of ungrazed eliminative areas in fields used by horses. *Applied Animal Ethology* 3, 27–34.

Oikawa, M., Hobo, S., Oyomada, T. and Yoshikawa, H. (2005) Effects of orientation, intermittent rest and vehicle cleaning during transport on development of transport-related respiratory disease in horses. *Journal of Comparative Pathology* 132, 153–168.

Oliver, J.E. and Lorenz, M.D. (1993) *Handbook of Veterinary Neurology*, 2nd edn. W.B. Saunders, Philadelphia, Pennsylvania.

Orsini, J. and Divers, T. (1998) *Manual of Equine Emergencies, Treatment and Procedures*. W.B. Saunders, Philadelphia, Pennsylvania.

Owen, R.A., Fullerton, J. and Barnum, D.A. (1983) Effects of transportation, surgery, and antibiotic therapy in ponies infected with *Salmonella*. *American Journal of Veterinary Research* 44, 46–50.

Palmer, A.C. (1976) *Introduction to Animal Neurology*, 2nd edn. Blackwell, Oxford.

Palmer, A.C. and Rossdale, P.D. (1976) Clinical studies on the newborn thoroughbred foal. *Research in Veterinary Science* 20, 267–275.

Palmer, J.E. (2007) Neonatal foal resuscitation. *Veterinary Clinics of North America: Equine Practice* 23, 159–182.

Panksepp, J. (1998) *Affective Neuroscience*. Oxford University Press, New York.

Pavord, T. and Pavord, M. (2002) *The Complete Equine Veterinary Manual*. David and Charles, Newton Abbot, UK.

Pearson, A.J. (1997) Anatomy and physiology. In: Lane, D.R. and Cooper, B. (eds) *Veterinary Nursing*. Butterworth–Heinemann, Oxford.

Pellis, S.M. and Pellis, V.C. (1998) The structure function interface in the analysis of play-fighting. In: Bekoff, M. and Byers, J.A. (eds) *Animal Play: Evolutionary, Comparative and Ecological Perspectives*. Cambridge University Press, Cambridge, UK, pp. 115–140.

Peterson, P.K., Chao, C.C., Molitor, T., Murtaug M., Strogar, F. and Sharp, B.M. (1991) Stress and pathogenesis of infectious disease. *Review of Infectious Diseases* 13, 710–720.

Pilliner, S. and Davies, Z. (2004) *Equine Science*, 2nd edn. Blackwell, Oxford.

Podberscek, A.L. (2006) Positive and negative aspects of our relationship with companion animals. *Veterinary Research Communication* 30 (Suppl.1), 21–27.

Price, E.O. (2002) *Animal Domestication and Behaviour*. CAB International, Wallingford, UK.

Prosser, C.L. (ed.) (1991) Environmental and metabolic animal physiology: neural and integrative animal psychology. In: *Comparative Animal Physiology*, 4th edn. John Wiley, Chichester, UK.

Pryse-Phillips, W. (2009) *Companion to Clinical Neurology*, 3rd edn. Oxford University Press, Oxford.

Pycock, J.F. (2001) Reproduction. In: Coumbe, K.M. (ed.) *The Equine Veterinary Nursing Manual*. Blackwell Science Ltd, Oxford, pp. 81–100.

Quinn, P.J., Markey, B.K., Carter, M.E., Donnelley, W.J. and Leonard, F.C. (2000) *Veterinary Microbiology and Microbial Diseases*. Blackwell, Oxford.

Radostits, O.M., Gay, C.C., Blood, D.C. and Hinchcliff, K.W. (2000) *Veterinary Medicine: a Textbook of the Diseases of Cattle, Sheep, Pigs, Goats and Horses*, 9th edn. W.B. Saunders, London.

Rifa, H. (1990) Social facilitation in the horse (*Equus caballus*). *Applied Animal Behaviour Science* 25, 167–176.

Riolo, R.L., Cohen, M.D. and Axeford, R. (2001) Evolution of cooperation without reciprocity. *Nature* 414, 441–443.

Roberts, M. (1996) *The Man Who Listens to Horses*. Hutchinson, London.

Roberts, W.A. (2000) *Principles of Animal Cognition*. McGraw-Hill, Boston, Massachusetts.

Robinson, N.E. (2007) Respiratory Function (Section VIII) and Homeostasis (Section IX). In: Cunningham, J.G. and Klein, B.G. (eds) *Veterinary Physiology*. Saunders Elsevier, Amsterdam.

Rollin, B.E. (ed.) (1995) *The Experimental Animal in Biomedical Research*, Vol. II. CRC Press, Boca Raton, Florida.

Rossdale, P.D. (1999) Birth trauma in newborn foals. *Equine Veterinary Journal* 31, 92.

Ruckebusch, Y. (1972) The relevance of drowsiness in farm animals. *Animal Behaviour* 20, 637–643.

Russell, C.M. and Wilkins, P.A. (2006) Evaluation of the recumbent neonate. *Clinical Techniques in Equine Practice* 5, 161–171.

Sambraus, H.H. (1985) Mouth-based anomalous syndromes. In: Fraser, A.F. (ed.) *Ethology of Farm Animals, World Animal Science*, A5. Elsevier, Amsterdam, pp. 381–411.

Samper, J. (2000) *Equine Breeding Management and A.I.* W.B. Saunders, Philadelphia, Pennsylvania.

Sappington, B.F. and Goldman, L. (1994) Discrimination learning and concept formation in the Arabian horse. *Journal of Animal Science* 72, 3080–3087.

Schneider, K.M. (1930) Das flehmen. *Zoologischer Garten Leipzig* 4, 183–198.

Schorr, E.C. and Arnason, B.G.W. (1999) Interactions between the sympathetic nervous system and the immune system. *Brain, Behaviour and Immunity* 13, 271–278.

Schulkin, J. (1999) *Neuroendocrine: Regulation of Behaviour*. Cambridge University Press, Cambridge, UK.

Seaman, S.C., Davidson, H.P.B. and Waran, N.K. (2002) How reliable is temperament assessment in the domestic horse (*Equus caballus*)? *Applied Animal Behaviour Science* 78, 157–191.

Simpson, B.S. (2002) Neonatal foal handling. *Applied Animal Behaviour Science* 78, 303–317.

Singer, J.W., Babsin, N., Bamka, W.J. and Kluchinski, D. (1999) Horse pasture management. *Journal of Equine Veterinary Science* 19, 540–592.

Smolensky, M.H. (2001) Circadian rhythms in medicine. *CNS Spectrums* 6, 467–482.

Sondergaard, E. and Ladewig, J. (2004) Group housing exerts a positive effect on the behaviour of young horses in training. *Applied Animal Behaviour Science* 87, 105–118.

Soulsby, Lord and Morton, D. (eds) (2001) Pain: its nature and management in man and animals. *Royal Society of Medicine International Congress Symposium* Series 246, 17–25.

Spier, S.J., Pusterla, J.B., Villarroel, A. and Pusterla, N. (2004) Outcome of tactile conditioning or 'imprint training' on selected handling measures in foals. *Veterinary Journal* 168(3), 252–258.

Spiers, V.C. (1997) *Clinical Examination of Horses*. W.B. Saunders, Philadelphia, Pennsylvania.

Spruijt, B.M., van der Bos, R. and Pijlman, F.T.A. (2001) A concept of welfare based on reward evaluating mechanisms in the brain: anticipatory behaviour as an indicator for the state of neuronal systems. *Applied Animal Behaviour Science* 72, 145–171.

Stafford, C. and Oliver, R. (1991) *Horse Care and Management*. J.A. Allen, London.

Stoneham, S.J. (2001) Foal nursing. In: Coumbe, K.M. (ed.) *The Equine Nursing Manual*. Blackwell Science Ltd, Oxford, pp. 284–297.

Timney, B. and Keil, K. (1992) Visual acuity in the horse. *Vision Research* 32, 2289–2293.

Toates, F. (2002) Physiology, motivation and the organization of behaviour. In: Jensen, P. (ed.) *Ethology of Domestic Animals – an Introduction*. CAB international, Wallingford, UK.

Treves, A. (2000) Theory and methods in studies of vigilance and aggregation. *Animal Behaviour* 60, 711–722.

Valla, W.E. (1994) Perinatology. *Veterinary Clinics of North America: Equine Practice* 10, 1.

Van Dierendonck, M.C., De Vries, H., Schilder, M.B.H., Colenbrander, B., Goran, A. and Sigurjonsdottir, J. (2009) Interventions in social behaviour in a herd of mares and geldings. *Applied Animal Behaviour Science* 116, 67–73.

Vandenbergh, J.C. (ed.) (1983) *Pheromones and Reproduction in Mammals*. Academic Press, London.

Visser, E.K., Van Reenen, C.G., Schilder, M.B.H., Barneveld, A. and Blokhuis, H.J. (2003) Learning performances in young horses using two different learning tests. *Applied Animal Behaviour Science* 80, 311–326.

Visser, E.K., Ellis, A.D. and Van Reenen, C.G. (2008) The effect of two different housing conditions on the welfare of young horses stabled for the first time. *Applied Animal Behaviour Science* 114, 521–533.

Wall, P.D. (1992) Defining 'pain in animals'. In: Short, C.E. and van Poznak, A. (eds) *Animal Pain.* Churchill Livingstone, New York, pp. 63–79.

Waran, N.K., Clarke, N. and Farnworth, N. (2008) The effects of weaning on the domestic horse (*Equus caballus*). *Applied Animal Behaviour Science* 110, 42–57.

Warbel, H. (2009) Ethology applied to animal ethics. *Applied Animal Behaviour Science* 118, 118–127.

Waring, G.H. (2003) *Horse Behaviour,* 2nd edn. Noyes Publications, New Jersey, 292 pp.

Webster, J. (1994) *Animal Welfare: a Cool Eye towards Eden.* Blackwell, Oxford.

Wentink, G. (1978) Biokinetical analysis of the movements of the pelvic limb of the horse and the role of the muscles in the walk and the trot. *Anatomical Embryology* 152, 261–272.

Whitten, W.K. (1985) Vomeronasal organ and the accessory olfactory system. *Applied Animal Behaviour Sciences* 14, 105–109.

Wiepkema, P.R. (1985) Abnormal behaviour in farm animals. Ethological implications. *Netherlands Journal of Zoology* 35, 279–289.

Wiepkema, P.R. (1987) Behavioural aspects of stress. In: Wiepkema, P.R. and van Adrichem, P.W.M. (eds) *Biology of Stress in Farm Animals: an Integrative Approach. Current Topics in Veterinary Medicine and Animal Science* 42. Martinus Nijhoff, The Hague, the Netherlands, pp. 113–183.

Wiepkema, P.R., Broom, D.M., Duncan, I.J.H. and van Putten, G. (1983) *Abnormal Behaviours in Farm Animals.* Commission of the European Communities, Brussels.

Willeberg, P. (1997) Epidemiology and animal welfare. *Epidemiologie. Santé Animale* 31, 3–7.

Williams, J.L., Friend, T.H., Toscano, M.J., Collins, M.N., Sisto-burt, A. and Nevill, C.H. (2002) The effects of early training sessions on the reactions of foals at 1, 2, and 3 months of age. *Applied Animal Behaviour Science* 77, 105–114.

Wolski, T., Houpt, K. and Alonson, R. (1980) The role of stress in mare–foal recognition. *Applied Animal Ethology* 6, 121–138.

Wong, R. (2000) *Motivation: a Biobehavioural Approach.* Cambridge University Press, Cambridge, UK.

Wright, R., Cruz, A.M. and Kenney, D. (2002) Congenital anomalies and inherited disorders. *Equine Ranching* (spring issue). North American Equine Ranching Information Council, Kentucky and Saskatchewan, pp. 18–20.

Wyatt, T.D. (2003) *Pheromones and Animal Behaviour.* Cambridge University Press, Cambridge, UK.

Yang, E.V. and Glasser, R. (2000) Stress-induced immunomodulation: impact on immune defenses against infectious disease. *Biomedical Pharmacotherapy* 54, 245–250.

Youatt, W. (1858) Vices. In: *The Horse.* Longman, Brown, Green & Longmans, London, pp. 440–456.

Zayan, R. and Dantzer, R. (eds) (1990) *Social Stress in Domestic Animals.* Kluwer Academic Publishing, Dordrecht, the Netherlands.

Zentall, T.R. (1996) The analysis of initiative learning in animals. In: Hayes, C.M. and Galef, B.G. (eds) *Social Learning of Animals: the Roots of Culture.* Academic Press, San Diego, California, pp. 221–243.

Index

Note: page numbers in *italics* refer to figures and tables.

hypothermia 78, 228
    see also chilling

Icelandic mares 134–135, 138–139
Icelandic photoperiod 134, 135, *136*
idling *110*, 229
illness, recovery 7, 8
imitation 14, 16
immunity 155–157
immurement 4, 195, 216
    dysphoria 4, 203, 212–213, 217
impact, shoulder muscle action 79, *80*
imprinting 13, 229
incident frequencies 8
individual distance 98, 101
individual space 99, 100, 101
    violation 179
infections
    control 193, 194
    foals 157
    neonatal 166–167
    umbilical cord 157, 166–167
ingestion 48–49, 229
ingestive welfare 58–67
inherent behaviour 6, 12
innate behaviour 12, 14
innate releasing mechanism (IRM) 12
innate response release 12
inner ear 27–28
insemination 128, 129
instincts 12
integumental areas, friction 68, *69*
intelligence 17–19, 25, 229
internal parasites 103, 193, 194, 218–219
    see also worming
interneurons 28, 38, 39
intestinal accidents 65
investigatory activities 17, 217, 229
iron deficiency 198
isolation 16, *105*, 180
    distress 203–204
    stress 210

Jacobson's organ 23
Jamaican mares/photoperiod 134, 135, 136
jibbing 207, *208*
joints 93
    neonates 160
    pandiculation 74
jumping 86–87

kicking 177
    abnormal reactions 206, *207*, *208*
    double-legged 206, *207*, 219

mares 123
stallions 206
territoriality 56, 97, 100
kinesis 227
    neonatal 40
kinetic activity 51, 170, 229
kinetic behaviour 79–88
kinetic drive 106
kinetic need 93

labour
    fetal posture 138, 142
    onset 140, 141
    second stage 141–143
    third stage 143–144,
        145–146
lameness 11
laminitis 10, 65, 229
language 47–48
large intestine blockage 162
leadership 102, 177, 229
learning 3–4, 24–25, 229
    conditioning 15–16
    foals 17
    inherent capability 4–5
    initial 2
    investigatory activities 17
    routine 16
    social relationships 178
leaves, eating 60, *62*
legs
    deformities 168
    foreleg motion 79, *80*
    injuries 10
    restraint 186–187, *188*
    support apparatus 109–110
    wet horse 116
    see also hindlimbs
lenitive activity 216–217, 229
lethargic behaviour 184
licking, mare of neonatal
        foal 143
light stimulus 134–136
limbic system 30–31, 43, 46
limbs *see* foot; hoof; joints; legs
Lipizzaner stallions 87
litter-eating 198, *200*
loading 119–120
loafing 220
locomotion 11–12, 33, 80, 229
locus ceruleus 29
lounging phases 97, 109,
        110, 220
lumbo-sacral joint 89
lungeing 94
lupins 63